T0331147

THE PROSPECT OF INDUSTRY 5.0 IN BIOMANUFACTURING

THE PROSPECT OF INDUSTRY 5.0 IN BIOMANUFACTURING

Edited by
Pau Loke Show
Kit Wayne Chew
Tau Chuan Ling

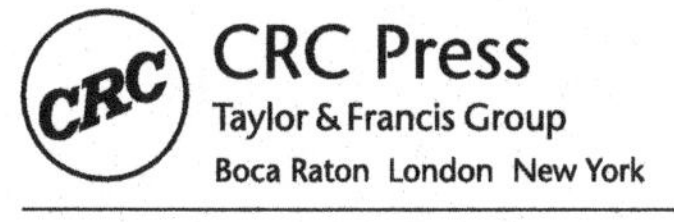

CRC Press is an imprint of the
Taylor & Francis Group, an informa business

First edition published 2022
by CRC Press
6000 Broken Sound Parkway NW, Suite 300, Boca Raton, FL 33487-2742

and by CRC Press
2 Park Square, Milton Park, Abingdon, Oxon, OX14 4RN

Library of Congress Cataloging-in-Publication Data
Names: Show, Pau Loke, editor. | Chew, Kit Wayne, editor. | Ling, Tau Chuan, editor.
Title: The prospect of industry 5.0 in biomanufacturing / edited by Pau Loke Show, Kit Wayne Chew, Tau Chuan Ling.
Description: First edition. | Boca Raton, FL : CRC Press, [2021] | Includes bibliographical references and index. | Summary: "This is the first book to present the idea of Industry 5.0 in biomanufacturing and bioprocess engineering, both upstream and downstream. It details the latest technologies and how they can be used efficiently and explains process analysis from an engineering point of view. In addition, it covers applications and challenges. This work enables readers in industry and academia working in the biomanufacturing engineering sector to understand current trends and future directions in this field"-- Provided by publisher.
Identifiers: LCCN 2021004341 (print) | LCCN 2021004342 (ebook) |
ISBN 9780367493783 (hardback) | ISBN 9781003080671 (ebook)
Subjects: LCSH: Biochemical engineering. | Biological products. | Industry 4.0.
Classification: LCC TP248.3 .P76 2021 (print) | LCC TP248.3 (ebook) |
DDC 660.6/3--dc23
LC record available at https://lccn.loc.gov/2021004341
LC ebook record available at https://lccn.loc.gov/2021004342

ISBN: 978-0-367-49378-3 (hbk)
ISBN: 978-0-367-53144-7 (pbk)
ISBN: 978-1-003-08067-1 (ebk)

Typeset in Times
by MPS Limited, Dehradun

Contents

Preface

The fast-growing and ever-changing digital age has brought many great advances in technologies and artificial intelligence–based results. The rapid transformation in digital sectors, mass customization, and commercial manufacturing have opened up prospects of the human-robot collaboration for better and more efficient systems. Industry 5.0 takes the concept of customization and personalization to another level. In biomanufacturing, the possibility of creating intellectual systems that can customize and personalize products according to the specific needs of consumers is a strong basis for the development of Industry 5.0. A relationship where humans work with robots as collaborators instead of competitors will be the key to the successful evolution of this Industry 5.0, which will bring an abundance of technological advancement for improving the human quality of life and creation of the future society. This book's target can provide the knowledge on Industry 5.0 to help readers understand the basic principles of the concept, the struggles of previous revolutions, current applications of this concept in biomanufacturing, and the challenges ahead of this concept implementation. The progress in Industry 5.0 is unavoidable and industries must prepare for it by finding opportunities to utilize automation to support human labor in biomanufacturing. The balance between efficiency and productivity will be essential to maximize the process performance efficiency and lead to an optimized production system that will fully exploit the benefits of Industry 5.0. This book is expected to encourage biomanufacturing industries to understand and create flexibility for the collaborative robotic system to aid people in the manufacturing of customized products.

This book is organized into chapters expressing the significant aspects of Industry 5.0, its potential adaptation, the applications in biomanufacturing, and challenges associated with the industrial concept. The first section provides the understandings and visions of previous Industry 1.0, 2.0, 3.0, and 4.0, which includes the principles, technological developments, and biotechnological advances of the respective Industrial Revolution. The processing techniques developed during the previous IRs are explained, along with their role in contributing to urbanization. The second section describes the fundamentals of emerging Industry 5.0, and outlines the significance of this paradigm. This section contains several chapters on the ideology of this industrial concept, the challenges faced post–Industry 4.0, as well as the impact of the transition from IR 4.0 to 5.0, from different viewpoints and sources. The third section evaluates the biomanufacturing practices and industrial production potential of Industry 5.0 in various industries type, including medicine and pharmaceuticals, food and beverage, fuels and biofuels, fruits and vegetables, and fine chemicals and biopolymers. The chapters in this section focus on the creation of flexibility in processing to supply the specialized customization of products to suit the needs of customers. The strategies to implement and commercialize Industry 5.0 in these industries are also part of the key points in the chapters. The fourth section explores the technologies and challenges in Industry 5.0, which includes the state-of-the-art technologies and sustainability and development of biomanufacturing processes in Industry 5.0. The cooperation between human and machine, and our ability to work in harmony with artificial intelligence are part of the developments for this concept realization. The fifth section summarizes the industry perspective of Industry 5.0, providing thoughts on the community demand for mass customization, the cost-benefit of product personalization and the potential need of worker upskilling to bring Industry 5.0 to the industries.

The content in this book comprehensively summarizes the prospects of Industry 5.0 in biomanufacturing and important findings concerning the adaptation and application of this industrial concept. The major changes of the shift in Industrial revolutions involves the new skills and structures of the workforce, need for human-robot collaboration, advancements in cyber security and protection, in addition to higher investments and costs. The early preparation and support would be vital to ensure the smooth transition, as the workforce of the future generation would be very different from that of today. The information provided in this book will open up future possibilities of incorporating Industry 5.0 into existing biomanufacturing practices and processing, in order to improve the product quality and cost efficiency of the process.

Editors

Pau Loke Show is the director of Sustainable Food Processing Research Centre and co-director of the Future Food Malaysia, Beacon of Excellence, at the University of Nottingham, Malaysia. He is a full professor at the Department of Chemical and Environmental Engineering, Faculty of Science and Engineering, University of Nottingham, Malaysia. He earned a PhD in two years' time after earning a bachelor's degree at Universiti Putra Malaysia. He is currently a professional engineer registered with the Board of Engineers Malaysia, Chartered Engineer of the Engineering Council UK, and a professional technologist registered from the Malaysia Board of Technologists. Prof. Ir. Ts. Dr. Show obtained a Post Graduate Certificate of Higher Education (PGCHE) in 2014 and is now a fellow of the Higher Education Academy UK. Since 2012 he has received numerous prestigious domestic and international academic awards, including the ASPIRE Malaysia Award 2020, Nation Young Scientist 2019 Award, ASEAN-India Research and Training Fellowship 2019, the DaSilva Award 2018, JSPS Fellowship 2018, Top 100 Asian Scientists 2017, Asia's Rising Scientists Award 2017, and Winner of Young Researcher in IChemE Award 2016. Prof. Dr. Show is also listed in the top 2% of scientists in the Stanford List and has published more than 350 journal articles and book chapters. He is a renowned expert in bioprocessing and biomanufacturing technologies.

Kit Wayne Chew is a lecturer at the School of Energy and Chemical Engineering, Xiamen University, Malaysia. He is an associate member (AMIChemE) of the Institution of Chemical Engineers (IChemE). Dr. Chew's research involves chemical engineering, biochemical engineering, optimization, and bioprocess engineering design. He has conducted various researches in bioseparation processing, waste management, algal cultivation, and biofuel and bioproducts applications. He is the winner for the Young Researcher of IChemE Global Awards 2020, Young Researcher for IChemE Malaysia Award 2020, and Rising Star Award 2019. Dr. Chew has published more than 80 journal papers, book chapters, and made several conference presentations. He has collaborated with international renowned researchers in the field of bioprocessing in Taiwan, India, Japan, and China.

Tau Chuan Ling earned a doctoral degree in 2002 in chemical engineering at the University of Birmingham, UK. He is a chartered engineer of the Engineering Council, United Kingdom (CEng) and fellow member of the Institution of Chemical Engineers (FIChemE). Since 2011 he has been a professor at the Institute of Biological Sciences, Faculty of Science, University of Malaya (UM). Prof. Dr. Ling is the editor-in-chief for the *Current Biochemical Engineering* journal, and he has more than 15 years of research experience in the field of downstream processing and bioprocess engineering. His current research mainly focuses on bioseparation, bioprocessing, green chemistry, and bioprospecting of microorganisms for useful biomolecules. Prof. Dr. Ling has published more than 280 international peer-reviewed journals and presented more than 100 conference papers. He is listed in the UM Researchers Top 2% Scientists by Stanford University, and he was awarded the Young Asian Biotechnologist Prize 2017 by the Society for Biotechnology, Japan. Prof. Dr. Ling has served as a visiting professor at several universities, including Nanjing Agricultural University, Tsinghua University, Xiamen University, Lund University, National Cheng Kung University, Canterbury University, and Kobe University.

Contributors

Nurul Natasha binti Azhar
Department of Chemical and Environmental Engineering
Faculty of Science and Engineering
University of Nottingham, Malaysia
Semenyih, Malaysia

Abdul Azim bin Azmi
Department of Chemical and Environmental Engineering
Faculty of Science and Engineering
University of Nottingham, Malaysia
Semenyih, Malaysia

Yee Ho Chai
Biomass Processing Laboratory
HICoE – Centre for Biofuel and Biochemical Research, and Department of Chemical Engineering
Universiti Teknologi Petronas
Seri Iskandar, Malaysia

Kit Wayne Chew
School of Energy and Chemical Engineering
Xiamen University Malaysia
Sepang, Malaysia

Shir Reen Chia
Department of Chemical and Environmental Engineering
Faculty of Science and Engineering
University of Nottingham, Malaysia
Semenyih, Malaysia

Wen Yi Chia
Department of Chemical and Environmental Engineering
Faculty of Science and Engineering
University of Nottingham, Malaysia
Semenyih, Malaysia

Meng-Choung Chiong
Department of Chemical and Environmental Engineering
Faculty of Science and Engineering
University of Nottingham, Malaysia
Semenyih, Malaysia

Deepshika Deepak
Department of Chemical and Environmental Engineering
Faculty of Science and Engineering
University of Nottingham, Malaysia
Semenyih, Malaysia

Vishno Vardhan Devadas
Department of Chemical and Environmental Engineering
Faculty of Science and Engineering
University of Nottingham, Malaysia
Semenyih, Malaysia

Omar Ashraf ElFar
School of Pharmacy
Faculty of Science and Engineering
University of Nottingham, Malaysia
Semenyih, Malaysia

Jilu Feng
Food Quality and Design Group
Wageningen University and Research
Wageningen, Netherlands

Bridgid Lai Fui Chin
Department of Chemical Engineering
Faculty of Engineering and Science
Curtin University
Miri, Malaysia

Khalisanni Khalid
Malaysian Agricultural Research and Development Institute (MARDI)
MARDI Headquarters, Serdang, Malaysia, and Department of Chemistry
Faculty of Science
University of Malaya
Kuala Lumpur, Malaysia

Kuan Shiong Khoo
Department of Chemical and Environmental Engineering
Faculty of Science and Engineering
University of Nottingham, Malaysia
Semenyih, Malaysia

Apurav Krishna Koyande
Department of Chemical and Environmental Engineering
Faculty of Science and Engineering
University of Nottingham, Malaysia
Semenyih, Malaysia

Yoong Kit Leong
Department of Chemical and Materials Engineering
College of Engineering
Tunghai University
Taichung, Taiwan

Tau Chuan Ling
Institute of Biological Sciences
Faculty of Science
University of Malaya
Kuala Lumpur, Malaysia

Xuwei Liu
INRAE, UMR408 Sécurité et Qualité des Produits d'Origine Végétale
Avignon, France

Adrian Chun Minh Loy
Chemical Engineering Department
Monash University
Victoria, Australia

Zahid Majeed
Department of Biotechnology
University of Azad Jammu and Kashmir
Muzaffarabad, Pakistan

Muhammad Mubashir
Department of Petroleum Engineering
School of Engineering
Asia Pacific
University of Technology and Innovation, 57000
Kuala Lumpur, Malaysia

Zahra Nashath
Department of Chemical and Environmental Engineering
Faculty of Science and Engineering
University of Nottingham, Malaysia
Semenyih, Malaysia

Saifuddin Nomanbhay
Institute of Sustainable Energy (ISE)
Universiti Tenaga Nasional (UNITEN)
Kajang, Malaysia

Mei Yin Ong
Institute of Sustainable Energy (ISE)
Universiti Tenaga Nasional (UNITEN)
Kajang, Malaysia

Angela Paul A/p Peter
Department of Chemical and Environmental Engineering
Faculty of Science and Engineering
University of Nottingham, Malaysia
Semenyih, Malaysia

Revathy Sankaran
Research and Knowledge Exchange Hub
Graduate School
University of Nottingham, Malaysia
Semenyih, Malaysia

Hui Shi Saw
School of Biosciences
Faculty of Science and Engineering
University of Nottingham, Malaysia
Semenyih, Malaysia

Pau Loke Show
Department of Chemical and Environmental Engineering
Faculty of Science and Engineering
University of Nottingham, Malaysia
Semenyih, Malaysia

Chung Hong Tan
Department of Chemical and Environmental Engineering
Faculty of Science and Engineering
University of Nottingham, Malaysia
Semenyih, Malaysia

Jian Hong Tan
Department of Chemical and Environmental Engineering
Faculty of Engineering
University of Nottingham, Malaysia
Semenyih, Malaysia

Doris Ying Ying Tang
Department of Chemical and Environmental Engineering
Faculty of Science and Engineering
University of Nottingham, Malaysia
Semenyih, Malaysia

Yang Tao
College of Food Science and Technology
Nanjing Agricultural University
Nanjing, China

Guo Yong Yew
Department of Chemical and Environmental Engineering
Faculty of Science and Engineering
University of Nottingham, Malaysia
Semenyih, Malaysia

Kai Ling Yu
Institute of Biological Sciences
Faculty of Science
University of Malaya
Kuala Lumpur, Malaysia

Suzana Yusup
Biomass Processing Laboratory
HICoE – Centre for Biofuel and Biochemical Research, and Department of Chemical Engineering
Universiti Teknologi Petronas
Seri Iskandar, Malaysia

1.1 Industrial Revolution 1.0 and 2.0

Adrian Chun Minh Loy, Bridgid Lai Fui Chin, and Revathy Sankaran

CONTENTS

1.1.1 INDUSTRIAL REVOLUTION 1.0

The First Industrial Revolution (IR) was a new transition (760–1830s) in Europe and United States to a manufacturing era. Aware of the head start, the British forbade the export of machinery, skilled workers, and manufacturing equipment to other Europe countries. However, the monopolies could not last a long period due to high profitable industrial opportunities abroad, while many European businessmen sought to lure British know-how to their countries. Thus, it leads to an unprecedented rise in the population growth rate and standard of living in the Europe Continental as claimed by many economies. The major effect of IR 1.0 was that the increase of living standard for the Western colonization for the first time in history (Szreter and Mooney 1998). This is because the GDP per capita growth significantly throughout the revolution and emergence into a modern capitalist economy. Thus, most of the economic historians are in a good agreement that the onset of the revolution is the most glorious event in the history of humanity since the domestication of animals and plants (Hirschman and Mogford 2009; Clark 2014; Akhter and Ormerod 2015).

1.1.2 INDUSTRIAL REVOLUTION 2.0

The Second IR is commonly known as the Technological Revolution, which is said to begin between the year of 1870 and 1914s; although number of major breakthrough events can be dated to the 1850s. However, it was seen that swift rate of pioneering inventions were dawdled after year 1825 and accelerated in the last third of the century (Mokyr 2000). In this revolution, the invention moved toward micro invention instead of macro invention which focused mainly on the productivity, and product quality improvements rather than path breaking invention.

It was observed that the inventions after 1870s were different compared to the First IR and it was found that the innovations were more productive and denser (Mowery and Rosenberg 1991). One of the aspects during this revolution is that people viewed useful knowledge can be mapped into new technology. This can be further explained that during the previous IR i.e., First IR, most people are unable to understand how certain things do not function and hardly understood why it could work for certain inventions from engineering, medical technology, to agriculture (Mokyr 2000). Hence, the people's viewpoint of technology is knowledge and considerable feedback from technology to science that lead to outcomes of technology improvement and novel invention during this revolution. The second aspect during this revolution is the changing nature of the organization of production (Mokyr 2000). This has resulted in a massive boost in the economic scale in terms of manufacturing and organizational, and marketing factors involved. A typical example in manufacturing is providing storage for chemicals, which involves the construction of storage containers which correlated to the surface area and the volume of the chemicals interrelates with the capacity of storage. As for the organizational factor, an example can be the mass production via interchangeable parts technology involved. As for the involvement of the marketing side, it was observed that big U.S. companies such as Dupont, General Electric, and others were involving a small portion of the labor force and emphasized flexibility and targeting to a more general market (Floud 2004).

There were also some consequences faced during this revolution phase when alteration was made on the production technology, which was attributed to the increasing technological system (Hughes 1983). This IR had converted large technological system from unique to ordinary (Mokyr 2000). This happened because the system involved a large amount of synchronization that free market finds it difficult to supply, and therefore this involved either the government or leading organizations to make a decision on standards for railroad gauges, electricity voltages, road regulations, and many more. The idea of producing separate components in a technology that could be optimized separately did not came to realization after year 1870.

1.1.3 TECHNOLOGY DEVELOPMENT IN INDUSTRIAL 1.0 AND 2.0

Many new technologies have been discovered during the transition, not limited to hand production to machines, new machine tools manufacturing, and power generation using steam as well as iron ore production processes as shown in Table 1.1.1. The following sections will be discussing the major developments during the First and Second IRs which consist of steel, chemicals, electricity, and transportation, agriculture, and food engineering.

1.1.3.1 Textile

During IR 1.0, textiles were the dominant industry in terms of employment and capital market cap (Ayres 1990). By 1750s, Britain has imported more than 2.5 million pounds of raw cotton, in which most of them were spun and woven. Most of the work was performed by hand in home or master weaver's shops. In 1800, the usage of cotton in the British textile industry was 52 million pounds and increased more than tenfold in 1850 (Hopkins 2000). Besides that, the value share added by the cotton textile industry in Britain was also increased gradually from 2.6% to 22.4%.

The movement of cotton textile prices was also known as the indicator of the expansion or diffusion of the cotton's technology. During the middle of the 19th century, the substitution of spinning to power weaving has causes the prices of cotton goods to decrease significantly as documented in the history (Harley 1998). When the innovation was confined to spinning, a huge impact on fine yarns and on warps was resulted. Nevertheless, all yarn prices started to decline significantly from the mid-1780s as shown in Table 1.1.2.

Meanwhile, the first invention of textile machine which known as flying shuttle was invented by John Kay in 1733. Subsequently in 1764, James Hargreaves has invented the spinning jenny, which patented in 1770 to substitute the flying shuttle (Lawrence 2010). It was the first practical spinning frame with multiple spindles. Although the textile mechanization has significantly decreased the operating cost of cotton cloth, by the mid-1900s, machine-woven cloth still could not compete with hand-woven Indian cloth in terms of quality such as fineness of thread. Nevertheless, the high productivity of British textile manufacturing allowed coarser grades of British cloth to undersell hand-spun and woven fabric in low-wage India.

1.1.3.2 Steam Engine

The development of the steam engine was a key element of the IR to replace water and wind energies. In 1815s, a 210,000-horsepower steam engine was developed, which helped out many small industrials in power generation. Basically, a steam engine is a heat engine where the working fluid (steam) perform mechanical works, as the force of the steam pressure pushes the piston back and forth inside a cylinder. This pushing force is then transformed by a connecting rod and flywheel into

TABLE 1.1.1
The Technologies Discovered in Industrial Revolution 1.0 and 2.0

Technology Development	Remarks	References
Textile	1. Development of mechanized cotton spinning powered by steam or water, enhancing the worker output by a factor of around 500. 2. Highest productivity was cotton, followed by wool and linen.	Harley (2012); Nuvolari (2019)
Steam power	1. The invention of the stationary steam engine was one the key element for the IR. 2. In 1800s, approximately 10,000 horsepower was being supplied by steam in Britain. 3. Ease the transportation as the high-pressure engine has a higher power to weight ratio. 4. Enable a large production of iron by countering the water power limitation using steam engine.	Bruland and Smith (2013); Amengual Matas (2007)
Iron making	1. The iron bar commodity has been used as the feedstock for making hardware goods. 2. Part of the iron bars are converted into kitchen utensils such as steel pots and stoves. 3. The iron bars were made by the bloomery process – a predominant iron smelting process developed in IR 1.0. 4. Reduction the fuel cost of iron production through substitution of coke for charcoal.	Bottomley (2014); B.J. Spear (2019)
Invention of machine tools	1. During 1798s, paper machine was patented by a French guy known as Nicholas Louis Robert. 2. During 1832s, glass making machine was developed in Europe by the Chance Brothers to create sheet glass.	Clapperton (1967); Hounshell (1984); Hopkins (2013)
Mining	1. Before development of the steam engine, removal of water is an issue. The introduction of the steam pump engine in 1712s overcome the problem of water removal, enabling more coal to be extracted and mining become more profitable.	B. Spear (2008)

TABLE 1.1.2
Yarn Prices, Nominal and Deflated, 5-Year Averages from 1769–1809 (Harley 1998)

	Current Prices (pence per lb)			Deflated Prices (pence per lb)		
	18 weft	40 warp	100 twist	18 weft	40 warp	100 twist
33						
1778	34					
1780/1784	33	122		47	168	
1785/1789	33	99	532	47	142	761
1790/1794	27	74	240	36	97	318
1795/1799	33	71	104	36	77	112
1800/1804	31	62	92	27	55	80
1805/1809	22	46	78	19	39	66
1810/1804	21	42	69	15	30	50
1815/1809	18	35	72	15	30	62

rotational force for mechanical work. The first commercially workable coal-powered steam pump was invented by Thomas Savery in 1698. It has a low lift combined with a vacuum and pressure water pump which generates approximately one horsepower (Figure 1.1.1). The main disadvantages were the restricted lift height and heating properties. Alas, small engines were effective, but larger models were problematic and prone to boiler explosions (Hills 1989).

Until the early of 1700s, a commercially power engine that could transmit continuous power to a machine was successfully invented around 1712 (Breeze 2018). It was known as the atmospheric engine which have vast improvement on the Savery's steam pump. It worked by creating a partial vacuum by condensing steam under a

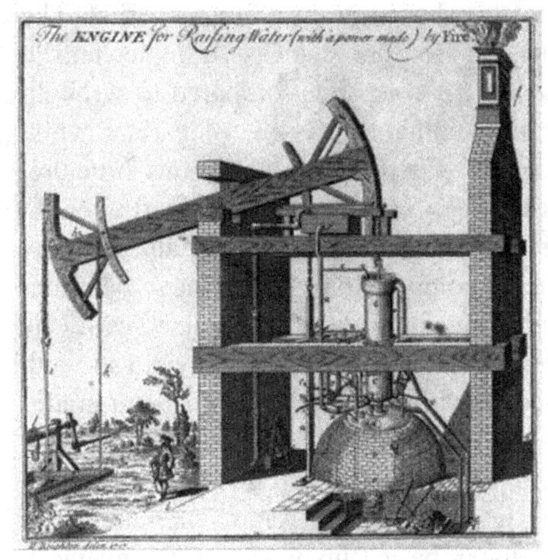

FIGURE 1.1.1 Newcomen engine (B. Spear 2008).

piston within a cylinder. The development of steam piston engines continued until mid-1900s with designers such as James Watt, who developed a more effective version of the Newcomen's engine. In early stage, all steam engines used low-pressure but gradually as technology improved, higher pressure was introduced into the system. The use of high-pressure steam allowed smaller advances of high-speed engines to be built, yielding a compact engine and boiler that can be easily applied on mobile automotive Britannica, The Editors of Encyclopaedia 2019.

1.1.3.3 Iron Production

In 1806, the charcoal cast iron production and coke cast iron were 7,800 tons and 250,000 tons, respectively. The significant change in the iron industries during the era of the IR 1.0 was the replacement of wood with coal. In the same amount of heat given, coal required much lesser preparation compared to wood. This is because wood needs to undergo a series of pre-treatments such as cutting and heating to convert it into charcoal; just before it can be utilized as a source of energy while coal is abundantly available and can be used instantly without any pre-treatment process. By 1750, coke has generally replaced charcoal in smelting and refining of iron with the advantage of less impurities (e.g., sulfur ash) in the coke migrate into the metal steel.

During the Second IR, steel has become one of the key inventions where it was invented by Sir Henry Bessemer using Bessemer process in year 1856 (Mokyr 2000). The Bessemer process is said to be the first cheaper alternative for the mass production of steel from molten pig iron prior to the open-hearth furnace (Lundén and Paulsson 2009). The key principle is to eliminate the impurities from the iron via oxidation process with air flowing pass the molten iron. The condition of the molten iron mass is maintained through oxidation process by increasing the temperature. Countries in East Asia region had used this process with the presence of air for iron purification in a non-industrial scale since the 11th century (Hurt and Schrock 2016). This steel was developed to find a substitution for the frequent wear and tear occurring in the machine parts and rails that was commonly made from wrought iron during that time, which is costly when used in a longer period. The advantages of steel over wrought iron and cast iron are steel has a higher tensile strength and possesses more vulnerability toward corrosion compared to wrought iron (Hurt and Schrock 2016). The cast iron contains 2%–4% of carbon while wrought iron <0.05% carbon with a presence of slag rolled into a fibrous structure. Meanwhile, the carbon content of steel is between both the cast iron and wrought iron and the presence of small percentage of manganese in it (Hurt and Schrock 2016). There are several types in the precise composition of steel have been developed over the years. In the earliest of the 20th century, the steel named as A7 by the American Society for Testing and Materials (ASTM) consists of a yield strength of 33 kpsi, and the contemporary A709 steel is widely available in different grades of 36, 50, 70, and 100 (Hurt and Schrock 2016).

The remaining methods involved for producing a steel is either removing impurities from pig iron or a combination of pig iron and steel scrap. The removal of impurities can be either using an acid (siliceous) or basic (limey) slag (Cheremisinoff,

Rosenfeld, and Davletshin 2008). The acid slag and basic slag involved the usage of acid furnace lining of silica and basic lining of magnesite or dolomite respectively with line charge (Wang 2016). The presence of acid slag silicon will be removed the manganese and carbon meanwhile the basic slag will be removed the silicon, manganese, carbon phosphorus, and sulfur from the charge through oxidation process. The acid Bessemer in the acid open-hearth steel process is said to be less economical compared to the basic electric arc furnace coupled with vacuum degassing and also produce a hematite ore with low phosphorus content (Thomas 2020). Meanwhile, the basic Bessemer process produces iron ores with high phosphorus content.

Sidney Gilchrist Thomas had developed a patented process with his cousin, Percy Gilchrist, to remove the phosphorus from the iron in the year 1878 at Blaenavon Ironworks in Wales (Thomas 2020) and Bolckow Vaughan & Co. in Yorkshire was the first company to apply his patented process (Barraclough 1981). The Siemens-Martin process developed by Sir Charles William Siemens had developed a regenerative furnace for steel making in the year of 1850s. He claimed that his process is able to recover sufficient heat for fuel recovery of 70%–80% (Barraclough 1981). The technique involved in this process utilized hot waste gas for preheating the incoming fuel and air, and both cast iron and wrought iron are combined together in a specific proportion to obtain steel (Mokyr 2000). The high temperature is properly maintained with hearths lined with special silica brick linings. This process is found to be cheaper compared to the Bessemer process in a long-term industrial operation (Mokyr 2000). Furthermore, this open-hearth steel has better quality compared to the Bessemer, although longer time is required to produce it.

In 1865, a French engineer by the name of Pierre-Émile Martin was the pioneer to produce a license for the Siemens furnace and implemented the process for the steel production in the year 1865 (Barraclough 1981). The advantage of using this method is that it limits the nitrogen exposure toward the steel allowing the steel to be less brittle, easier product control, allows large volume of scrap steel during the smelting and refining process, and lowering both the production and recycling costs. This has resulted in this process to be a leading worldwide process by the early 20th century.

1.1.3.4 Chemicals

Although Germany took the lead in chemistry during the Second IR, however, a British man, William Perkin, had the first major discovery in modern chemistry by discovering a chemical process to produce a synthetic organic purple dye, and mauveine made from aniline at the age of 18 in 1856 (Mauveine The Discovery and Inventor 2006). At that time, he was currently pursuing his studies in London's Royal College of Chemistry. It was an accidental invention when his main intention was to produce an artificial quinine from Victorian gas lighting. He had previously failed to produce quinine for malaria treatment (Jacpo 2017). A red aniline was discovered three years later by Emanuel Verguin. Furthermore, there are a few German chemists who had successfully found other artificial dyes. Hofmann and Kekulé had formulated a dyestuff's molecules structure. A group of German chemists had successfully synthesized alizarin, a red dye from madder roots by defeating Perkin by producing a patent a day earlier. This resulted in a beginning process for Germany to unveil their hegemony in chemical discovery (Haber 1958). They also successfully produced indigotin, also known as synthetic indigo, sulfuric, and soda making in year 1897, 1875, and 1860s, respectively. Besides that, Alfred Nobel discovered dynamite which was used for tunnels, roads, oil wells, and quarries construction.

1.1.3.5 Electricity

In this IR, electricity is one of the main sources to advance this era of revolution. Before electricity was discovered, most industries are operated by using steam machines. Scientist Michael Faraday had first discovered electric current using a magnet by introducing movement into a wire coil (Electricity, n.d.). In the year 1808, Humphrey Davy had found a lighting potential based on the scientific discoveries by Dane Hans Oersted, Joseph Henry, and Michael Faraday on the invention of electric motor and dynamo in the years 1821 and 1831, respectively. Electricity application was applied to communication using the telegraph. It was documented that the first transcontinental telegram was transmitted from California to Washington on 24th October 1961. This invention had become revolutionary to construct an urgent telegraph line due to the Civil War. Before that, a post mail from Pony Express was the source of communication to deliver messages through letter from Sacramento to Missouri within ten days. The invention of the telegraph had eventually led to another communication invention known as the telephone. This invention was led by Alexander Graham Bell in the year 1876. It was reported that Bell had owned a telephone company with 5,000 shares that was issued by both his family members and partners.

The usage of electricity was said to expand swiftly in the 1870s. During the Berlin exhibition, a miniature electric railway was displayed in 1879. Meanwhile, electric blankets and hotplates were exhibited in one of Vienna's exhibitions four years later. Besides that, the modern light bulb was invented by both Joseph Swan and Thomas A. Edison from England and United States, respectively, in the 1880s. There are also other inventions such as alternating current built by Nikola Tesla in 1889 and the transformer by Lucien Gaulard and John D. Gibbs in the year 1884 (Hughes 1983).

1.1.3.6 Transportation

The steam power to train and factories was already well-established by the year 1870. During the Second IR, there was an improvement in the railroads to ensure the transportation could be faster, safer, and a smooth ride for the passengers. During this industrial era, the diesel engine was invented by Rudolf Diesel in the year 1897 (Mokyr 2000). He was known as an engineer trained in science by trying to include theoretical Carnot cycle to achieve a high efficiency through isothermal expansion in order to improve energy efficiency, and a source of cheaper fuel to boot since during that time Diesel had tried to utilize the coal dust into the engine instead. Unfortunately, Diesel discovered that the isothermal expansion method was not possible. However, he had found a compression-induced combustion method for the diesel engine that is still used until today through his unexpected discovery.

Ships made by steel were becoming popular after 1870. This is because larger ships were made of iron and steel compared to ships made of wood. Hence, the development of better performance ships in terms of speed, power, and size improved at exceptional rates (Mokyr 2000). Gustave de Laval and Charles Parson had invented a steam turbine in 1884 that provided a solution to replace the reciprocating marine steam engines which had been long used since the 1900s. The steam turbine provided much more advantages compared to the steam engine in terms of delivering an improved efficiency performance, faster speed, cleaner energy source, and less noise to the ship (Mokyr 2000).

Cracking process for crude oil refining process was developed in the earliest 1860s. During this time, scientists were particularly interested in finding a suitable fuel for Otto's gas engine. In the year 1885, Gottlieb Daimler and Karl Benz from Germany had successfully constructed a four-stroke gasoline-burning with the Otto-type engine incorporating a basic carburettor for fuel and mixing. Benz had customized the electrical induction coil powered in the engine by an accumulator in producing a source of spark plug.

1.1.3.7 Agriculture and Food Engineering

During this IR, food supply and nutrition are the main factors that attributed to the living quality of the population. Farmers started to add nitrates, potassium, and phosphates into the fertilizers to increase the agricultural productivity. The agricultural sector in the European countries had switched from natural fertilizer such as the guano to chemical-produced fertilizer. Furthermore, the fungicides developed from the Bordeaux mixture invented by M. Millardet from France in 1885 were used to fight the diseases found in the potato plantation in Ireland (Mokyr 2000). The implementation of drainage and irrigation pipes, steam-operated threshers, seed drills, and mechanical reapers made of steel are the few technologies to enhance the agricultural production. Andrew Meikle from Scotland had invented a threshing machine in 1784 and James Sharp from London build a winnowing machine (Mokyr 2000). The steam engine were attached on both the threshing and winnowing machine in the first half of the 19th century. Before World War I, tractors and combines were starting to be built in the Atlantic. It is also documented that an average of 20 man-hours were required to harvest wheat from one acre of land in 1880. The man-hours required for harvesting wheat gradually reduced to 6.1 man-hours per acre by 1935 (Mokyr 2000).

In 1795, food canning was invented; however, the food was poorly processed. This is due to the lack of understanding of food processing in the industry during this time. Louis Pasteur had successfully resolved the food-canning issue by discovering the optimal cooking temperature, 240 °F. The canned-food industry played an important part during the American Civil War to cater foods for the armies and also meeting the increasing consumption demand for the fast-developing countries. In 1850, Gail Borden invented milk powder (Mokyr 2000). And also, dehydration process on both eggs and soups were successfully implemented at the end of this century (Mokyr 2000).

1.1.4 INDUSTRIALIZATION BEYOND BRITAIN

The revolution on Europe and Asia continental came a little later than in Britain. Most of the technology was purchased and shipped abroad in search of new opportunities in other regions. By late-1809, many countries governments (e.g., Sweden, Japan, and Belgium) provided huge amount of funding to learn and adopt new technologies into their countries.

1.1.4.1 Sweden

Between 1790–1815, Sweden has experienced two parallel economic movements: agricultural revolution and proto industrialization. This industrialization has led to an economical growth that benefited the growth of population as well as revolution. From 1815 and 1850, the proto industries changed into specialized and commercial industries, an increase of regional specialization specifically mining, and textile mills were witnessed. After that, Sweden experienced its "first" IR with a high demand in export, dominated by crops, forestry, and steel (Bengtsson et al. 2018). In addition, Sweden government also abolished most of the tariff and tax to lure large infrastructural investments, especially the transportation sector.

1.1.4.2 United States

Prior to the IR, the citizens were reared in isolated agricultural households and small towns with self-sufficient in food and essential daily goods (Olmstead and Rhode 2000). This norm changed dramatically with the revolution as many new manufacturing goods existed and a better transportation through rapid expansion of railways.

A rise of employment, investment, and productivity in the manufacturing sector was also discovered. Following with the technological revolutions, many workshops and small foundries were supplemented by many business opportunities from large factories. At the end of the 19th century, the electricity power supply started to be commercialized, enabling industries to increase their production in large cities. The changes can be seen through the rise in the share of manufacturing horsepower generated by electrical motors from 23% in 1909 to 77% in 1929 (Hirschman and Mogford 2009). Perhaps the most significant change of the revolution was the urbanization of society and the shift of labor from farms to factories (Guest 2005). For example, in 1880, the workers in agriculture outnumbered industrial workers; but by 1920, the numbers were almost same. Meanwhile, employment in the manufacturing sector also experienced the same scenario with the number of employee increasing four times from 1880 to 1920.

1.1.4.3 Japan

The IR started around 1870 as the Meiji leaders tried to catch up with the West. Japan's government had built many railways, roads, and inaugurated a land reformation for country development. A new Western-based education system was also introduced to all young Japanese; thousands of Japanese students had been sent out to other countries to adopt and learn the Western technologies. In 1871, Japanese politicians were also sent to Europe and the United States, resulting in a deliberate state-led industrialization policy and also enabled Japan to quickly catch up to the modern industrial age (History 2015).

1.1.4.4 Belgium

The two Britains, William and John Cockerill, brought the IR to Belgium by introducing machine shops, which resulted in Belgium becoming the first country to be transformed economically in continental Europe. Like its British progenitor, the Belgian IR centered on iron, coal, and textiles. This transition was ongoing from hand production methods to machines, new chemical and steel production processes, and the use of steam power. Between 1840 and 1880, the railway networks also expanded tenfold, which is much greater than Britain. The transport communications of the country have profited from trade with less-developed neighbors. Most Belgian investors and entrepreneurs made contribution to building up industrial activities along the rivers Ruhr und Emscher. Lastly, Belgium became a revolution gateway in Europe and changed the image of the world economy. It has proved to the world that a small country could spark worldwide economics.

1.1.5 SOCIAL EFFECTS OF THE INDUSTRIAL REVOLUTION

1.1.5.1 Factories and Labors

The IR has created a life changing deal in society. One major change was the shift from "work at home" to "work in factories". However, the working environments were harsh and unsafe in early 1800. The machines posed a significant threat to workers' lives, resulting in many workers dying, especially coal mining workers. The mine's owner had considerable control over the lives of laborers who worked long hours for low pay. For instance, an average worker needs to work more than 14 hours a day, six days a week. In order to secure their jobs, workers usually did not complain about the harsh conditions and low pay. In 1850, owners realized that the salary for women and children was even less than men. As a result, the demand of child labor increased to lower the production costs and enhance the profit.

1.1.5.2 Social Effect for Women

A dramatic change for women can be seen in the IR. This is because most of them entered the work society for the first time and needed to compete with men for jobs. Female factory workers often made only one-third as much as men. By the 1918s, women started to be involved in politics and demand suffrage, the right to vote. With the hardship and lastly, Britain granted women over 30 to have the right to vote; meanwhile the United States also granted women suffrage with the passing of an amendment in 1920.

1.1.5.3 Urbanization

The IR has shown a positive effect in urbanization such as an increase in wealth, the quantity and quality of products, and uplifting the living standard. More people realized the importance of education and started to attend classes in school. Moreover, the invention of the smallpox vaccine also brought positive perspectives to the healthcare field. Mostly the middle and upper classes straightforward benefited from the IR as compared to the skilled workers.

1.1.6 CONCLUSION

The insights of IR 1.0 and 2.0 are discussed as follows: 1) The main contributions of these two revolutions to mankind are "mechanization, steam power and weaving loom" (IR 1.0) and "mass production, assembly line and electrical energy" (IR 2.0). 2) The IR started in Britain and soon became a significant event in world history. 3) The IR marked a significant change in Europe, followed by Asia and the United States and led to the creation of the modern world.

REFERENCES

Akhter, Majed, and Kerri Jean Ormerod. 2015. "The Irrigation Technozone: State Power, Expertise, and Agrarian Development in the U.S. West and British Punjab, 1880–1920." *Geoforum* 60 (March): 123–132. doi:10.1016/j.geoforum.2015.01.012.

Amengual Matas, Rubén. 2007. "Reseñas." *Investigaciones de Historia Económica* 3 (9): 186–187. doi:10.1016/S1698-6989(07)70225-4.

Ayres, Robert U. 1990. "Technological transformations and long waves. Part I." *Technological Forecasting and Social Change* 37 (1): 1–37. doi:10.1016/0040-1625(90)90057-3.

Barraclough, K.C. 1981. "*Steel Processes – An Essay in the History of Technology*." University of Sheffield.

Bengtsson, Erik, Anna Missiaia, Mats Olsson, and Patrick Svensson. 2018. "Wealth inequality in Sweden, 1750–1900." *The Economic History Review* 71 (3): 772–794. doi:10.1111/ehr.12576.

Bottomley, Sean. 2014. "Patenting in England, Scotland and Ireland during the Industrial Revolution, 1700–1852." *Explorations in Economic History* 54 (October): 48–63. doi:10.1016/j.eeh.2014.08.002.

Breeze, Paul. 2018. "An Introduction to Piston Engine Power Plants." In *Piston Engine-Based Power Plants*, 1–11. Elsevier. doi:10.1016/B978-0-12-812904-3.00001-X.

Britannica, The Editors of Encyclopaedia. 2019. "Industrial Revolution." In *Encyclopædia Britannica*. Encyclopædia Britannica, Inc. https://www.britannica.com/event/Industrial-Revolution.

Bruland, Kristine, and Keith Smith. 2013. "Assessing the role of steam power in the first Industrial Revolution: The early work of Nick von Tunzelmann." *Research Policy* 42 (10): 1716–1723. doi:10.1016/j.respol.2012.12.008.

Cheremisinoff, Nicholas P., Paul Rosenfeld, and Anton R. Davletshin. 2008. "P2 and best management practices in different industries." In *Responsible Care*, 435–476. Elsevier. doi:10.1016/B978-1-933762-16-6.50011-6.

Clapperton, R.H. 1967. "The First British Paper-Making Machine Patent." In *The Paper-Making Machine*, 24–33. Elsevier. doi:10.1016/B978-0-08-001975-8.50007-2.

Clark, Gregory. 2014. "The Industrial Revolution." In *Handbook of Economic Growth*, edited by Philippe Aghion and Steven Durlauf 217–262, Elsevier. doi:10.1016/B978-0-444-53538-2.00005-8.

Eric Hopkins. 2000. "*Industrialisation and Society A Social History*," *1830–1951*. London: Routledge.

Floud, Roderick. 2004. "*The Cambridge Economic History of Modern Britain": Volume 2. Growth and Decline, 1870 to the Present*, 2nd edition, edited by Paul Johnson, Nicholas Crafts, and Kevin O'Rourke. Cambridge University Press.

Guest, Avery M. 2005. "Frontier and urban-industrial explanations of US occupational mobility in the late 1800s." *Social Science Research* 34 (1): 140–164. doi:10.1016/j.ssresearch.2004.01.001.

Haber, L.F. 1958. *The Chemical Industry during the Nineteenth Century*. Oxford: Clarendon Press.

Harley, C. Knick. 1998. "Cotton textile prices and the Industrial Revolution." *The Economic History Review* 51 (1): 49–83. doi:10.1111/1468-0289.00083.

Harley, C. Knick. 2012. "Was technological change in the early Industrial Revolution Schumpeterian? Evidence of cotton textile profitability." *Explorations in Economic History* 49 (4): 516–527. doi:10.1016/j.eeh.2012.06.004.

Hills, Richard L. 1989. *Power from Steam: A History of the Stationary Steam Engine*. Cambridge: Cambridge University Press.

Hirschman, Charles, and Elizabeth Mogford. 2009. "Immigration and the American Industrial Revolution from 1880 to 1920." *Social Science Research* 38 (4): 897–920. doi:10.1016/j.ssresearch.2009.04.001.

History. 2015. "Bank of Japan." https://www.boj.or.jp/en/about/outline/history/index.htm/.

Hopkins, Eric. 2013. *Industrialisation and Society*. Routledge. doi:10.4324/9780203130896.

Hounshell, David A. 1984. *From the American System to Mass Production, 1800–1932: The Development of Manufacturing Technology in the United States*. Baltimore: Johns Hopkins University Press. http://hdl.handle.net/2027/heb.04049.0001.001.

Hughes, Thomas Parke. 1983. *Networks of Power: Electrification in Western Society, 1880–1930*. Baltimore: Johns Hopkins Press.

Hurt, Mark, and Steven D. Schrock. 2016. "Bridge Elements and Materials." In *Highway Bridge Maintenance Planning and Scheduling*, 31–98. Elsevier. doi:10.1016/B978-0-12-802069-2.00002-7.

Jacpo, Prisco. 2017. The color purple: How an accidental discovery changed fashion forever. https://edition.cnn.com/style/article/perkin-mauve-purple/index.html.

Lawrence, C.A. 2010. "Overview of Developments in Yarn Spinning Technology." In *Advances in Yarn Spinning Technology*, 3–41. Elsevier. doi:10.1533/9780857090218.1.3.

Lundén, R., and B. Paulsson. 2009. "Introduction to Wheel–Rail Interface Research." In *Wheel–Rail Interface Handbook*, 3–33. Elsevier. doi:10.1533/9781845696788.1.3.

Mauveine The Discovery and Inventor. 2006. *Mauveine The Discovery and Inventor*. Royal Society of Chemistry. https://www.rsc.org/Chemsoc/Activities/Perkin/2006/minisite_perkin_mauveine_non_flash.html.

Mokyr, Joel. 2000. "Innovation and Its Enemies: The Economic and Political Roots of Technological Inertia." In *A Not-so-Dismal Science*, 61–91. Oxford University Press. doi:10.1093/0198294905.003.0003.

Mowery, D.C., and N. Rosenberg. 1991. *Technology and the Pursuit of Economic Growth*. Cambridge University Press. https://books.google.com.my/books?id=eU8FhP3_XrgC.

Nuvolari, Alessandro. 2019. "Understanding Successive Industrial Revolutions: A 'Development Block' Approach." *Environmental Innovation and Societal Transitions* 32 (September): 33–44. doi:10.1016/j.eist.2018.11.002.

Olmstead, Alan, and Paul Rhode. 2000. "The Transformation of Northern Agriculture, 1910–1990." In *The Cambridge Economic History of the United States: Volume 3: The*

Twentieth Century, edited by Robert E. Gallman and Stanley L. Engerman. Cambridge: Cambridge University Press.

Spear, B.J. 2019. "Iron and steel patents: The sinews of the GB Industrial Revolution." *World Patent Information* 58 (September): 101901. doi:10.1016/j.wpi.2019.101901.

Spear, Brian. 2008. "James Watt: The steam engine and the commercialization of patents." *World Patent Information* 30(1): 53–58. doi:10.1016/j.wpi.2007.05.009.

Szreter, Simon, and Graham Mooney. 1998. "Urbanization, mortality, and the standard of living debate: New estimates of the expectation of life at birth in nineteenth-century British cities." *The Economic History Review* 51(1). [Economic History Society, Wiley]: 84–112. http://www.jstor.org/stable/2599693.

Thomas, Sidney Gilchrist. 2020. "In Welsh Biography Online." Accessed March 20. https://biography.wales/article/s-THOM-GIL-1850.

Wang, George C. 2016. "Usability Criteria for Slag Use as a Granular Material." In *The Utilization of Slag in Civil Infrastructure Construction*, 185–199. Elsevier. doi:10.1016/B978-0-08-100381-7.00009-4.

1.2 Industry 3.0

Chung Hong Tan

CONTENTS

1.2.1 FROM INDUSTRY 1.0 TO INDUSTRY 3.0

Industry 1.0, or the First Industrial Revolution, was the transition of human production to machine production through the use of steam and water power. The implementation of steam technology took place between 1760 and 1820, or 1840 in the US and Europe. Steam technology transformed the industries, especially the textile industry and transportation sector (steam engines). Apart from these, other industries also adopted mechanized production using steam power, such as iron industry, mining, and agriculture (Berlanstein 2003).

Industry 2.0, or the Second Industrial Revolution, was the technological revolution where electricity permitted mass production in assembly lines. Other than improvements in industrialization, the establishment of vast railroad and telegraph systems also enabled swifter transfer of people and ideas. Industry 2.0 took place between 1870 and 1914, and marked an era of high productivity and economic growth. However, this had caused a rise in unemployment due to the replacement of numerous workers by machines in many factories (Bosch Sanayi Ve Ticaret A.Ş. 2017).

Industry 3.0, or the Third Industrial Revolution, was the digital revolution where information technology (IT) and computer advancement led to the spread of automation in many industries and factories. Industry 3.0 started in the late 20th century after the second world war (around 1970). Although computer and communication technologies were widely used in production processes without the need for human intervention, human operators were still required to monitor and control the automated processes (Bosch Sanayi Ve Ticaret A.Ş. 2017).

1.2.2 ERA OF MODERN GENETIC ENGINEERING

Around the time Industry 3.0 started to take off, in 1973, a major breakthrough in genetically modified organism (GMO) technology occurred when Herbert Boyer (from the University of California San Francisco, CA, USA) and Stanley Cohen (from Stanford University, Stanford, CA, USA) collaborated in successfully creating the first genetically engineered microorganism. Both scientists devised a technique to cut out a specific gene from one microorganism and insert it into another. By using this technique, they successfully transferred a gene that codes for antibiotic resistance from one bacterial strain into another, providing the latter strain with the same antibiotic resistance (Cohen et al. 1973). In the following year, Rudolf Jaenisch (from Massachusetts Institute of Technology, Cambridge, MA, USA) and Beatrice Mintz (from Fox Chase Cancer Center, Philadelphia, PA, USA) employed a similar technique in small animals, inserting foreign deoxyribonucleic acid (DNA) into mouse embryos (Jaenisch and Mintz 1974).

Shortly after the development of this new technology, the scientists, government officials, and media were anxious about the potential ramifications of this technology on human health and the Earth's ecosystems (Berg et al. 1974). By mid-1974, a universal agreement was reached to enforce a moratorium on all genetic engineering projects, so that experts could gather and contemplate the future directions of genetic engineering in the Asilomar Conference of 1975. At the end of the conference, it was decided that genetic engineering projects should be permitted to continue while adhering to safety guidelines that minimized risks of each experiments. In addition, the principal investigator in every lab was responsible for the safety of their researchers and updating the scientific community on important technological advances. The initial guidelines were set to be fluid, and could change as more knowledge was added in the field (Berg et al., 1974). Following the unprecedented transparency and cooperation at the Asilomar Conference, genetic engineering research was supported by government agencies around the world, thus began the era of modern genetic engineering.

The rapid advancement in automation, ever-improving computer processing power, and software engineering brought about by Industry 3.0 played a critical role in establishing the first genome sequence of a living microorganism, the bacterium *Haemophilus influenza*, in July 1995. Algorithms were constructed to re-create a full genome sequence based on fragmented and random DNA sequences (Fleischmann et al. 1995). The genome of another bacterium, *Mycoplasma genitalium,* was reported shortly after in October 1995 (Fraser et al. 1995). These two reports solidified the whole-genome shotgun sequencing and assembly method for the reconstruction of genome sequences. The methods for genome sequencing and assembly is continuously improved to obtain higher throughput and lower cost, which has allowed the sequencing of genomes of many different species as well as human individuals (Giani et al. 2020). This opened up the field of genomics, which is the study of the structure, function, and evolution, as well as the mapping of genomes. The genomes of non-genetically modified organisms can be used as references against their genetically modified counterparts to study the effects of modifying specific genes or ensure the correct gene expressions (National Academies of Sciences, Engineering, and Medicine, 2016).

1.2.3 WHAT IS BIOMANUFACTURING?

The majority of the general public is not well informed of just how deeply biotechnology, utilizing the fermentation of both natural and recombinant organisms, has influenced our daily lives and various consumer products. Many may be familiar with the common antibiotics (such as amoxicillin and azithromycin) or large recombinant pharmaceutical proteins (such as antibodies and insulin) produced through industrial (or large-scale) fermentation. However, the role of fermentation in small-molecule pharmaceuticals, flavors and fragrances, chemical industry, household items, and many other industries is largely unknown to the public (Hans-Peter, Wolfgang, and Diego 2016).

The term "fermentation" initially referred to the conversion of starch grains to alcohol under anaerobic conditions, which is a process still used today in synthesizing first-generation biofuels. This is the reason many textbooks refer to this definition as the origin of biotechnology. However, in modern biotechnology, fermentation refers to any submersed cultivation in a bioreactor under either aerobic or anaerobic conditions (Hans-Peter, Wolfgang, and Diego 2016). In our current world, most of the biotechnology products are manufactured using fermentation via the process called biomanufacturing.

Biomanufacturing, also known as biologics manufacturing, is a process that employs biological systems (like microbes, cells, enzymes, tissues, plants, animals, and in vitro synthetic biology systems) to create commercially important biomolecules which are useful in various industries such as food, agriculture, energy, materials, nutraceuticals, and pharmaceuticals (Michels and Rosazza 2009). The targeted biological products can be harvested from natural sources (like natural plant cells and animal cells, tissues, or blood) or dedicated cultivation environments (for instance, cells cultured in bioreactors or plants cultivated in sterile and controlled conditions). The cells, tissues, or enzymes employed in the biological systems may be natural or modified via genetic engineering, synthetic biology, metabolic engineering, or protein engineering (Vasic-Racki 2006). The realization and demonstration of concepts in recombinant organisms from the research bench is further studied by process and analytical groups, where scientific and engineering tools as well as regulatory experience will be utilized to determine efficient methods of scaling up and rigorous tests to ensure safe and high-quality products. Higher product yields will ensure a more stable supply to industries (which use enzymes or amino acids) and better support for clinical programs (which focuses on pharmaceuticals). Unlike traditional chemical manufacturing, the process for each biological system is complex and the biological products synthesized from living cells is not an exact science, different from the case of chemistry (Conner et al. 2014).

The long-standing model for biomanufacturing is "the process is the product" and that any alterations to the process could cause changes in the safety and efficacy of the products. Although current raw materials, process, and analytics are well defined and permit higher degree of flexibility in designing and developing different processes, alterations to the process could result in a product with completely different profile or affect the safety of the product (Conner et al. 2014). It has been shown that endogenous and adventitious viruses may contaminate the biological products due to process changes or infected raw materials (Barone et al. 2020). Thus, thorough analysis on the production processes and genetic makeup of the modified organisms or cell lines are necessary to understand the consequences of alterations in the production process.

1.2.4 FERMENTER – THE PRIMARY WORKHORSE OF BIOMANUFACTURING

The most common yet crucial piece of equipment in biomanufacturing facilities is a fermenter, which is a vessel for growing microorganisms. The fermenter is operated as a closed system to mitigate contamination risks while still have inlets to provide the necessary nutrients to culture broth. The fermenter is appropriately equipped to provide ideal culture conditions by allowing the control of pH, temperature, oxygen level, culture volume, nutrient levels, and other environmental conditions. In the chemical industry, vessels where reactions occur are known as reactors. In this sense, fermenters are also known as bioreactors (Nduka and Benedict 2017).

The culture in fermentations can be in liquid state, also known as submersed, or solid state, also known as surface. Majority of industrial fermentations are carried out as submersed processes due to lower space requirement, ease of parameter control, and greater flexibility in bioreactor design. Based on the intended application, the capacity of fermenters can range from 1 to 20 liters in laboratory-scale or 100,000 to 500,000 liters in factories. The capacity of pilot fermenters is normally observed between these two extremes. It is worth emphasizing that while fermenters are quantified by their total internal volume, only around 75% of that volume is normally used for the actual fermentation. The remaining volume acts as a buffer region for foaming and exhaust gases. There are several different kinds of fermenters that can be classified by their configurations, fermentation processes (aerobic or anaerobic), and operations (batch or continuous) (Nduka and Benedict 2017). The categorization of different fermenters is shown in Figure 1.2.1. The most commonly used fermenters include continuous stirred-tank, bubble column, airlift, packed bed, fluidized bed, membrane, and fermenter-type photobioreactor.

1.2.4.1 CONTINUOUS STIRRED-TANK FERMENTER

The most traditional fermenter found in industries is the stirred-tank fermenter, and is mainly utilized for generating highly valuable products such as fine chemicals

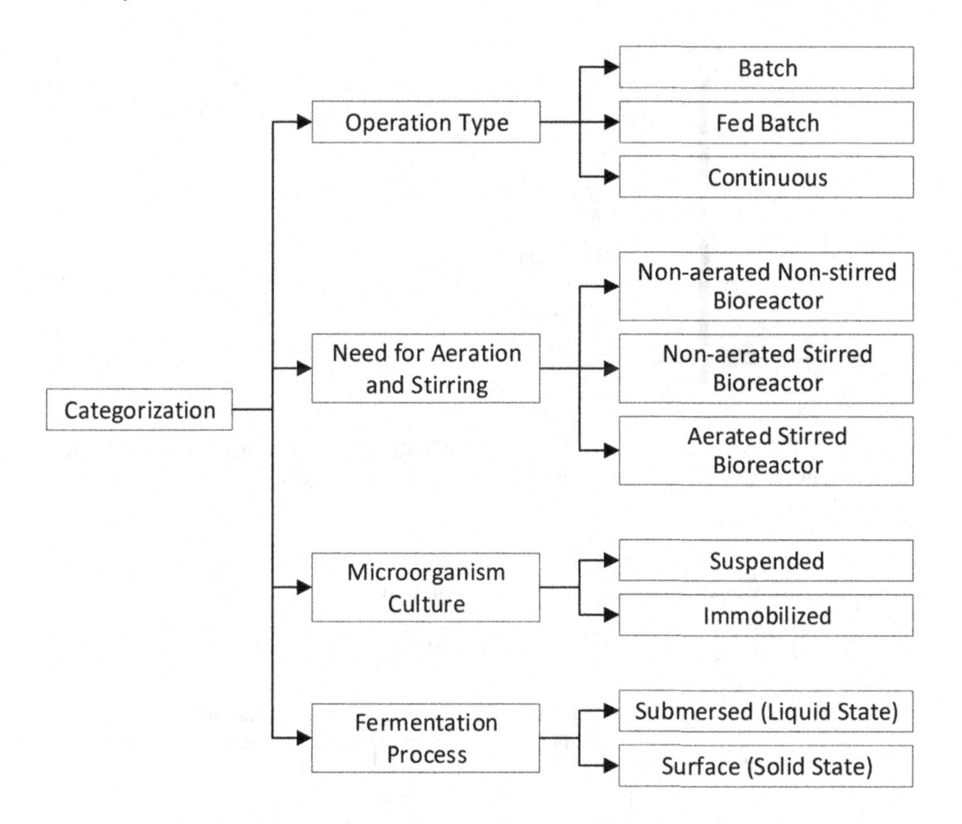

FIGURE 1.2.1 Categorization of different fermenters.

and pharmaceuticals (Mata, Martins, and Caetano 2010). In the stirred-tank fermenter, the culture broth is maintained in a precisely controlled environment, continuously stirred, and/or continuously aerated as shown in Figure 1.2.2. The continuous stirring ensures that the culture reaches homogeneity in a short time frame. For aerobic cultivation, oxygen can be supplied via bubbling from the base of the fermenter. These advantages are important for the production of high-value biological products (Lee et al. 2001).

1.2.4.2 Bubble Column Fermenter

A bubble column fermenter comprises vertical cylindrical columns where oxygen is usually pumped into the base of the column, as shown in Figure 1.2.3a. The advantages of a bubble column fermenter are low fabrication cost, high rates of mass and heat transfer, high surface area to volume ratio, and homogenous culture condition. Gaseous mass transfer and mixing is achieved by bubbling oxygen at the base of the fermenter (Kumar et al. 2011). The exhaust gases leave the culture into the freeboard region at the upper section of the fermenter, before escaping to the atmosphere through vents located at the top of the fermenter (Wang, Lan, and

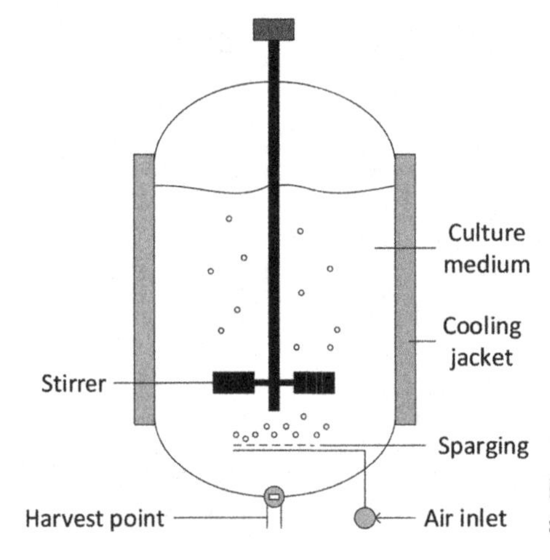

FIGURE 1.2.2 Schematic diagram aerated stirred-tank fermenter.

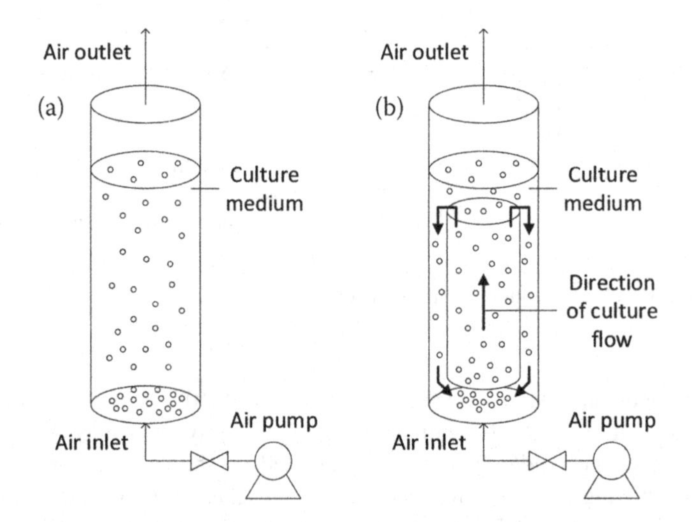

FIGURE 1.2.3 Schematic diagram of (a) bubble column bioreactor and (b) airlift bioreactor.

Horsman 2012). In a bubble column fermenter, the turbulence caused by the sparged gas can lead to random and erratic mixing conditions. As a result, cell sedimentation is more likely to occur. When scaling up, perforated plates can be installed inside the column to break up and redistribute coalesced bubbles, thereby enhancing turbulence and improving mixing of the culture (Halim et al. 2011; Miron et al. 1999; Wang, Lan, and Horsman 2012).

1.2.4.3 Airlift Fermenter

Airlift fermenters have two distinct regions, known as riser and downcomer, which are separated by a cylindrical baffle, as shown in Figure 1.2.3b. The riser (or inner zone of the cylindrical baffle) allows the sparged gas to travel upwards, inducing turbulence and causing the culture inside the riser to flow upward with the gas bubbles. The downcomer (or outer zone of the cylindrical baffle) allows the agitated culture from the riser to flow back down toward the base of the fermenter. In the riser, mixing is achieved purely by sparging gas and no physical stirring occurs (Kumar et al. 2011). The mixing in airlift fermenter is greatly affected by the gas hold-up of the downcomer. Upon reaching the top of the culture broth, the degassed culture circulates downward through the downcomer with defined and oriented motions. The difference in gas hold-up between the riser and downcomer presents one of the most important design parameters for airlift fermenters (Barbosa et al. 2003; Kumar et al. 2011; Singh and Sharma 2012). Airlift fermenters are typically considered for microbial cultures that are fragile and easily damaged by shear stress. Although mixing can be done efficiently by raising the rate of aeration, care must be taken so as to prevent cell damage (Ugwu and Aoyagi 2012).

Compared to bubble column fermenters, airlift fermenters enable higher microbial growth rates owing to better mixing patterns. Airlift fermenters have the benefit of creating circular and homogeneous mixing patterns. This occurs when the culture continually circulates through riser and downcomer zones (Monkonsit, Powtongsook, and Pavasant 2011; Xu et al. 2009). In addition, the residence time of the sparged gas in different zones of the airlift fermenter can greatly influence important parameters such as heat and mass transfer, turbulence, and mixing (Chisti and Moo-Young 1993).

1.2.4.4 Packed Bed Fermenter

A packed bed reactor, also known as a fixed bed reactor, is commonly employed in classical chemical engineering for catalytic reactions. The packed bed reactor is a two-phase system that consists of a reaction mixture (liquid or gas stream) flowing continuously across a stationary bed of catalytic particles or pellets. Packed bed reactors usually have one or more columns loaded with catalytic pellets of varying shapes and sizes and operated in a vertical configuration (Levenspiel 1998). Utilizing the same operating concepts, packed bed fermenters can be designed to use a bed of immobilized microbial cells or enzymes as the biocatalyst. The most frequently used configuration of packed bed fermenter is a cylindrical tube design, as shown in Figure 1.2.4 (Aragon et al. 2013). As fluid passes through the packed bed, the fluid becomes well-mixed in the radial direction but little mixing occurs in the axial direction. Majority of bioreactions in packed bed fermenters occur under isothermal conditions, thus the removal or addition of heat is not mandatory in these fermenters. By employing proper immobilization methods, biocatalysts with suitable sizes (1–3 mm) can be made by immobilizing enzymes or whole cells in appropriate matrices (Clark and Blanch 1997; Doran 2013).

One of the design parameters for a packed bed fermenter is the direction of substrate flow through the packed bed. There are three different ways for substrate flow, namely upward, downward, and recycling. The packed bed fermenter is usually designed for single pass operation. However, when single pass operation could not achieve the targeted conversion rate, feed recycling operation is employed

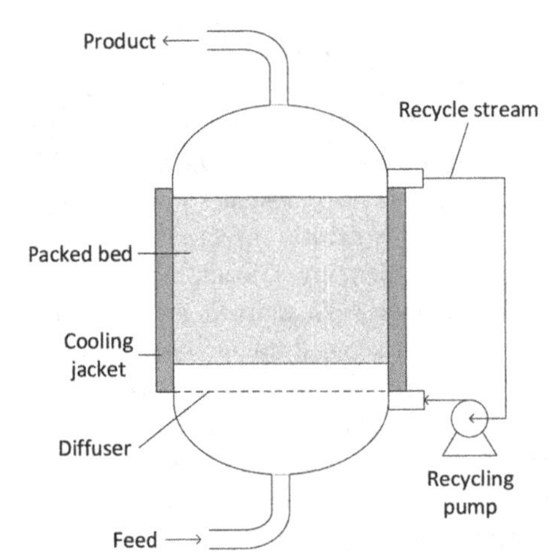

FIGURE 1.2.4 Schematic diagram of packed bed fermenter with upward flow and recycling.

(Aragon et al. 2013; Özdural et al. 2001). The recycling operation permits re-circulation of the feed stream back through the packed bed, increasing the rate of conversion. The velocity of the feed stream can also be controlled via the recycling operation, increasing the residence time and thus the conversion rate of substrates in the fermenter. For industrial application, upward flow is more favorable compared to downward flow. This is because feed streams flowing upward does not compress the packed beds and result in low flow rates. In addition, upward flow can also aid in transporting gases produced by bioreactions out of the fermenter (Bohmann, Pörtner, and Märkl 1995).

Apart from catalyzing bioreactions, packed bed fermenters can be used to culture and promote high cell densities from low concentration of free cells suspended in nutrient medium. This advantage in cultivation is due to low shear forces in the packed bed system. These fermenters have been utilized to culture and synthesize a diverse range of cell lines and biological products such as monoclonal antibodies, antileukemic factors from stromal cells, and retrovirus vectors. These biologics are important materials used in pharmaceuticals and genetic engineering researches (Sen, Nath, and Bhattacharjee 2017).

1.2.4.5 Fluidized Bed Fermenter

A fluidized bed fermenter makes use of fluidization principles whereby a fluid (in this case the culture medium) moves upward through a stationary bed of immobilized cells (either in capsules or on carriers) and suspends them, creating fluid-like behavior in the stationary bed (Kunii and Levenspiel 1991). The advantage of this design is the high degree of mixing achieved due to the continuous circulation of fluid (culture medium and/or air) through the solids (immobilized cells) (Wang and Zhong 2007). In addition, this design also provides high heat and mass transfer rates as well as low hydrodynamic shear stress to the immobilized cells (Werther 2007). The main disadvantage is that the cells need to be immobilized onto suitable matrices before culturing, otherwise the cells would be elutriated from the fermenter

(Wu et al. 2003; Yang 2003). Immobilization creates a 3D structure for the whole cells but may impose restrictions on cell preparation. For instance, the chosen cells have to be non-adherent types and specific techniques have to be utilized to produce carriers that encourage cell adherence (Mendonça da Silva et al. 2020). Nonetheless, fluidized bed fermenters have become a relevant technology utilized in developing bioartificial liver devices, which are bioreactors consisting of immobilized hepatic cells capable of performing biochemical functions of the liver (Yu et al. 2014; Figaro et al. 2017; Li et al. 2018; Figure 1.2.5).

1.2.4.6 Membrane Fermenter

A membrane fermenter is a system that combines bioreactions and membrane operations in a singular unit. In the membrane fermenter, a synthetic membrane is used as a barrier to compartmentalize the primary biomolecules responsible for performing bioreactions as well as control the transport of substrates and products in and out of the reaction compartment. The implementation of membranes allows flexibility in the designs and bioreaction processes in these fermenters compared to traditional bioreactors. This is because the membranes can allow continuous operation as well as function as a reactant supplier and/or a product removal tool. The reactive biomolecules (such as enzymes or cells) can be immobilized onto the membrane that enables easy management and separation of the reactants and products. The membranes can be submerged within the reaction mixture or placed externally to the mixture (Giorno, De Bartolo, and Drioli 2011).

Biocatalytic membrane fermenters are attractive bioreactors, but to use them at a productive level, the stability of the biocatalyst needs to be improved. In this regard, immobilization has proved to be an effective solution, even though it may alter the catalytic activity and enantioselectivity of the biocatalysts. These alterations are related to the bonding or adherence of enzymes to the membranes. Immobilization results in a more rigid enzyme-matrix particle, thereby increasing its stability, but the loss in flexibility of the enzyme reduces its active sites, decreasing its catalytic activity and specificity. Thus, the challenge of immobilization is to develop

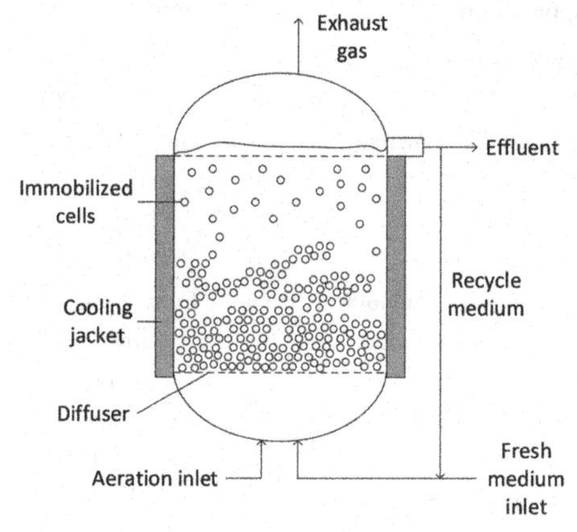

FIGURE 1.2.5 Schematic diagram of three-phase fluidized bed fermenter with medium recycling.

techniques that can achieve a balance among the stability, activity, and enantioselectivity of the biocatalyst (Giorno, De Bartolo, and Drioli 2011). For industrial application, the main technological hurdles with employing immobilized biological systems include the relatively short lifetime of the enzymes, the high cost of procuring pure enzymes, the low substrate concentration environment necessary for optimal operation of biocatalysts, risk of microbial contamination, and the need for trial and error to balance product yield with lifetime of biocatalysts. Despite these hurdles, biocatalytic membrane fermenters have been applied successfully in industries, as shown in Table 1.2.1.

1.2.4.7 Fermenter-Type Photobioreactor

A photobioreactor is a type of bioreactor used to culture phototrophic microorganisms (such as microalgae and cyanobacteria) in the presence of a light source. Phototrophic microorganisms undergo photosynthesis to create food in the form of glucose and starch using water, carbon dioxide, and light. The common configuration for fermenter-type photobioreactors is cylindrical vessels made of transparent materials (such as glass, acrylic, or plastic) which allows light penetration. Light sources are located at specified distances from the walls of the vessels to control the amount of light falling on the culture. The fermenter-type photobioreactor can perform open gas exchange, making it a suitable choice for culture optimization studies. The primary benefit of using fermenter-type photobioreactor is its ability to monitor and manage each operating parameter accurately (Carvalho, Meireles, and Malcata 2006; Dasgupta et al. 2010). However, its main drawback is the difficulty in scaling-up as the design is limited by low surface area to volume ratio (or limited light penetration into the culture broth) and high capital investment. In large-scale cultivation, one way to overcome the light penetration issue is to

TABLE 1.2.1
Examples of Industrial Applications of Biocatalysts

Biocatalyst	Immobilization Method	Application	Reference
Escherichia coli	Encapsulated in polyacrylamide	Synthesis of L-aspartic acid	Mazzei et al. (2009)
Pseudomonas dacunahe	Glutaraldehyde carrier	Synthesis of L-alanine	Giorno, Mazzei, and Piacentini (2013)
Amino acylase	DEAE-Sephadex carrier	Synthesis of L-amino acids from racemic mixtures	Carasik and Carroll (1983)
Lipase	Encapsulated in asymmetric membranes with hollow-fiber	Synthesis of isomer of methyl ester of 4-methoxyphenylglycidic acid	Takata and Tosa (1993)

provide internal illumination by inserting light sources into the fermenter and agitation by using stirrers (Dasgupta et al. 2010; Heining et al. 2014).

1.2.5 MODELING OF BIOREACTOR AND FERMENTATION

As our population continues to increase, the market demand on biotechnology products will also increase. There is a growing need to generate more products faster for the markets as these markets are getting larger and more competitive with time. Thus, from the industrial point of view, there is a strong need for higher research throughput in the laboratory, greater accuracy and predictability when scaling up and designing novel bioreactors, as well as faster and reliable generation of products in the factory. Historically, the trial and error method has provided success in scaling up bioreactors and fermentation process from the laboratory to pilot scale to large scale and, with some fine-tuning, to the factory. However, with rapid improvements in the processing power of computers, storage and speed of hard drives, as well as software engineering, it has become increasingly important to develop and improve modeling and simulation programs which can help to predict bioreaction processes and bioreactor behaviors upon scaling up (Mudde, Noorman, and Reuss 2017).

In bioreactor design, one of the most important mathematical model is computational fluid dynamics (CFD) models. The CFD models can estimate and simulate the behavior of fluids (liquids and gases) within the bioreactors by using governing equations for conservation of mass and momentum, turbulence models, as well as source and sink terms to calculate the substrate consumption and product generation kinetics. The CFD models have provided valuable insights to various industrial applications, but they are still restricted by the computational capabilities of current-generation computers and limited collaboration between the CFD and bioprocessing communities. In addition, data from industrial-scale bioreactors are scarce, making it difficult to verify the predictions of CFD models. However, in the near future, it is expected that new solutions for bioreactor modeling and greater computational power can significantly improve the usage of CFD modeling and simulation in the industries (Mudde, Noorman, and Reuss 2017).

In the fermentation process, different organisms require different environmental conditions to synthesize specific biological products. To obtain the highest yield for the targeted products, the culture conditions must be optimized. Some of the key variables that can be optimized include type of microorganisms, nutrient composition and concentration, biomass growth rate, stirring speed, aeration rate, residence time, pH, temperature, and type of fermentation process. These variables can be optimized using modeling and kinetics study (Olaoye and Kolawole 2013). Kinetics study is the analysis of the interpretations of experimental data and operating parameters influencing the fermentation process. This analysis can be performed by three main approaches, namely phenomenological, thermodynamic, and kinetic (Deindoerfer 1960). The main benefits of performing modeling and kinetics study on the fermentation process are reduced production cost, increased product yield, and improved understanding of the fermentation conditions and bioreactor performance (Nielsen and Villadsen 1992). Some commonly used software in fermentation processes are listed in Table 1.2.2.

TABLE 1.2.2
Examples of Common Software Used for Fermentation Process

Software	Application	Reference
Matlab	Data analysis, algorithm development, mathematical model creation	Nagy (2007)
Minifor	Visualization and monitoring of culture parameters	Cervinkova et al. (2013)
FNet	Ready-to-use software for Minifor bioreactors	Ménoret et al. (2015)
Process control software (PCS)	Allows automatic control, data recording, and real-time visualization of bioreactor parameters	Pasotti et al. (2017)

1.2.6 BIOTECHNOLOGY ENTREPRENEURSHIP

The huge markets for various biotechnology products has opened up countless business opportunities for biotechnology and biomanufacturing. This has given rise to biotechnology entrepreneurship, which is the construction of an enterprise through the integration of both scientific and business disciplines. An enterprise creates, develops, and eventually commercializes a new biotechnology product or a biosimilar drug. Some of the most innovative medical treatment and devices, advanced fuels, and efficient crops have been generated by biotechnology enterprises using biomanufacturing (Shimasaki 2014a).

A competent and seasoned leader is necessary for a company to have any hope of becoming successful in the competitive markets. However, if there is no entrepreneur, there will be no company. For instance, without Rob Swanson and Herb Boyer, there would be no Genentech. For any company or organization to be successful, it is essential to round up diverse teams of individuals. However, if there is no vision, leadership, and driving force of an entrepreneur, biotechnology products would never be created (Shimasaki 2014a).

Biotechnology entrepreneurs represent the backbone of the biotechnology and biomanufacturing industries as well as the source for their future inventions. Biotechnology entrepreneurs are passionate leaders with visions who start companies for various reasons. But universally, they believe that their services or products can improve the well-being of the society and even extend these benefits to poorer parts of the world. Majority of biotechnology entrepreneurs start companies with a large dose of altruism, and these beliefs are often the driving force for them to tirelessly pursue their goals. It is no doubt that biotechnology entrepreneurs also believe in financial gains and that their inventions can be both commercialized and useful to the public. But it is worth noting that financial prosperity is not the main motivator for these individuals. If financial success is the main goal, there are other easier and faster career paths compared to starting a biotechnology company. Ultimately, the sense of altruism in biotechnology entrepreneurs can be advantageous when confronting challenging financial circumstances without giving up, but can also be detrimental when determining sound business decisions. The struggles of a biotechnology entrepreneur can best be explained as a challenging journey toward a rewarding and satisfying destination. Since better-equipped biotechnology entrepreneurs will have less difficulty in succeeding, the majority of biotechnology entrepreneurs are usually scientists, engineers, physicians, or experts with technical knowledge in specific biotechnology disciplines (Shimasaki 2014a; Collins 2001).

1.2.7 BIOTECHNOLOGY PRODUCT SECTORS

The term "biotechnology industry" is a broad reference to a diverse range of biologics, medical treatments, diagnostics, medical devices, clinical tests, as well as industrial, agricultural, and biofuel applications. The biotechnology industry, as well as its portfolio of products and services, continues to expand as new scientific and technical inventions are developed and new applications are discovered. The research in biotechnology industry may seem complicated due to the seemingly countless and diverse range of products that can be manufactured. However, upon closer inspection, it is surprising how every sector employs many similar methods and techniques to create and develop various products (Shimasaki 2014b).

The development of all biotechnology products to the point of commercialization is an expensive undertaking and there is no way to avoid the high cost of investment. Many biotechnology companies were created with ingenious technological concepts and novel product ideas, but the lack of funding at critical time periods have dissolved the development of these inventions. The reasons for this unfortunate event may be poor financial planning, lack of knowledge in development costs, and less focus on consistent fundraising. No one should be committed to starting up a biotechnology company without first understanding the total development costs to bring any product to the market (Shimasaki 2014b). An estimation of the development costs for biotechnology products in different sectors can be found in Table 1.2.3.

TABLE 1.2.3
Estimation of Development Costs for Biotechnology Products (DiMasi and Grabowski 2007)

Product Type	Estimated Development Cost (USD)
Biologics and vaccines	\$250 million–\$1.5 billion
Therapeutics	\$250 million–\$1.5 billion
In vitro diagnostics and personal medical diagnostic kit	\$5–\$100 million
Medical devices	\$15–\$100 million
Digital health monitoring devices	\$250k–\$15 million
Industrial products	\$15–\$75 million
Agricultural sector	\$75–\$200 million
Biofuel sector	\$50–\$150 million

1.2.8 CONCLUSIONS

With the advent of Industry 3.0 and the current move toward Industry 4.0, we have enjoyed many benefits and conveniences brought forth by advancements in automation and information technology (IT). The vast digital network allows the connection of people and industries to share and transfer ideas and technological knowledge around the world. One of the many rising industries utilizing these technological advances is the biomanufacturing industry. The main workhorse in biomanufacturing is the fermenter, and current generation fermenters are well-equipped with an array of sensors that can accurately measure the culture conditions. Computer software can then utilize this information to monitor the culture conditions and make adjustments automatically if needed. The rapid increase in processing power of computers have increased the industrial usage of mathematical (computational fluid dynamics (CFD)) models and simulations to predict and simulate different bioreactor designs at various capacities. It is expected that new solutions to the mathematical models and advancement in computer technology will see greater applications of CFD models at the industrial level. Given the large number of products that biotechnology and biomanufacturing can offer, it is imperative for any biotechnology company to have an adept, passionate, and visionary leader-cum-biotechnology-entrepreneur who can guide the future directions of the company and development of novel inventions. The biotechnology and biomanufacturing sectors will no doubt continue to contribute valuable products and services that can benefit the human population.

REFERENCES

Aragon, Caio C., Andrea F. Santos, Ana I. Ruiz-Matute, Nieves Corzo, Jose M. Guisan, Rubens Monti, and Cesar Mateo. 2013. "Continuous production of xylooligosaccharides in a packed bed reactor with immobilized–stabilized biocatalysts of xylanase from *Aspergillus versicolor*." *Journal of Molecular Catalysis B: Enzymatic* 98: 8–14. doi: https://doi.org/10.1016/j.molcatb.2013.09.017.

Barbosa, Maria J., Marcel Janssen, Nienke Ham, Johannes Tramper, and René H. Wijffels. 2003. "Microalgae cultivation in air-lift reactors: Modeling biomass yield and growth rate as a function of mixing frequency." *Biotechnology and Bioengineering* 82 (2): 170–179. doi: https://doi.org/10.1002/bit.10563.

Barone, Paul W., Michael E. Wiebe, James C. Leung, Islam T. M. Hussein, Flora J. Keumurian, James Bouressa, Audrey Brussel, Dayue Chen, Ming Chong, Houman Dehghani, Lionel Gerentes, James Gilbert, Dan Gold, Robert Kiss, Thomas R. Kreil, René Labatut, Yuling Li, Jürgen Müllberg, Laurent Mallet, Christian Menzel, Mark Moody, Serge Monpoeho, Marie Murphy, Mark Plavsic, Nathan J. Roth, David Roush, Michael Ruffing, Richard Schicho, Richard Snyder, Daniel Stark, Chun Zhang, Jacqueline Wolfrum, Anthony J. Sinskey, and Stacy L. Springs. 2020. "Viral contamination in biologic manufacture and implications for emerging therapies." *Nature Biotechnology* 38 (5): 563–572. doi: https://doi.org/10.1038/s41587-020-0507-2.

Berg, Paul, David Baltimore, Herbert W. Boyer, Stanley N. Cohen, Ronald W. Davis, David S. Hogness, Daniel Nathans, Richard Roblin, James D. Watson, and Sherman Weissman. 1974. "Potential biohazards of recombinant DNA molecules." *Science* 185 (4148): 303. doi: https://doi.org/10.1073/pnas.71.7.2593.

Berg, Paul, David Baltimore, Sydney Brenner, Richard O. Roblin, and Maxine F. Singer. 1975. "Summary statement of the Asilomar conference on recombinant DNA molecules."

Proceedings of the National Academy of Sciences of the United States of America 72 (6):1981. doi: https://doi.org/10.1073/pnas.72.6.1981.

Berlanstein, Lenard R. 2003. *The Industrial Revolution and Work in Nineteenth Century Europe*: Routledge.

Bohmann, A., R. Pörtner, and H. Märkl. 1995. "Performance of a membrane-dialysis bioreactor with a radial-flow fixed bed for the cultivation of a hybridoma cell line." *Applied Microbiology and Biotechnology* 43 (5): 772–780. doi: https://doi.org/10.1007/BF02431907.

Bosch Sanayi Ve Ticaret, A.Ş. 2017. *A Brief History of Industry*. Available from https://www.sanayidegelecek.com/en/sanayi-4-0/tarihsel-gelisim/.

Carasik, William, and Carroll J.O. 1983. "Development of immobilized enzymes for production of high-fructose corn syrup." *Food Technology* 37: 85–91.

Carvalho, Ana P., Luís A. Meireles, and F. Xavier Malcata. 2006. "Microalgal reactors: A review of enclosed system designs and performances." *Biotechnology Progress* 22 (6): 1490–1506. doi: https://doi.org/10.1021/bp060065r.

Cervinkova, Dana, Vladimir Babak, Durdica Marosevic, Iva Kubikova, and Zoran Jaglic. 2013. "The role of the qacA gene in mediating resistance to quaternary ammonium compounds." *Microbial Drug Resistance* 19 (3): 160–167. doi: https://doi.org/10.1089/mdr.2012.0154.

Chisti, Yusuf, and Murray Moo-Young. 1993. "Improve the performance of airlift reactors." *Chemical Engineering Progress* 89, 38–45.

Clark, Douglas S., and Harvey W. Blanch. 1997. *Biochemical Engineering*: CRC Press.

Cohen, Stanley N., Annie C.Y. Chang, Herbert W. Boyer, and Robert B. Helling. 1973. "Construction of biologically functional bacterial plasmids in vitro." *Proceedings of the National Academy of Sciences of the United States of America* 70 (11): 3240–3244. doi: https://doi.org/10.1073/pnas.70.11.3240.

Collins, Jim. 2001. "*Why Some Companies Make the Leap ... and Others Don't. Good to Great*." New York: Harper Business.

Conner, John, Don Wuchterl, Maria Lopez, Bill Minshall, Rabi Prusti, Dave Boclair, Jay Peterson, and Chris Allen. 2014. "The Biomanufacturing of Biotechnology Products." In *Biotechnology Entrepreneurship*, edited by Craig Shimasaki, 351–385. Boston: Academic Press.

Dasgupta, Chitralekha Nag, J. Jose Gilbert, Peter Lindblad, Thorsten Heidorn, Stig A. Borgvang, Kari Skjanes, and Debabrata Das. 2010. "Recent trends on the development of photobiological processes and photobioreactors for the improvement of hydrogen production." *International Journal of Hydrogen Energy* 35 (19): 10218–10238. doi: https://doi.org/10.1016/j.ijhydene.2010.06.029.

Deindoerfer, Fred H. 1960. "Fermentation Kinetics and Model Processes." In *Advances in Applied Microbiology*, edited by Wayne W. Umbreit, 321–334. Academic Press.

DiMasi, Joseph A., and Henry G. Grabowski. 2007. "The cost of biopharmaceutical R&D: Is biotech different?" *Managerial and Decision Economics* 28 (4–5): 469–479. doi: https://doi.org/10.1002/mde.1360.

Doran, Pauline M. 2013. *Bioprocess Engineering Principles*. 2nd ed.: Academic Press.

Figaro, Sarah, Ulysse Pereira, Hiram Rada, Nicolas Semenzato, Dominique Pouchoulin, Patrick Paullier, Murielle Dufresne, and Cécile Legallais. 2017. "Optimizing the fluidized bed bioreactor as an external bioartificial liver." *The International Journal of Artificial Organs* 40 (4): 196–203. doi: https://doi.org/10.5301/ijao.5000567.

Fleischmann, Robert D., Mark D. Adams, Owen White, Rebecca A. Clayton, Ewen F. Kirkness, Anthony R. Kerlavage, Carol J. Bult, Jean-Francois Tomb, Brian A. Dougherty, and Joseph M. Merrick. 1995. "Whole-genome random sequencing and assembly of *Haemophilus influenzae* Rd." *Science* 269 (5223): 496–512. doi: https://doi.org/10.1126/science.7542800

Fraser, Claire M., Jeannine D. Gocayne, Owen White, Mark D. Adams, Rebecca A. Clayton, Robert D. Fleischmann, Carol J. Bult, Anthony R. Kerlavage, Granger Sutton, and Jenny M. Kelley. 1995. "The minimal gene complement of *Mycoplasma genitalium*." *Science* 270 (5235): 397–404. doi: https://doi.org/10.1126/science.270.5235.397

Giani, Alice Maria, Guido Roberto Gallo, Luca Gianfranceschi, and Giulio Formenti. 2020. "Long walk to genomics: History and current approaches to genome sequencing and assembly." *Computational and Structural Biotechnology Journal* 18: 9–19. doi: https://doi.org/10.1016/j.csbj.2019.11.002.

Giorno, L., L. De Bartolo, and E. Drioli. 2011. "Membrane Bioreactors." In *Comprehensive Biotechnology*, 2nd edition, edited by Murray Moo-Young, 263–288. Burlington: Academic Press.

Giorno, Lidietta, Rosalinda Mazzei, and Emma Piacentini. 2013. "Biocatalytic membrane reactors for the production of nutraceuticals." In *Integrated Membrane Operations: In the Food Production*, edited by Alfredo Cassano and Enrico Drioli.

Halim, Ronald, Brendan Gladman, Michael K. Danquah, and Paul A. Webley. 2011. "Oil extraction from microalgae for biodiesel production." *Bioresource Technology* 102 (1): 178–185. doi: https://doi.org/10.1016/j.biortech.2010.06.136.

Hans-Peter, Meyer, Minas Wolfgang, and Schmidhalter Diego. 2016. "Industrial-Scale Fermentation." In *Industrial Biotechnology: Products and Processes*, edited by Wittmann Christoph and C. Liao James, 3–54. John Wiley & Sons.

Heining, M., A. Sutor, S.C. Stute, C.P. Lindenberger, and R. Buchholz. 2014. "Internal illumination of photobioreactors via wireless light emitters: A proof of concept." *Journal of Applied Phycology* 27 (1): 59–66. doi: https://doi.org/10.1007/s10811-014-0290-x.

Jaenisch, Rudolf, and Beatrice Mintz. 1974. "Simian virus 40 DNA sequences in DNA of healthy adult mice derived from preimplantation blastocysts injected with viral DNA." *Proceedings of the National Academy of Sciences of the United States of America* 71 (4): 1250–1254. doi: https://doi.org/10.1073/pnas.71.4.1250.

Kumar, Kanhaiya, Chitralekha Nag Dasgupta, Bikram Nayak, Peter Lindblad, and Debabrata Das. 2011. "Development of suitable photobioreactors for CO_2 sequestration addressing global warming using green algae and cyanobacteria." *Bioresource Technology* 102 (8): 4945–4953. doi: https://doi.org/10.1016/j.biortech.2011.01.054.

Kunii, Daizo, and Octave Levenspiel. 1991. *Fluidization Engineering*. Butterworth-Heinemann.

Lee, Dong-Woo, Hack-Woo Kim, Keun-Wook Lee, Byoung-Chan Kim, Eun-Ah Choe, Han Seung Lee, Doo-Sik Kim, and Yu-Ryang Pyun. 2001. "Purification and characterization of two distinct thermostable lipases from the gram-positive thermophilic bacterium *Bacillus thermoleovorans* ID-1." *Enzyme and Microbial Technology* 29 (6–7): 363–371. doi: http://doi.org/10.1016/S0141-0229(01)00408-2.

Levenspiel, Octave. 1998. *Chemical Reaction Engineering*, 3rd edition. Wiley.

Li, Yi, Qiong Wu, Yujia Wang, Chengxin Weng, Yuting He, Mengyu Gao, Guang Yang, Li Li, Fei Chen, and Yujun Shi. 2018. "Novel spheroid reservoir bioartificial liver improves survival of nonhuman primates in a toxin-induced model of acute liver failure." *Theranostics* 8 (20): 5562. doi: https://doi.org/10.7150/thno.26540.

Mata, Teresa M., António A. Martins, and Nidia S. Caetano. 2010. "Microalgae for biodiesel production and other applications: A review." *Renewable and Sustainable Energy Reviews* 14 (1): 217–232. doi: https://doi.org/10.1016/j.rser.2009.07.020.

Mazzei, R., L. Giorno, E. Piacentini, S. Mazzuca, and E. Drioli. 2009. "Kinetic study of a biocatalytic membrane reactor containing immobilized β-glucosidase for the hydrolysis of oleuropein." *Journal of Membrane Science* 339 (1–2): 215–223. doi: https://doi.org/10.1016/j.memsci.2009.04.053.

Mendonça da Silva, Joana, Eloy Erro, Maooz Awan, Sherri-Ann Chalmers, Barry Fuller, and Clare Selden. 2020. "Small-scale fluidized bed bioreactor for long-term dynamic culture of 3D cell constructs and in vitro testing." *Frontiers in Bioengineering and Biotechnology* 8 (895). doi: https://doi.org/10.3389/fbioe.2020.00895.

Ménoret, Séverine, Anne De Cian, Laurent Tesson, Séverine Remy, Claire Usal, Jean-Baptiste Boulé, Charlotte Boix, Sandra Fontanière, Alison Crénéguy, and Tuan H Nguyen. 2015. "Homology-directed repair in rodent zygotes using Cas9 and TALEN engineered proteins." *Scientific Reports* 5 (1): 1–15. doi: https://doi.org/10.1038/srep14410.

Michels, P., and J. Rosazza. 2009. "The evolution of microbial transformations for industrial applications." *SIM News*, 36–52.

Miron, Asterio Sanchez, Antonio Contreras Gomez, Francisco Garcıa Camacho, Emilio Molina Grima, and Yusuf Chisti. 1999. "Comparative evaluation of compact photobioreactors for large-scale monoculture of microalgae." *Journal of Biotechnology* 70 (1): 249–270. doi: https://doi.org/10.1016/S0168-1656(99)00079-6.

Monkonsit, Saranya, Sorawit Powtongsook, and Prasert Pavasant. 2011. "Comparison between airlift photobioreactor and bubble column for *Skeletonema costatum* cultivation." *Engineering Journal* 15 (4): 53–64. doi: https://doi.org/10.4186/ej.2011.15.4.53.

Mudde, Rob, Henk Noorman, and Matthias Reuss. 2017. "Bioreactor Modeling." In *Industrial Biotechnology*, edited by Christoph Wittmann and James C. Liao, 81–128, Wiley.

Nagy, Zoltan Kalman. 2007. "Model based control of a yeast fermentation bioreactor using optimally designed artificial neural networks." *Chemical Engineering Journal* 127 (1–3): 95–109. doi: https://doi.org/10.1016/j.cej.2006.10.015.

National Academies of Sciences, Engineering, and Medicine. 2016. "Future Genetic-Engineering Technologies." In *Genetically Engineered Crops: Experiences and Prospects*, 353–404. National Academies Press.

Nduka, Okafor, and C. Okeke Benedict. 2017. "Fermentors and Operation of Fermentation Equipment." In *Modern Industrial Microbiology and Biotechnology*, edited by Okafor Nduka and C. Okeke Benedict, 149–170. Boca Raton: CRC Press.

Nielsen, Jens, and John Villadsen. 1992. "Modelling of microbial kinetics." *Chemical Engineering Science* 47 (17–18): 4225–4270. doi: https://doi.org/10.1016/0009-2509(92)85104-J.

Olaoye, O.S., and O.S. Kolawole. 2013. "Modeling of the kinetics of ethanol formation from glucose biomass in batch culture with a non structured model." *International Journal of Engineering Research and Application* 3 (4): 562–565.

Özdural, Ahmet R., Deniz Tanyolaç, Zafer Demircan, İsmail H. Boyaci, Mehmet Mutlu, and Colin Webb. 2001. "A new method for determination of apparent kinetics parameters in recirculating packed-bed immobilized enzyme reactors." *Chemical Engineering Science* 56 (11): 3483–3490. doi: https://doi.org/10.1016/S0009-2509(01)00049-5.

Pasotti, Lorenzo, Susanna Zucca, Michela Casanova, Giuseppina Micoli, Maria Gabriella Cusella De Angelis, and Paolo Magni. 2017. "Fermentation of lactose to ethanol in cheese whey permeate and concentrated permeate by engineered *Escherichia coli*." *BMC Biotechnology* 17 (1): 48. doi: https://doi.org/10.1186/s12896-017-0369-y.

Sen, P., A. Nath, and C. Bhattacharjee. 2017. "Packed-Bed Bioreactor and Its Application in Dairy, Food, and Beverage Industry." In *Current Developments in Biotechnology and Bioengineering*, edited by Christian Larroche, Maria Ángeles Sanromán, Guocheng Du, and Ashok Pandey, 235–277. Elsevier.

Shimasaki, Craig. 2014a. "Chapter 4 – What is Biotechnology Entrepreneurship?" In *Biotechnology Entrepreneurship*, edited by Craig Shimasaki, 45–56. Boston: Academic Press.

Shimasaki, Craig. 2014b. "Chapter 9 – Understanding Biotechnology Product Sectors." In *Biotechnology Entrepreneurship*, edited by Craig Shimasaki, 113–138. Boston: Academic Press.

Singh, R.N., and Shaishav Sharma. 2012. "Development of suitable photobioreactor for algae production – A review." *Renewable and Sustainable Energy Reviews* 16 (4): 2347–2353. doi: https://doi.org/10.1016/j.rser.2012.01.026.

Takata, Isao, and Tetsuya Tosa. 1993. "Production of L-Malic Acid." In *Industrial Application of Immobilized Biocatalysts*, edited by Atsuo Tanaka, Tetsuya Tosa, and Takeshi Kobayashi, 53–66. Marcel Dekker, Inc.

Ugwu, Charles U., and Hideki Aoyagi. 2012. "Microalgal culture systems: An insight into their designs, operation and applications." *Biotechnology* 11 (3): 127. doi: https://doi.org/10.3923/biotech.2012.127.132.

Vasic-Racki, Durda. 2006. "History of Industrial Biotransformations—Dreams and Realities." *Industrial Biotransformations* 40: 1–36, Wiley-VCH. doi: https://doi.org/10.1002/3527608184.

Wang, Bei, Christopher Q. Lan, and Mark Horsman. 2012. "Closed photobioreactors for production of microalgal biomasses." *Biotechnology Advances* 30 (4): 904–912. doi: https://doi.org/10.1016/j.biotechadv.2012.01.019.

Wang, Si-Jing, and Jian-Jiang Zhong. 2007. "Bioreactor Engineering." In *Bioprocessing for Value-Added Products from Renewable Resources*, edited by Shang-Tian Yang, 131–161. Elsevier.

Werther, Joachim. 2007. "Fluidized-Bed Reactors." *Ullmann's Encyclopedia of Industrial Chemistry*, Wiley. doi: https://doi.org/10.1002/14356007.b04_239.pub2.

Wu, Jane-Yii, Kuo-Cheng Chen, Chun-Ting Chen, and Sz-Chwun John Hwang. 2003. "Hydrodynamic characteristics of immobilized cell beads in a liquid–solid fluidized-bed bioreactor." *Biotechnology and Bioengineering* 83 (5): 583–594. doi: https://doi.org/10.1002/bit.10710.

Xu, Ling, Pamela J. Weathers, Xue-Rong Xiong, and Chun-Zhao Liu. 2009. "Microalgal bioreactors: Challenges and opportunities." *Engineering in Life Sciences* 9 (3): 178–189. doi: https://doi.org/10.1002/elsc.200800111.

Yang, Wen-ching. 2003. *Handbook of Fluidization and Fluid-Particle Systems*: CRC Press.

Yu, Cheng-Bo, Xiao-Ping Pan, Liang Yu, Xiao-Peng Yu, Wei-Bo Du, Hong-Cui Cao, Jun Li, Ping Chen, and Lan-Juan Li. 2014. "Evaluation of a novel choanoid fluidized bed bioreactor for future bioartificial livers." *World Journal of Gastroenterology* 20 (22): 6869. doi: https://doi.org/10.3748/wjg.v20.i22.6869.

1.3 Industry 4.0

Khalisanni Khalid, Shir Reen Chia, Kit Wayne Chew, and Pau Loke Show

CONTENTS

1.3.1 INTRODUCTION

The Fourth Industrial Revolution (Industry 4.0) or Industry Revolution 4.0 (IR 4.0) is a technical advance that changes and improves the way of productivity. IR 4.0 comprises cyber security, augmented reality, industrial internet of things (IIoT), and other technologies. As a consortium of key technologies, IR 4.0 is a driver to the fast route of modernization. For instance, GPS (global positioning system) suggest the route of destination, Apple's Siri artificial intelligence as an activated voice assistant, and handphone ability to perform user's face recognition. As a result of the fast emergence and advance technologies, IR 4.0 has transformed the world technologies and triggered a paradigm shift for every business sector, especially manufacturing industries as well as the lifestyle of modern society.

The pavement of manufacturing evolution from the 1800s is beneficial towards the understanding of the emergence of IR 4.0. Four distinct Industrial Revolutions have occurred or continue to the present day; namely the First, Second, Third, and Fourth Industrial Revolutions. In the late 1700s to early 1800s, the timeline for the First Industrial Revolution (IR 1.0) has evolved. The manufacturing encompasses the utilization of animals, water, and steam engines to assist the human labor on machines. Early in the 1920s is the era of the Second Industrial Revolution (IR 2.0) where the use of electricity and steel in the factories are practiced for the mass manufacturing of products. The manufacturers able to increase the efficiency of the productions and make factory machinery more mobile by using electricity and the productivity has increased through the mass production concept. Manufacturers have started to incorporate computer technology into productions around 1950s. This is when the Third Industrial Revolution (IR 3.0) slowly began to emerge and manufacturers started to shift to digital technologies and automotive productions. For the past few decades, IR 4.0 began to emerge. IR 4.0 emphasizes the application of digital innovation and leveling the IoT (Internet of Things), real-time data, and cyber systems for every sector. The present Industrial Revolution offers more comprehensive, interconnectivity, and holistic approach within the manufacturing system. It empowers the business tools, design, and leverage the productivity and process of manufacturing. Thus, the present chapter will discuss the IR 4.0 key technologies, challenges, future perspectives, and impact on the biomanufacturing industry.

1.3.2 KEY TECHNOLOGIES FOR IR 4.0

The key technologies of IR 4.0 will transform the process of production to be more efficient and productive as shown in Figure 1.3.1. The advance digital technology also changes the production relationship between suppliers-producers-customers and human-machines.

1.3.2.1 SIMULATION

Simulation is known as the synthetic operation of a real-world practice or structure over time. Hence, it is an important aspect for engineering and industrial system to obtain real-time process analysis. It also provides an opportunity for the experts to presume the process control of imitated system's environment. Simulation is used extensively in plant operation to determine the physical world through virtual model and leverage the real-time data of the operations for machines, processes, and humans. It enables the manufacturers to predict and optimize the operational cost includes costs of laboring, raw materials, and electricity. It also assists the production executive to set the machine settings for the next production in line, thereby increasing the quality of productivity. The usage of computer simulation with the application of mathematical modeling as an indispensable tool is an innovation driven for better understanding to the dynamics of business systems. The challenges faced by the manufacturing industries can be overcome through the present technology.

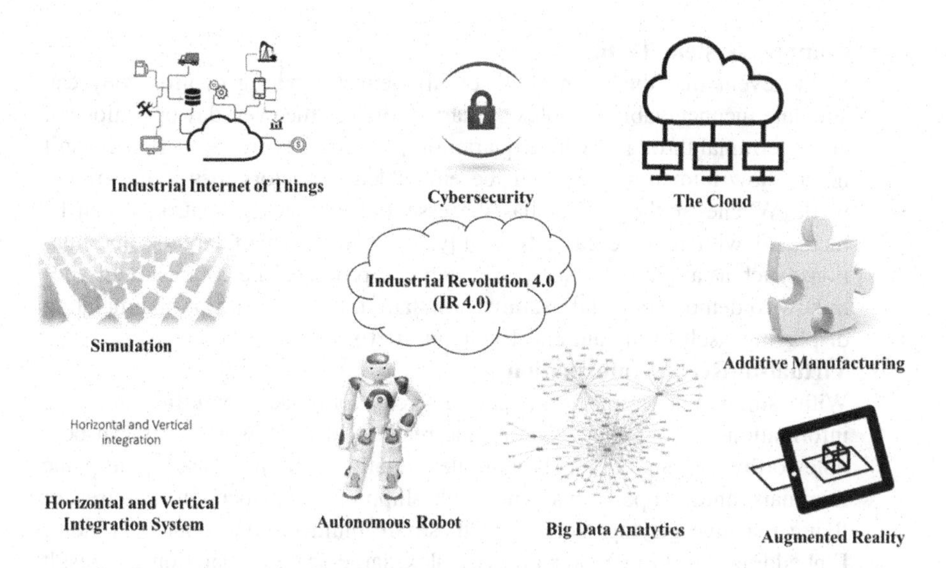

FIGURE 1.3.1 Nine technology trends of Industry 4.0.

Simulation modeling is able to gain insight information of the complex systems and test new policies, new concepts, or new operations preceding its actual implementations to obtain important information and knowledge (cost, product losses, energy, and human capital) prior to the real operation. A high reliability re-creation of fabricating production line is characterized as virtual factory (VF). The collaborative manufacturing surroundings focusing on virtual reality (VR) demonstration is called VF. VF is envisioned to imitate approved genuine manufacturing plants re-creation models to produce information and designs of original conditions of production line. Digital Twin (DT) is a conceptual framework inspired by the latest simulation modeling (Cheng et al. 2020). This super reliable concept by DT plays a role of critical insight in IR 4.0. DT has expanded the innovations of overall items in lifecycle stages, integrating significant information and modernization frameworks for improved presentation efficiency and maintenance created by practical information. Thus, the innovations based on re-creation are the center part within the advanced manufacturing plant approach, permitting tests, and approval upon distinctive fabricating framework designs, formations, and itemizations such as distinguish fabrication.

Uses, Applications, and Benefits of Industrial Simulations

- **Flexibility**
  Individuals can mimic numerous distinctive objects and process. Started from commerce setups to preparing airplane pilots, there is no deficiency of current and potential applications for simulating frameworks. When it comes to simulation framework, individuals can utilize it to capture bits of knowledge in mining, fabricating, retail, supply chain administration, coordination, and numerous others. It is industry rationalist and pertinent to endless use-cases (Shan, Guo, and Gill 2020).

- **Complex System Testing**
  In the event that the partners have sufficient computing control, they can simulate inconceivably complex scenarios, such as the everyday operations of an air terminal through a whole quarter or a city activity framework. It doesn't matter how numerous rules will be embedded or factors toss at the framework. Whenever the partner has the essential computing control, it can be recreated with relative ease. Currently, the simulation of large-scale situations, such as airplane terminals is a standard process. The contrast really lies in how to demonstrate and examine simulation, not the concept of simulation displaying itself (Vulpiani and Baldovin 2020).
- **Virtual-to-Reality Information**
  With simulation framework, partners can produce bountiful sums of information without ever touching the real-world framework. This can be a noteworthy advantage for large-scale situations. In the case of airplane terminals, mining operations, worldwide shipping and dispersion exercises, or flying machine get together; all of these are multi-billion-dollar operations. Embedding indeed one alter in a complex, large-scale preparation can result in delays and quality disconfirmation issues to the tens or hundreds of millions of dollars values of business. With simulation framework, the stakeholders can field-test the changes before applying to the real condition. The stakeholder can obtain the knowledge for potential risk and prepare for them (Eem, Koo, and Jung 2019).
- **Address Theoretical information**
  Whether it's way for better knowledge the antiquated developments or building-up commerce insights, the stakeholders can utilize simulation modeling to produce information for the knowledge (Popova Zhuhadar and Thrasher 2019).
- **Analysis of Distinctive and Interrelated Factors**
  It's common for the complex operations to include the numerous distinctive variables. In fabrication for instance, the stakeholders depend on hundreds or thousands of machines, logistics, providers, and employees. With simulation modeling, the secure understanding of operational fabrication will be understood as a result of a variable, such as climate change, political calamity in a nation that supplies raw materials, and others. These data are very important for decision-makers, officials, and shareholders to determine the extend recommendations and changes to their existing frameworks (Li et al. 2020).
- **Time Density**
  If the stakeholders need the data traversing months or more, they cannot bear to hold up that long. Instead of obtaining the actual data in long-term period, for example, 12 months, simulation able to generate the required information rapidly, such as within 1 day (Lan et al. 2017).
- **Test for Problems**
  For the acceptance of a modern instrument in a plant or a new process, the stakeholders can examine whether it works as expected through the simulation modeling. In expansion, they can distinguish the potential complications and consolidate the arrangements for the problems (and retest) before

actualizing the information to the system or process (Wang *et al.,* 2017). The simulation modeling gives a wide extend of commerce benefits. It is impartially anticipating information about the process prior to implementation.

1.3.2.2 Industrial Internet of Things (IIoT)

Industrial Internet of Things (IIoT) is a quickly progressing sector for the greatest connection within the worldwide IoT investment. The beginning of the term, IIoT was more of an empowering innovation for computerized changes. IIoT can also be pertained as savvy actuators and devices utilization to upgrade fabrication with mechanical processes. The control of shrewd machines and real-time analytics are required for the advantage of the information, in which inefficient machines can be leveraged through IIoT. The driving logic behind IIoT is that the machines are better at communicating critical data that can be utilized to drive trade choices quicker and more precisely.

Client IoT is driven by the indecisive interface of people and might have unstable buying patterns. IIoT is much diverse and includes the endorsement by the choice of stakeholders who require a clear advantage and comparable commerce case. The support system often examines and decides how the advantage will be determined and incorporates IIoT in a proposition. By using IIoT, the administration surveys either to endorse or deny the venture which leads to a judicious and business-driven choice. IIoT also includes ventures with clear commerce benefits. Subsequently, the design for IIoT can be disentangled into three major components:

- **Data procurement from different frameworks, hardware, gadgets or sensors:**
  Within the case of an owner/operator, the information comes from the previous operator or standard operation database. For an undertaking chief observing its installed system, the sensor is a smart device with processor, memory, and computer program. In both cases, the information can be prepared values (weight, temperature, stream, electric current, and etc.) as the resource for optimization of system data (Zhang et al. 2019).
- **Infrastructures, networking and security:**
  Ordinarily, hierarchical exchange of data happens from sensor to control framework and finally to cloud applications. Nevertheless, peer-to-peer communications among machinery tools has excitingly conceivable outcomes for administration and coordination) (Al-Turjman and Alturjman 2018).
- **Cloud applications:**
  Presently, the utilization of the information includes big data analytics to anticipate hardware catastrophe to repair unscheduled downtime of manufacturing process. A few applications of the cloud such as infrastructure as a service (IaaS) and platform as a service (PaaS) recognize generation or working issues that require consideration. When conditions in these services warrant, an alarm goes to operations or support to be concerned (Aazam, Zeadally & Harras, 2018).

Uses, Application and Benefits of Industrial IoT:

- **Digital factory**
  IIoT empowered tools to transmit its operational data to the stakeholders such as unique equipment producers and field engineers. This will empower operation supervisors and plant heads to remotely oversee the production line units and take advantage to prepare mechanization and optimization process. Aside of this, a carefully associated interlinked system can be developed to recognize key results for managers (Tirabeni et al. 2019).
- **Facility management**
  The use of IIoT in sensors fabricating hardware permits the application of maintenance alarms. Various simple devices are developed to operate in the selected conditions such as different vibration ranges and temperature. IIoT sensors can efficiently screen the machineries and send an alert for the hardware veers off from its endorsed parameters. To ensure the endorsed working environment for apparatus, the producers can preserve vitality, diminish costs, dispense with machine interruption, and increase operational proficiency through IIOT (Mouratidis and Diamantopoulou 2018).
- **Manufacturing flow monitoring**
  IIoT in fabrication can empower the monitoring of generation lines from the beginning of refining handle down to the bundling of last item. The observation of the whole process in real-time has given the superior administrators to prescribe alterations in operations which directly affect the operational cost of the factories. In addition, the near observation highlights deficiency in productivity, and hence, dispensing the squanders and pointless work in advance inventory (Al-Rubaye et al. 2019).
- **Inventory administration**
  IIoT applications allow the checking of occasions over a supply chain. Utilizing these frameworks, the inventory is followed and trailed universally on a line-item level. Subsequently, the clients are informed of any noteworthy deviations from the plans. This gives cross-channel occurrence into inventories and supervisors are given real-time estimation, advance information, and evaluated entry time of new materials. Eventually, the supply is improved and the shared costs within the value chain are diminished (Paul, Chatterjee, and Guha 2019).
- **Plant safety and security**
  IIoT has combined huge information to improve workers' security and the security within the plant. By observing the Key Performance Index (KPI) of health and security, just like the number of wounds and ailment rates, near-misses, nonattendances, vehicle occurrences, and property harm or misfortune amid day-by-day operations. Hence, viable observation guarantees a better security for both workers and plants. Lagging indicators which measure specified results after the process such as number of incidents and injuries can be used as a way to guarantee the optimal health, security, and environment (HSE) issues (Mondal 2019).

- **Quality control**
  IIoT sensors collect total item and other third-party information from different stages of the product cycle. The information collected is related to the composition of crude materials utilized, temperature and working environment, wastes, as well as the effect of transportation on the ultimate products. Moreover, in the event that utilized the item, the IIoT gadget can give information to the stakeholders' opinions on utilizing the item. All of these inputs can be analyzed afterward to distinguish and redress the quality issues (Aazam, Harras, and Zeadally 2019).
- **Packaging optimization**
  By utilizing IIoT sensors in items and products, producers can obtain information from the utilization designs and deal with the item from different clients. Intelligent tracking mechanism can trace the product disintegration amid travel and other environment factors on the item. This function will offer information that can be utilized to re-engineer the items and packaging of items for superior execution in both client involvement and packaging cost reduction (Liu et al. 2019).
- **Logistics and supply chain optimization**
  The IIoT can give real-time supply chain data by tracing materials, gear, and items as they move through the supply chain. Successful detailing empowers producers to gather and nourish conveyance data into business systems. By interfacing plants to providers, all the stakeholders within the supply chain can track interdependencies, fabric stream, and fabrication cycle. The information gained will offer assistance to the producers to anticipate issues, reduce inventory, and possibly decrease the capital prerequisites (Neto et al., 2017).

1.3.2.3 Cybersecurity

The IR 4.0 brings features such as modern operational networking system, smart productivity and computerized supply cyber systems. The cyber networking system environment of IR 4.0 operation and computerized changes increase the risk of cyber-attacks far more distance than we could imagine. To secure the network of the cyber system in the era of IR 4.0, cybersecurity procedures and measurements must be up to date, powerful and strong, as well as completely coordinates into organizational and data innovation procedure from the beginning.

As an important aspect of the IR 4.0, the manufacturing industry is encouraged to fortify its security frameworks to reassure savvy internet connectivity within the system of manufacturing. The manufacturing system was previously not associated as they are managed in separated manufacturing environment where its prime concern is security. IR 4.0 features modern age of associated, savvy fabricating, responsive supply systems, and custom-fitted administrations. By using smart technologies, IR 4.0 attempts integrating digitalized sphere and corporate feature to realize virtual industry with capabilities of progressive manufacturing.

Previous study in 2009 reported the manipulation of malware for the out-of-control centrifuges speed in a nuclear enrichment plant (Tian et al. 2020). This Stuxnet malware infected the nuclear plant system through single network drives which spread throughout the system. This is an example of cyber-attack weapons in the established networking system factories.

Uses, Applications, and Benefits of Cybersecurity

- **Business protection**
  The major benefit is cyber security enables inclusive digital defense to the company. It allows the employees to surf the Internet connection in secure mode, hence reduces potential threats (Berry and Berry 2018).
- **Personal information protection**
  The most valuable information in the present era is private data. For instance, the virus that gets into personal data eventually increases the risk of leaking information or cyber hacking (Kshetri 2017).
- **Safety of devices**
  Employees' cyber devices are constantly at the high risk of cyber attacks if the cybersecurity is not well maintained. If the computer system is infected, the productivity of the work will be decreased and high risk of computer replacements (Leuprecht, Skillicorn, and Tait 2016).
- **Productivity protection**
  Malware and viruses can reduce the speed of computers and it will become difficult to be dealt with especially during the working period. This situation will result in data losses and reduction of profits due to the time consumed for fixing the system (Grocke 2017).
- **Website breakdown prevention**
  For a businessman, hosting website is a part of the strategies. However, the business website is forced to shut down if the system is infected and caused losing customer trust and missed transaction (Kiradoo 2019).
- **Spyware prevention**
  The virus is developed to infiltrate others network and transmit the data to the cybercriminal. The confidentiality and employees private information can be kept in safe through a comprehensive cyber security system (Kashif et al. 2018).
- **Adware prevention**
  This form of cyber virus affects the computer through advertisement. However, these advertisements can harm the computer if the user has accidently clicked on them and released the virus into the personalize computer system, which subsequently impacted the work productivity (Zhang-Kennedy, Chiasson, and Biddle 2016; Bitam, Zeadally, and Mellouk 2016; Bustos 2017).
- **Increase customers' confidence**
  If the company can prove to the customer that they are secured from all kinds of cyber attacks and stimulate belief to the stakeholders, the confidence levels of customers to purchase the products will be increased (Henriques de Gusmão et al., 2018).

1.3.2.4 The Cloud

The cloud is a superb integration of technologies which transforms the edge of information administration. Manufacturers are willing to share data, rather than accumulating and obscuring it from their contenders. These endeavours will create the opportunity of communication between the businesses and an added advantage to general industries pacing up faster and more sophisticated. The cloud has boundless capacity proficiencies. Thus, high data is procured representing more prominent requirements for appropriate institutes to ensure the data is open and noteworthy. This will create high-speed process and system that makes differences in trade and all business adjustments through cloud technologies. Cloud platforms able to optimize commerce forms, empower more effective supply chain and give perceptive support. Inventive modern applications on coordinated cloud platform administrations are versatile to the stakeholders. They are expected to process the information rapidly and able to do service when adapting to a sum of information. The cloud will proceed to be a tool for the medium and huge businesses to outperform through advancement. The cloud will be driven by the combination of new technologies and resources such as big data, cybersecurity, and simulation. Thus, the cloud produces outcome for the realization in commerce driven by technology frontier (Goddard 2016; Kalra et al. 2019).

Uses, Applications, and Benefits of the Cloud

- **Cost savings**
  Twenty percent of the companies are concerned about the cost of actualizing cloud technology in their company. Considering the return of investment (ROI) is an essential factor for the endeavouring companies that are preferred to apply cloud in their companies. The cloud will ensure the significance of access of data, time savvy, and cost reduction for the initialization of project (Chen and Benusa 2017).
- **Security**
  Many companies are concerned about cloud computing arrangement especially cyber attacks by the hackers or viruses. However, encryption technologies and powerful security system are required to prevent the cyber attacks. For better security measurement, different security can be established to the cloud system to ensure all data is safe (Kuratko, Holt, and Neubert 2020).
- **Flexibility**
  The cloud offers more adaptable business by facilitating on the servers. If the stakeholder wished for additional transfer speed, a cloud-based service can meet the requirement immediately, instead of experiencing a complex (and costly) upgrade to the existing IT facilities (Janaki 2017).
- **Mobility**
  The cloud permits portable entree to business information through phones and gadgets where 3 billion of smart phones are utilized and inclusive nowadays. It may be a remarkable pace to guarantee that nobody was left out throughout this progression. Employees with active plans, or far away from meeting

location and unable to attend the meeting, can utilize the technology to keep in touch with the stakeholders. Through the cloud, the company is able to offer open data to deal with staff who is traveling, independent workers, or inaccessible workers, for better working adjustments (Bittencourt et al. 2017).

- **Insight**
  In the progression to advanced era, it's getting to be significant that the ancient maxim "knowledge is power" are started to be in advanced and precise frame: "Data is money". Covering up the tonnes of bits information that encompass the client exchanges and trade, the information is chunks of important, significant data fair holding up to be distinguished and acted upon. Of course, filtering that information to discover the essential parts can be exceptionally troublesome, unless the expert gets to the correct cloud-computing arrangement. Numerous cloud-based capacity arrangements initiate the cloud analysis integration for the company information. Along with the data in the cloud, the IT experts effectively actualize following instruments and construct customized reports to analyze the data of organization (Senyo, Addae, and Boateng 2018).
- **Increased collaboration**
  Collaboration is making its point in case the trade has two representatives or more. Cloud computing makes collaborations of companies or individuals easier where group individuals can see and share data effectively and safely over a cloud-based stage. A few cloud-based administrations indeed give collaborative social spaces to associate representatives over the organization, in this manner expanding intrigued and engagement of organizations (Ning et al. 2019).
- **Quality control**
  Many aspects are hindering the victory of commerce such as low quality and fluctuation in announcement. In a cloud-based framework, all archives are put in single arrangement. With everybody getting to the same data, the stakeholder will be able to keep up consistency in information, maintain a strategic distance from human mistake, and have a clear record of any corrections or overhauls. Alternately, overseeing data in silos can lead to inadvertently sparing diverse forms of records, which leads to disarray and weakened information (Wei et al. 2018).
- **Recovery of disaster**
  Apart of the variables that initiate the successful of a trade is controlled, there will be continuous out of control and contribute to negative impact no matter how in control of the organization for the real process. Downtime in the administrations leads to erroneous efficiency, income, and brand notoriety. Cloud-based administrations give fast information for all sorts of crisis scenarios, from normal calamities to control blackouts (Liu et al. 2018).
- **Loss prevention**
  Cloud computing restores valuable data within the cyber system accompanied with networking security. This advance system prevents data losses during hardware and software malfunction for many reasons (Stergiou and Psannis 2017).

- **Automatic software updates**
Compelling an IT section to execute a manual organizational updated data is quite troublesome. Through cloud technology, the software automatically updates the data itself. It saves the expenditure of cyber security maintenance and software breakdown (Abdelghader Morsi et al. 2020).
- **Competitive edge**
The cloud technology will gives a competitive edge to the conventional competitor where report has showed that 77% of commerce thought cloud technology gives them an economical benefit (Akinrolabu, New, and Martin 2017).
- **Sustainability**
Cloud framework supports ecological proactivity, productivity, and powering virtual services; reduce paper waste and energy consumption. Pike Research reported that the energy consumption reduced to 31% from 2010 to 2020 through the application of cloud-based technology (de Bruin and Floridi 2017).

1.3.2.5 Additive Manufacturing

In additive manufacturing (AM), a 3D item is made by placing materials layer-by-layer. This is different with customary subtractive fabricating which expels fabric to form a certain item. The examples of customary subtractive production are processing, drilling, and computer numerical control (CNC) machining. In layman perspectives, the terms "additive manufacturing" and "3D printing" are ordinarily used. Comparing AM to the routine technique, AM is predominant in terms of its plan requirements. When manufacturing of objects utilizes customary strategies, numerous plans need to be considered. Jigs and installations of objects make a difference to control the area of items and to hold the item separately. The plan consolidation of these fabrications limits the geometry complexity of the objects. But with AM, any plan or shape is conceivable at zero imperatives. The machines regulate to the plan. In this way, creating objects with cavities or objects inside objects is more than possible.

Uses, Applications, and Benefits of Additive Manufacturing

- **Healthcare**
AM is getting to be essential in the IR 4.0. It will permit the real-time formation of tailor-made organs implanted into the patient bodies. However, the foremost difficult application of AM is bioprinting (Özceylan et al. 2018). Application of bioprinting in healthcare industries are tailored human organs and transplants. It creates living tissue by putting living cells layer upon layer in a three-dimensional framework (Chimene, Kaunas, and Gaharwar 2020).
- **Aerospace**
A second sector that benefited from the AM technology is aerospace engineering. In the year 2014, the National Aeronautics and Space Administration (NASA) announced the 3D printed part had been produced using 3D printer on International Space Station (ISS) (Attaran 2017). AM has become more important since NASA and other space agencies are planning for human trip to Mars and improves space exploration.

1.3.2.6 Augmented Reality

The last 20 years have perceived great advances in research and development for Augmented Reality (AR). AR technology is a knowledge that associates virtual – reality information. AR technology and knowledge incorporate clients to be involved in expanded world by overlaying virtual data within the real world. Thus, the clients can experience both the real and virtual world while perceiving real-time information. The applications of AR comprise 3D modeling, sensor, real-time tracking, multimedia, and more. For the principle, 3D models, music, video, text, images, and slides, are applied to the virtual information to the real world after simulation. Two kinds of information complement each other and enhance the reality (Papagiannakis, Singh, and Magnenat-Thalmann 2008; Enyedy et al. 2012).

Uses, Applications, and Benefits of Augmented Reality Technology

- **Intelligent display technology**
  Concurring to important information, more than 65% of the data obtained by humans comes from their vision, which has ended up the foremost instinctive way for human to connect with the real environment (Lv et al. 2015). With the advancement of innovation, AR gets to be believable, which is a boost to the different sorts of gadgets produced by brilliant technology (Behringer, Klinker, and Mizell 1999; Nayyar et al. 2018; Chakravarthula et al. 2018).
- **3D registration technology**
  As one of the foremost basic advances within the AR framework, 3D technology enables virtual pictures to be superimposed precisely within the reality. The stream of 3D enlistment innovation has two steps. To begin with, decide the relationship between the virtual picture, the framework, and the course and position data of the camera or gadget. Later, the virtual extracted picture and framework are precisely projected into the reality, so the virtual picture and model can be combined with the reality (Talaat et al. 2020).
- **Intelligent interaction technology**
  Smart interactive technology is closely related to brilliant innovation, 3D registration innovation, ergonomics, cognitive brain research, and other disciplines. In AR frameworks, there are assortments of cleverly intelligent, smart gadget, intuitive analytics, tag-based, or other information-based intelligence. With the improvement of cleverly interaction innovation, AR realizes the interaction between individuals and virtual objects in genuine scenes (Han, Claudia tom Dieck & Jung, 2018).

1.3.2.6.1 Other Areas of Applied Technology

AR innovation is regularly utilized in archaeological ponders to zoom in on relics in reality to guarantee that archaeologists can pinpoint their area more precisely. AR innovation permits customers to see almost everything without opening its bundle (Han et al. 2019). AR technology plays an important role in public security as well. It can be used to integrate the input data such as camera to the real scene for better understanding in investigating the criminal cases (Bottani and Vignali 2019).

1.3.2.7 Big Data and Analytics

Big data contains greater information at higher volume, velocity, and variety. It is also known as 3 Vs (volume, velocity, and variety). Big data is more complex than traditional data processing software especially from new data sources (Nasim et al. 2018). IR 4.0 big data comes from many and diverse sources, as shown below:

- Threshold specifications from product and/or machine design data
- Control systems machine-operation data
- Manufacturing execution systems
- Manufacturing and operational costs information
- Staff's records and manual operations
- Fault-detection and system-monitoring deployments
- Process and product quality data
- Third-party logistics information
- Product usage and feedback from customer

Big data is segregated into structured (chemical sensor signals), semi-structured (records), and unstructured (image file) data sources (Yang et al. 2017). The corporations need to empower the application of big data analytics through AI, expert systems, and forecast analysis. In the year 2018, PWC piloted a study among 3,600 individuals regarding the adaptation and adoption of IR 4.0 in industrial sectors, namely chemicals, metals, aerospace, automotive, and electronic on the expectation of cost reduction in next 5 years. It was anticipated that the IR 4.0 usage in year 2020 counting enormous information analytics with the highest cost reduction predicted in aerospace and automotive sectors, 4.3% of operation cost for cumulative benefits of digitalization (Tuffnell et al. 2019).

Uses, Applications, and Benefits of Big Data Analytics

- **Improve production quality**
  A semiconductor producer started to connect single-chip information captured within the testing stage at the final stage of the manufacturing where the data is collected prior process. The producer then recognized the flawed chips earlier and significantly improved the quality of the manufacturing process.
- **Empowered customers**
  The vehicle industry is excited grasping IR 4.0 in arranging the cost-effective strategies to meet customer desires for more reasonable and intelligent system associated cars. The big data connected the enormous information between manufacturers and smart vehicles.
- **Reduced downtime**
  The big data analytics can predict process failure of the machine or manufacturing process. The flow or process supervisor can assess the machine at instance and reduce the downtime analytics.

1.3.2.8 Autonomous Robots

Autonomous robots are similar to humans. Robots are able to make their own decision and perform actions accordingly. It can manipulate and actuate itself within the environment through the program installed in the autonomous robotic system (Indri, Grau, and Ruderman 2018). In the case of mobility, the decision making is incorporated with the maneuvering decision-based support systems such as stop, start, and manipulate the dynamic of its surrounding. AI technology is installed in the robotic system network to ensure autonomous decision making is applicable. Autonomous robots is use to execute routine work, high-risk schedule, complex programming, and repetitive assignments in the manufacturing and production process where the tasks are hardly executed by human (Benotsmane, Kovács, and Dudás 2019).

Autonomous robots have been applied in the area of medicine and health in Thailand as an interphase for the medical officers and patients during Covid-19 pandemic to reduce the potential of infection. These robots are also use in Malaysian food and agricultural industries to do routine and labor-intensive handling task. With the application of these modern robots, the labor cost and probability of product defects can be reduced with less supervision. It drives the supply chain at a high success rate and ensures the sustainable production process (Hahn 2020). Autonomous robots bring beneficial insight in manufacturing industries through IR 4.0 and deliver specific value through:

- Increasing productivity and efficiency in mass-production process
- Reducing rate and error in manufacturing process
- Decreasing health, safety, and environmental (HSE) issues among workers
- Enhancing the revenue by increasing customer perception through sustainable production
- Adding efficiency through human–robotic collaborative working strategies
- Enhanced employee value by focusing on strategic work instead of mundane tasks

1.3.2.9 Horizontal and Vertical System Integration

Horizontal integrated system activities are surrounded by its core competencies and partnerships to develop an end-to-end value chain, while the vertical system contains its in-house value chain from product development to production, sales, and marketing up to the distribution process (Wang et al. 2016). The best way to explain horizontal and vertical integration is through an example of expanding a coffee shop business. Horizontal integration would be partnering or buying other coffee shops competing in the market as well as indirect competition such as stores that sell drinks. Through horizontal integration, the company can control more of the market competition and set barriers of entry. Example of the company practices in a horizontal integration system is L'Oreal where they own Maybelline, Kiehl's, Lancôme, Biotherm, and more. For vertical integration, the company would partner or buy the flow of supply chain up and down streams that include the distributor who supplies coffee beans, the milk, and the source of raw materials. By doing this, the company controls the unit economics of the product and can have much more control on the profit margin of products as well as the time needed to get products through for consumers to enjoy their coffees. Examples of a company that practices vertical integration system is Zara, who own the supply of fabric, manufacturer, transportation, and all the way to the physical stores.

1.3.2.9.1 Horizontal Integration IR 4.0

IR 4.0 envisions interconnected cyber networks and enterprise systems through the introduction of mechanization, flexibility, and operating efficiency translated into manufacturing practices in horizontal system such as (Saucedo-Martínez et al. 2018):

- On the **production floor**: Production network with the interconnectivity of machines and production units (controller) are being constantly communicate about the performance status to respond autonomously for effectively producing process and reduce costly downtime.
- Through multiple **manufacture services**: IR 4.0 encourages horizontal system across plant-level business system for the distributed manufacture facilities enterprise industries. For the horizontal integration system, all the production and facility data will be shared with the entire stakeholders and the respond time is increased for the production parameters.
- Through the **holistic supply chain**: IR 4.0 recommends data transparency and automated system of collaboration integrating upstream and downstream supply as well as logistic chain.

1.3.2.9.1.1 Horizontal Integration Strategies

Horizontal integration may be an effective strategy when the institution rivals a rising of manufacturing where the competitor has a lack of particular resources, capabilities and competencies capabilities, competencies, skills, or resources. The horizontal integration would champion the industry through a legal pathway. Horizontal integration strategies would be implied when the economic contributes to the significance effect and the organization has sufficient resources of mergers and acquisition (M&A).

1.3.2.9.1.2 Vertical Integration IR 4.0

The purpose of vertical integration in IR 4.0 is to connect the working stages within the manufacturing or business level from the research and development sector, production stages, sales, and marketing to distribution stage (Wollschlaeger, Sauter, and Jasperneite 2017). Data flows transparently throughout the stages and action time is increased such as product recall if necessary. The vertically integrated IR 4.0 enterprise gains a crucial competitive edge by being able to respond appropriately and with agility to change market signals and provide new opportunities.

1.3.2.9.1.3 Vertical Integration Strategies

Vertical system integrates IT business through supplying raw materials (backward integration) or distributing products to end consumers (forward integration).

For instance, the supermarket may acquire vegetables from suppliers (backward integration) or buy machines like vehicles to smoothen its product distributions (forward integration). However, the third type of vertical integration, namely balanced integration, is a judicious mix of backward and forward integration strategies (Sony 2018). As the organization's IT systems and production processes become more integrated and complex, enterprises will need to adopt strong orchestration platforms that can provide end-to-end visibility and actionable insights across diverse, distributed systems and entities (Xu, Xu, and Li 2018).

Uses, Applications, and Benefits of Horizontal and Vertical System Integration
Horizontal System Integration Companies

- Economies scale: Horizontally integrated company should be in high competent to achieve a higher production than the companies merged at a lower cost.
- Increased differentiation: Ensure company offers dynamic product feature to customers.
- Increased market power: The new company will become a big company through the merger of companies for their old suppliers. It will command a bigger end-product market and greater power over distributors.
- Ability to enter new markets: If the merger is collaborating with an organization abroad, the new company will have an additional foreign market.

Vertical System Integration Companies

- Able to smoothen the supply chain by ensuring the readiness of product components that acquire specification
- Opening the showroom to ensure efficient aftersales services
- Able to absorb downstream and upstream profits to increase revenue
- Able to reduce operational cost to increase entry barriers for new competitors
- Able to develop core competencies by investing in specific functions such as tire-making

1.3.3 BIOMANUFACTURING OF INDUSTRY REVOLUTION 4.0

Biomanufacturing emerged a long time ago, when fermentation and vaccination became important to our daily needs. However, the modern biomanufacturing began in 1970s where it was applied in the healthcare sector, related to recombinant DNA (Zhang, Sun, and Ma 2017). A decade later, business strategized biomanufacturing in agricultural and food industries through a molecular biology approach. Finally, biologists have started to utilize the biomanufacturing approach to study and modify the genes to create good microorganisms that benefit humankind. These microorganisms are capable of producing a variety of chemicals with industrial importance, including dicarboxylic acids (succinic acid and adipic acid), diols (1,3-propanediol and 1,4-butanediol), and diamines (putrescine and cadaverine). Some of the microbes, such as yeast, have been known to be bioengineered for the mass production of biofuel precursors. Moreover, contemporary biomanufacturing

TABLE 1.3.1
Types of Major Technologies in Biomanufacturing Industries

Biomanufacturing Industry	Major Technology
Food and beverage industry	• Radio-frequency identification (RFID)
	• Real-time production control
	• Digital technology
	• Intelligent labeling
	• Touch interface system
Medicine	• Robotic
	• Sensor
	• Precision medicine
	• Genetic engineering
	• 3D printing
	• Biosecurity and biosafety
Industrial application	• Digital biotechnology
	• DNA digital data storage
	• Digital gene circuit

has produced biomaterials including polysaccharides (microbial cellulose), proteins (spider silk), and even formerly synthetic polymers (polylactate and poly[lactate-co-glycolate]) through the fermentation of engineered microorganisms (Kusiak 2018).

An underlying theme in IR 4.0 for industrial players in biomanufacturing industries is the acceleration of innovation and applications of major technologies related to IR 4.0 that have impacted the business. These major technologies for each business industry are tabulated in Table 1.3.1.

1.3.3.1 Food and Beverage

Food and beverage industries will transform into better manufacturing production systems through IR 4.0. IR 4.0 enables these industries to save money, increase customer perception, reduce product loss, and increase productivity by incorporating smart technologies into their systems. Tracing product defects through RFID and sensor technology has reduced the tracking time and time consumed for the product recall process (Majeed and Rupasinghe 2017). Data collection through the cloud and big data analytics will give the company advantages in responding to these problems faster at real time and pull back the items before shipping out the goods. The prediction of customer preferences through the online shopping database is essential information for the manufacturer and business stakeholders. The capability of equipment maintenance and progression of production have been enhanced through simulation process where the prediction of productivity at different parameters (time, cost, etc.) during real time has become significance. Cyber security secures the cyber system of the production and manufacturing process where autonomous robots are utilized to assist the human labor (Lin et al. 2016).

1.3.3.2 Medicine

Medicine and healthcare industries should be prioritized to ensure the sustainable well-being and prosperity among the society. IR 4.0 gives the opportunities to these industries to boost their technologies technically. For instance, robotic surgical method is implemented in routine surgery, has decreased the implication for the patients, and reduced the infection of surgical wounds. By using this method, the patients will recover at a faster rate with low cost required (Vuong et al. 2019).

IR 4.0 significantly contributes to the precise diagnosis and treatments for genomic testing and radiological imaging. New medical devices such as sensor and detection are moving forward to IIoT and cyber systems where information is transferred through the Internet and mobile phone to the patient and medical officer from the laboratory testing. In addition, the laboratory information system (LIM) technology allows the cloud and big data to secure the information of diagnosis and patients (Salter and Salter 2017; Eggert and Hutmacher 2019; Mosharraf et al. 2019; Fatorachian and Kazemi 2018; Bauer 2018).

Currently, the pandemic coronavirus (COVID-19) has hit most of the countries around the world. IR 4.0 has played a pivotal role to assist the frontliners such as medical officers and local authorities to prevent the emergence of infection. In Thailand, autonomous robots have been developed as an interphase for the medical officers and patients to reduce the risk of infection. The autonomous robots deliver the information from/to the doctors-patients and collect data of patients' body temperature. Malaysia companies have developed the sensor technology to determine the infected person through DNA-based aptamer against the novel coronavirus.

1.3.3.3 Industrial Applications

- **Digital biotechnology**
  Recombinant and synthetic biology have become digitalized in the era of IR 4.0. The discreet information of living cells and biologics intermediate part has intrigued the biotechnology firm to approach the digital transformation such as a simulation system to build living structures by components and promote high density data storage for nucleic acid information (Scheitz, Peck, and Groban 2018).
- **DNA digital data storage**
  Development of computing device based on deoxyribonucleic acid (DNA) molecules information has intrigued the biologist to utilize the technologies in IR 4.0. Mathematical modeling and molecular mean of DNA have been utilized for the DNA digital data storage (Ceze, Nivala, and Strauss 2019).
- **Digital gene circuits**
  The synthetic gene circuit technology has been used in the research of metabolic engineering to study the interaction of cells towards the dynamic of environment. This information is a huge advantage for the bio-production process prior to the upscaling process (Xie and Fussenegger 2018; Valasek and Repa 2005; Caicedo and Brady 2016).

1.3.4 CHALLENGES

Many challenges are faced by the biomanufacturing industries through IR 4.0, especially from the industrial perspectives and contract-based manufacturing organization. The biomanufacturing process is complex because the industries mainly cooperated with cells, microorganisms, and living resources. For example, in the biomanufacturing of fermentation, the production system requires specific human capital knowledge, particularly professionals with basic backgrounds of biotechnology and microbiology, equipped with the understanding of IR 4.0 insight. However, with the IR 4.0 coming to the edge, the engineer or biologist must catch up with the revolution of IR 4.0 technologies such as DNA circuit, simulation modeling, and integrated system. Prior to the knowledge in the production process, the technical expert should be well versed with the good manufacturing practice (GMP) for the requirement of licensing and authority purposes. The technical expert must understand the application of the cloud, big data analytics, and cyber security to foresee the holistic understanding of the manufacturing process as the applications are very essential to apply for a certificate related to the industry. The other issue for biomanufacturing is the low rate of technology transfer between manufacturers and research entities (universities and research institutions). Towards IR 4.0, the technologies, namely simulation, the cloud, big analytics, additive manufacturing, and etc. should be integrated in the transfer of knowledge to empower the manufacturing strategies and leverage the productivity. It can be ensured that the commercial technology is driven by IR 4.0 for the benefits of the industries.

1.3.5 FUTURE PERSPECTIVES

IR 4.0 has a big impact in biomanufacturing industries, especially in healthcare, food, beverage, and agricultural businesses. However, the assurance to meet the productivity and capacity for consumer demands can be only achieved through the right timing, right location, with the right solution since the cost of production (labor, raw materials, and machineries) is increasing from time to time. IR 4.0 technologies ensure the manufacturing process is paced with the needs and the scale volume of production through the integration of multiple technology (simulation, big data analytics, and the cloud). The integration of biomanufacturing and IR 4.0 technologies will increase the annual revenue, improve the productivity, and reduce operational cost for industries.

In healthcare industries, IR 4.0 offers the opportunities for patient care through sustaining the medical supplies chain by securing the manufacturing production process that produces drugs in a reliable and cost-effective way. IR 4.0 can also ensure the availability, assessment, utilization, and self-sufficiency level (SSL) for food and beverage supplies is achieved. Due to the importance of IR 4.0, the government, industrial players, and stakeholders should invest in the IR 4.0–related industries to ensure the sustainability of production process and competitiveness in the global platform.

REFERENCES

Aazam, M., K.A. Harras, and S. Zeadally. 2019. "Fog computing for 5G tactile Industrial Internet of Things: QoE-aware resource allocation model." *IEEE Transactions on Industrial Informatics* 15 (5): 3085–3092. doi: 10.1109/TII.2019.2902574.

Aazam, M., S. Zeadally, and K.A. Harras. 2018. "Deploying fog computing in Industrial Internet of Things and Industry 4.0." *IEEE Transactions on Industrial Informatics* 14 (10): 4674–4682. doi: 10.1109/TII.2018.2855198.

Abdelghader Morsi, Mohame, Eman Naji Mahmoud Fadoul, Esraa Mohammed Eshag Ibrahim, and Mehad Mohammed Ibrahim Mohammed. 2020. "Cloud computing challenges and opportunities." *University of Khartoum Engineering Journal* 10 (1).

Akinrolabu, O., S. New, and A. Martin. 2017. "Cyber supply chain risks in cloud computing – Bridging the risk assessment gap." *Open Journal of Cloud Computing* 5 (1): 1–19.

Al-Rubaye, S., E. Kadhum, Q. Ni, and A. Anpalagan. 2019. "Industrial Internet of Things driven by SDN platform for smart grid resiliency." *IEEE Internet of Things Journal* 6 (1): 267–277. doi: 10.1109/JIOT.2017.2734903.

Al-Turjman, F., and S. Alturjman. 2018. "Context-sensitive access in Industrial Internet of Things (IIoT) healthcare applications." *IEEE Transactions on Industrial Informatics* 14 (6): 2736–2744. doi: 10.1109/TII.2018.2808190.

Attaran, Mohsen. 2017. "The rise of 3-D printing: The advantages of additive manufacturing over traditional manufacturing." *Business Horizons* 60 (5): 677–688. doi: https://doi.org/10.1016/j.bushor.2017.05.011.

Bauer, Greg. 2018. "Delivering value-based care with e-health services." *Journal of Healthcare Management* 63 (4): 251–260. doi: 10.1097/jhm-d-18-00077.

Behringer, Reinhold, G. Klinker, and D. Mizell. 1999. "Augmented reality." In *Encyclopedia of Computer Science and Technology* vol. 45 (supplement 30): 45–57.

Benotsmane, Rabab, György Kovács, and László Dudás. 2019. "Economic, social impacts and operation of smart factories in Industry 4.0 focusing on simulation and artificial intelligence of collaborating robots." *Social Sciences* 8 (5): 143.

Berry, Christine T., and Ronald L. Berry. 2018. "An initial assessment of small business risk management approaches for cyber security threats." *International Journal of Business Continuity and Risk Management* 8 (1): 1–10.

Bitam, S., S. Zeadally, and A. Mellouk. 2016. "Bio-inspired cybersecurity for wireless sensor networks." *IEEE Communications Magazine* 54 (6): 68–74. doi: 10.1109/MCOM.2016.7497769.

Bittencourt, L.F., J. Diaz-Montes, R. Buyya, O.F. Rana, and M. Parashar. 2017. "Mobility-aware application scheduling in fog computing." *IEEE Cloud Computing* 4 (2): 26–35. doi: 10.1109/MCC.2017.27.

Bottani, Eleonora, and Giuseppe Vignali. 2019. "Augmented reality technology in the manufacturing industry: A review of the last decade." *IISE Transactions* 51 (3): 284–310. doi: 10.1080/24725854.2018.1493244.

Bustos, Rod A. 2017. "Facilitating support of cyber: Toward a new liaison model with cybersecurity education at Augusta University." *Journal of Business & Finance Librarianship* 22 (1): 24–31. doi: 10.1080/08963568.2016.1258935.

Caicedo, Hector Hugo, and Scott T. Brady. 2016. "Microfluidics: The challenge is to bridge the gap instead of looking for a 'killer app'." *Trends in Biotechnology* 34 (1): 1–3.

Ceze, Luis, Jeff Nivala, and Karin Strauss. 2019. "Molecular digital data storage using DNA." *Nature Reviews Genetics* 20 (8): 456–466. doi: 10.1038/s41576-019-0125-3.

Chakravarthula, P., D. Dunn, K. Aksit, and H. Fuchs. 2018. "FocusAR: Auto-focus augmented reality eyeglasses for both real world and virtual imagery." *IEEE Transactions on Visualization and Computer Graphics* 24 (11): 2906–2916. doi: 10.1109/TVCG.2018.2868532.

Chen, Jim Q., and Allen Benusa. 2017. "HIPAA security compliance challenges: The case for small healthcare providers." *International Journal of Healthcare Management* 10 (2): 135–146. doi: 10.1080/20479700.2016.1270875.

Cheng, Jiangfeng, He Zhang, Fei Tao, and Chia-Feng Juang. 2020. "DT-II: Digital twin enhanced Industrial Internet reference framework towards smart manufacturing." *Robotics and Computer-Integrated Manufacturing* 62: 101881. doi: https://doi.org/10.1016/j.rcim.2019.101881.

Chimene, David, Roland Kaunas, and Akhilesh K. Gaharwar. 2020. "Hydrogel bioink reinforcement for additive manufacturing: A focused review of emerging strategies." *Advanced Materials* 32 (1): 1902026. doi: 10.1002/adma.201902026.

de Bruin, Boudewijn, and Luciano Floridi. 2017. "The ethics of cloud computing." *Science and Engineering Ethics* 23 (1): 21–39. doi: 10.1007/s11948-016-9759-0.

Eem, Seung-Hyun, Jeong-Hoi Koo, and Hyung-Jo Jung. 2019. "Feasibility study of an adaptive mount system based on magnetorheological elastomer using real-time hybrid simulation." *Journal of Intelligent Material Systems and Structures* 30 (5): 701–707. doi: 10.1177/1045389x18754347.

Eggert, Sebastian, and Dietmar W. Hutmacher. 2019. "In vitro disease models 4.0 via automation and high-throughput processing." *Biofabrication* 11 (4): 043002.

Enyedy, Noel, Joshua A. Danish, Girlie Delacruz, and Melissa Kumar. 2012. "Learning physics through play in an augmented reality environment." *International Journal of Computer-Supported Collaborative Learning* 7 (3): 347–378. doi: 10.1007/s11412-012-9150-3.

Fatorachian, Hajar, and Hadi Kazemi. 2018. "A critical investigation of Industry 4.0 in manufacturing: Theoretical operationalisation framework." *Production Planning & Control* 29 (8): 633–644. doi: 10.1080/09537287.2018.1424960.

Goddard, Phil. 2016. "Quantum computing: Implications for portfolio managers." *The Journal of Investing* 25 (3): 81. doi: 10.3905/joi.2016.25.3.081.

Grocke, Derek. 2017. "Emerging cybersecurity threats in large and small firms." *Bulletin (Law Society of South Australia)* 39 (3): 20.

Hahn, Gerd J. 2020. "Industry 4.0: A supply chain innovation perspective." *International Journal of Production Research* 58 (5): 1425–1441. doi: 10.1080/00207543.2019.1641642.

Han, Dai-In, M. Claudia tom Dieck, and Timothy Jung. 2018. "User experience model for augmented reality applications in urban heritage tourism." *Journal of Heritage Tourism* 13 (1): 46–61. doi: 10.1080/1743873X.2016.1251931.

Han, Young-Soo, Jaejoon Lee, Jungmin Lee, Wonhyuk Lee, and Kyungho Lee. 2019. "3D CAD data extraction and conversion for application of augmented/virtual reality to the construction of ships and offshore structures." *International Journal of Computer Integrated Manufacturing* 32 (7): 658–668. doi: 10.1080/0951192X.2019.1599440.

Henriques de Gusmão, Ana Paula, Maisa Mendonça Silva, Thiago Poleto, Lúcio Camara e Silva, and Ana Paula Cabral Seixas Costa. 2018. "Cybersecurity risk analysis model using fault tree analysis and fuzzy decision theory." *International Journal of Information Management* 43: 248–260. doi: https://doi.org/10.1016/j.ijinfomgt.2018.08.008.

Indri, M., A. Grau, and M. Ruderman. 2018. "Guest Editorial Special Section on recent trends and developments in Industry 4.0 motivated robotic solutions." *IEEE Transactions on Industrial Informatics* 14 (4): 1677–1680. doi: 10.1109/TII.2018.2809000.

Janaki, M. 2017. "Real world tour of cloud computing for family." *International Journal of Education and Management Engineering* 7 (6): 24.

Kalra, Amolak Ratan, Navya Gupta, Bikash K. Behera, Shiroman Prakash, and Prasanta K. Panigrahi. 2019. "Demonstration of the no-hiding theorem on the 5-Qubit IBM quantum computer in a category-theoretic framework." *Quantum Information Processing* 18 (6): 170. doi: 10.1007/s11128-019-2288-4.

Kashif, Muhammad, Sheraz Arshad Malik, Muhammad Tahir Abdullah, Muhammad Umair, and Prince Waqas Khan. 2018. "A systematic review of cyber security and classification of attacks in networks." *International Journal of Advanced Computer Science and Applications* 9 (6): 201–207.

Kiradoo, Giriraj. 2019. "The impact of e-commerce in the entrepreneurship and the obstacles faced by the domestic enterprise." *International Journal of Management* 10 (5): 154–164.

Kshetri, Nir. 2017. "Blockchain's roles in strengthening cybersecurity and protecting privacy." *Telecommunications Policy* 41 (10): 1027–1038. doi: https://doi.org/10.1016/j.telpol.2017.09.003.

Kuratko, Donald F., Harrison L. Holt, and Emily Neubert. 2020. "Blitzscaling: The good, the bad, and the ugly." *Business Horizons* 63 (1): 109–119. doi: https://doi.org/10.1016/j.bushor.2019.10.002.

Kusiak, Andrew. 2018. "Smart manufacturing." *International Journal of Production Research* 56 (1–2): 508–517. doi: 10.1080/00207543.2017.1351644.

Lan, Mai Thi, Tran Thuy Duong, Toshiaki Iitaka, and Nguyen Van Hong. 2017. "Computer simulation of $CaSiO_3$ glass under compression: Correlation between Si–Si pair radial distribution function and intermediate range order structure." *Materials Research Express* 4 (6): 065201. doi: 10.1088/2053-1591/aa70d1.

Leuprecht, Christian, David B. Skillicorn, and Victoria E. Tait. 2016. "Beyond the Castle Model of cyber-risk and cyber-security." *Government Information Quarterly* 33 (2): 250–257. doi: https://doi.org/10.1016/j.giq.2016.01.012.

Li, Mengheng, Siem Jan Koopman, Rutger Lit, and Desislava Petrova. 2020. "Long-term forecasting of El Niño events via dynamic factor simulations." *Journal of Econometrics* 214 (1): 46–66. doi: https://doi.org/10.1016/j.jeconom.2019.05.004.

Lin, C., D. Deng, Z. Chen, and K. Chen. 2016. " Key design of driving industry 4.0: Joint energy-efficient deployment and scheduling in group-based industrial wireless sensor networks." *IEEE Communications Magazine* 54 (10): 46–52. doi: 10.1109/MCOM.2016.7588228.

Liu, Sen, Felix T.S. Chan, Junai Yang, and Ben Niu. 2018. "Understanding the effect of cloud computing on organizational agility: An empirical examination." *International Journal of Information Management* 43: 98–111. doi: https://doi.org/10.1016/j.ijinfomgt.2018.07.010.

Liu, Y., K. Wang, Y. Lin, and W. Xu. 2019. "A lightweight blockchain system for Industrial Internet of Things." *IEEE Transactions on Industrial Informatics* 15 (6): 3571–3581. doi: 10.1109/TII.2019.2904049.

Lv, Zhihan, Alaa Halawani, Shengzhong Feng, Shafiq ur Réhman, and Haibo Li. 2015. "Touch-less interactive augmented reality game on vision-based wearable device." *Personal and Ubiquitous Computing* 19 (3): 551–567. doi: 10.1007/s00779-015-0844-1.

Majeed, Aabid Abdul, and Thashika D. Rupasinghe. 2017. "Internet of things (IoT) embedded future supply chains for industry 4.0: An assessment from an ERP-based fashion apparel and footwear industry." *International Journal of Supply Chain Management* 6 (1): 25–40.

Mondal, Debasish. 2019. "The internet of thing (IOT) and industrial automation: A future perspective." *World Journal of Modelling and Simulation* 15 (2): 140–149.

Mosharraf, Sakib, Mohammad Salim Hossain, Md Abdul Barek, Hrishov Das, and Md Abdur Rahman Ripon. 2019. "A review on revolution of pharmaceutical sector in Bangladesh after Liberation War and future prospects and challenges." *International Journal of Pharmaceutical Investigation* 9 (3): 89–92.

Mouratidis, H., and V. Diamantopoulou. 2018. "A security analysis method for Industrial Internet of Things." *IEEE Transactions on Industrial Informatics* 14 (9): 4093–4100. doi: 10.1109/TII.2018.2832853.

Nasim, Saiful Farik Mat Yatin Ahmad, Mohd Sidek, Hanis Zawani Mobidin, and Siti Nurul Atiqah Adam. 2018. "Big data towards decision-making culture in organization." *Development* 7 (3): 103–115.

Nayyar, Anand, Bandana Mahapatra, D. Le, and G. Suseendran. 2018. "Virtual reality (VR) & augmented reality (AR) technologies for tourism and hospitality industry." *International Journal of Engineering & Technology* 7 (2.21): 156–160.

Neto, Albino Ribeiro, Maira Fernanda Gizotti Ribeiro, Gerson Gomes Cunha, and Luiz Landau. 2017. "The industrial internet of things and technological innovation in its applications for resources optimisation." *International Journal of Simulation and Process Modelling* 12 (6): 525–534.

Ning, Z., X. Kong, F. Xia, W. Hou, and X. Wang. 2019. "Green and sustainable cloud of things: Enabling collaborative edge computing." *IEEE Communications Magazine* 57 (1): 72–78. doi: 10.1109/MCOM.2018.1700895.

Özceylan, Eren, Cihan Çetinkaya, Neslihan Demirel, and Ozan Sabirlioglu. 2018. "Impacts of additive manufacturing on supply chain flow: A simulation approach in healthcare industry." *Logistics* 2 (1): 1.

Papagiannakis, George, Gurminder Singh, and Nadia Magnenat-Thalmann. 2008. "A survey of mobile and wireless technologies for augmented reality systems." *Computer Animation and Virtual Worlds* 19 (1): 3–22. doi: 10.1002/cav.221.

Paul, Souvik, Atrayee Chatterjee, and Digbijay Guha. 2019. "Study of smart inventory management system based on the Internet of Things (IOT)." *International Journal on Recent Trends in Business and Tourism* 3 (3): 27–34.

Popova Zhuhadar, Lily, and Evelyn Thrasher. 2019. "Data analytics and its advantages for addressing the complexity of healthcare: A simulated Zika case study example." *Applied Sciences* 9 (11): 2208.

Salter, Brian, and Charlotte Salter. 2017. "Controlling new knowledge: Genomic science, governance and the politics of bioinformatics." *Social Studies of Science* 47 (2): 263–287.

Saucedo-Martínez, Jania Astrid, Magdiel Pérez-Lara, José Antonio Marmolejo-Saucedo, Tomás Eloy Salais-Fierro, and Pandian Vasant. 2018. "Industry 4.0 framework for management and operations: A review." *Journal of Ambient Intelligence and Humanized Computing* 9 (3): 789–801. doi: 10.1007/s12652-017-0533-1.

Scheitz, Cornelia Johanna Franziska, Lawrence J. Peck, and Eli S. Groban. 2018. "Biotechnology software in the digital age: Are you winning?" *Journal of Industrial Microbiology & Biotechnology* 45 (7): 529–534. doi: 10.1007/s10295-018-2009-5.

Senyo, Prince Kwame, Erasmus Addae, and Richard Boateng. 2018. "Cloud computing research: A review of research themes, frameworks, methods and future research directions." *International Journal of Information Management* 38 (1): 128–139. doi: https://doi.org/10.1016/j.ijinfomgt.2017.07.007.

Shan, Minghe, Jian Guo, and Eberhard Gill. 2020. "An analysis of the flexibility modeling of a net for space debris removal." *Advances in Space Research* 65 (3): 1083–1094. doi: https://doi.org/10.1016/j.asr.2019.10.041.

Sony, Michael. 2018. "Industry 4.0 and lean management: A proposed integration model and research propositions." *Production & Manufacturing Research* 6 (1): 416–432. doi: 10.1080/21693277.2018.1540949.

Stergiou, Christos, and Kostas E. Psannis. 2017. "Recent advances delivered by Mobile Cloud Computing and Internet of Things for Big Data applications: A survey." *International Journal of Network Management* 27 (3): e1930. doi: 10.1002/nem.1930.

Talaat, Sameh, Ahmed Kaboudan, Omar Abdelbary, Katherine Kula, Ahmed Ghoneima, Reinhard Klein, and Christoph Bourauel. 2020. "3D superimposition of dental casts based on coloured landmark detection using combined computer vision and 3D computer graphics techniques." *Computer Methods in Biomechanics and Biomedical Engineering: Imaging & Visualization* 8 (1): 87–93. doi: 10.1080/21681163.2019.1585295.

Tian, J., R. Tan, X. Guan, Z. Xu, and T. Liu. 2020. "Moving target defense approach to detecting Stuxnet-like attacks." *IEEE Transactions on Smart Grid* 11 (1): 291–300. doi: 10.1109/TSG.2019.2921245.

Tirabeni, Lia, Paola De Bernardi, Canio Forliano, and Mattia Franco. 2019. "How can organisations and business models lead to a more sustainable society? A framework from a systematic review of the Industry 4.0." *Sustainability* 11 (22): 6363.

Tuffnell, Caryl, Pavol Kral, Anna Siekelova, and Jakub Horak. 2019. "Cyber-physical smart manufacturing systems: Sustainable industrial networks, cognitive automation, and data-centric business models." *Economics, Management and Financial Markets* 14 (2): 58–63.

Valasek, Mark A., and Joyce J Repa. 2005. "The power of real-time PCR." *Advances in Physiology Education* 29 (3): 151–159.

Vulpiani, Angelo, and Marco Baldovin. 2020. "Effective equations in complex systems: From Langevin to machine learning." *Journal of Statistical Mechanics: Theory and Experiment* 2020 (1): 014003. doi: 10.1088/1742-5468/ab535c.

Vuong, Quan-Hoang, Manh-Tung Ho, Thu-Trang Vuong, Viet-Phuong La, Manh-Toan Ho, Kien-Cuong P. Nghiem, Bach Xuan Tran, Hai-Ha Giang, Thu-Vu Giang, Carl Latkin, Hong-Kong T. Nguyen, Cyrus S.H. Ho, and Roger C.M. Ho. 2019. "Artificial intelligence vs. natural stupidity: Evaluating AI readiness for the Vietnamese Medical Information System." *Journal of Clinical Medicine* 8 (2): 168.

Wang, Carolyn L., Sankar Chinnugounder, Daniel S. Hippe, Sadaf Zaidi, Ryan B. O'Malley, Puneet Bhargava, and William H. Bush. 2017. "Comparative effectiveness of hands-on versus computer simulation-based training for contrast media reactions and teamwork skills." *Journal of the American College of Radiology* 14 (1): 103–110.e3. doi: https://doi.org/10.1016/j.jacr.2016.07.013.

Wang, Shiyong, Jiafu Wan, Di Li, and Chunhua Zhang. 2016. "Implementing smart factory of Industrie 4.0: An outlook." *International Journal of Distributed Sensor Networks* 12 (1): 3159805. doi: 10.1155/2016/3159805.

Wei, Nai-Chieh, Chiao-Ping Bao, Tai-Lioan Chen, Shun-Yuan Yao, and Yan-Yu Chen. 2018. "Cloud service based quality control circle." *International Journal of Organizational Innovation (Online)* 11 (2): 65–83.

Wollschlaeger, M., T. Sauter, and J. Jasperneite. 2017. "The future of industrial communication: Automation networks in the era of the Internet of Things and Industry 4.0." *IEEE Industrial Electronics Magazine* 11 (1): 17–27. doi: 10.1109/MIE.2017.2649104.

Xie, Mingqi, and Martin Fussenegger. 2018. "Designing cell function: Assembly of synthetic gene circuits for cell biology applications." *Nature Reviews Molecular Cell Biology* 19 (8): 507–525. doi: 10.1038/s41580-018-0024-z.

Xu, Li Da, Eric L. Xu, and Ling Li. 2018. "Industry 4.0: State of the art and future trends." *International Journal of Production Research* 56 (8): 2941–2962. doi: 10.1080/00207543.2018.1444806.

Yang, Chaowei, Qunying Huang, Zhenlong Li, Kai Liu, and Fei Hu. 2017. "Big Data and cloud computing: Innovation opportunities and challenges." *International Journal of Digital Earth* 10 (1): 13–53. doi: 10.1080/17538947.2016.1239771.

Zhang-Kennedy, Leah, Sonia Chiasson, and Robert Biddle. 2016. "The role of instructional design in persuasion: A comics approach for improving cybersecurity." *International Journal of Human–Computer Interaction* 32 (3): 215–257. doi: 10.1080/10447318.2016.1136177.

Zhang, Y., H. Huang, L. Yang, Y. Xiang, and M. Li. 2019. "Serious challenges and potential solutions for the Industrial Internet of Things with edge intelligence." *IEEE Network* 33 (5): 41–45. doi: 10.1109/MNET.001.1800478.

Zhang, Yi-Heng Percival, Jibin Sun, and Yanhe Ma. 2017. "Biomanufacturing: History and perspective." *Journal of Industrial Microbiology & Biotechnology* 44 (4): 773–784. doi: 10.1007/s10295-016-1863-2.

2.1 What Is Industry 5.0?

Omar Ashraf ElFar, Angela Paul A/p Peter, Kit Wayne Chew, and Pau Loke Show

CONTENTS

2.1 WHAT IS INDUSTRY 5.0?

2.1.1.1 The Implementation of a New Industrial Revolution

The Industrial Revolution involves industrial and transportation improvements, which started with fewer handcrafts, consequently using computers, machines, and advanced technology in macro production scale with advanced facilities. The focus has changed to a modernized manufacturing facility with the implementation of the most efficient new techniques. This transformation benefits most industries as all the previous limitations will be rectified.

Industrialization generates employment, offers schooling, promotes change and creativity, and allows efficient use of capital. All these benefits, and more, are highly beneficial to the community and to the local economy. The creation and growth of industry within a country is industrial development. Mass manufacturing, scientific advancements, and other resources cover these sectors. Within an urban region or market, the living standards, job development, and efficiency rise while sustaining production. There are many more opportunities as efficiency in a field improves.

Industrial development's economic growth is a positive growth that will change an economy. These go hand in hand with manufacturing production and economic development. When a business expands, industries prosper as development in the market means more employment, more capital, and more opportunity. The manufacturing sector produces more capital and more productive resources that contribute to more revenue per capita and further worker efficiency. Industrial development has a regular correlation with higher incomes. When industry increments and widens, the standard of living increases. The possibilities will change an environment and encourage endless development (Why Is Industrialization & Industrial Development Important? 2020).

It is also widely known that industrial growth gives the environment infinite opportunity. In this 21st century, the development and advances in the industrial sector are unstoppable, hence it is more likely to be called the era of technology. It is genuinely an industrial development, which provides an incentive for more progress. The developments in the market are thrilling as they open several doors and chances to societies. Economic growth pushes change; the greater the customer appetite, the more goods and services are produced (Gesrepair 2021).

The previous industrializations act as references to the economy to refer back to fill missing gaps and to avoid previous mistakes. The rising market for products and services is generating a population and a growing business; therefore, bringing further creativity and financial incentives. Many of us benefit from industrialization as the society thrives (Gesrepair 2021).

In the relevant literature, the community does not fully understand the rates of change from the effect of industrialization at which newly skilled employees are employed and whether job diversity was the most prevalent among local and newcomers, on technical growth and demand for skills; hence, this might be because there is no transparency between the government and its community. However, the effect of change might also not be transparent to the government itself, which leads to the miscommunication between the government and its community. This can be explored with related census statistics, where shifts in a worker's job can be studied over time. The benefits to the community out of this industrialization might be beneficial to the economy by increasing the gross domestic product, which increases the employability rate that would surely increase the money income to the country. Because there are more modernized technologies applied in the manufacturing processes that increase the processing efficiency that reflects on the product's quality, this is one of the main goals for the industry for brand construction in the market, whether it is local or international.

In fact, this research adds to our interpretation of the effects of technological progress in the early 20th century's central economics. The example of Norway is interesting, as in Norway the amount of structured training and schooling is quite low; this is due to the social costs that are build up with a clear association between school dropout and higher criminality, health problems, alcohol, and drug abuse, and health problems (Leknes and Modalsli 2019). Dropping out is associated with lower government income from taxes, lower productive capacity, and higher spending on social security payments, health care, and criminal justice. While the scale of the problem varies from country to country, dropouts could represent a heavy cost for Norway", in contrast with economies like Great Britain or the United States, though literacy levels were high and this is a comparative research study between economies on the effect of technological development correlation with the societies' literacy level (Why Is Industrialization & Industrial Development Important? 2020).

The Industrial Revolution commenced in Great Britain, and various technological innovations were of British origin. By the mid-18th century, Britain was the world's leading commercial nation. The enhancement of trade and the rise of business were among the major causes of the Industrial Revolution. The Industrial Revolution is a turning point that leaves a legacy to other generations to continue their footsteps, and results with unprecedented sustained growth. Some economists state that the enormous influence of the Industrial Revolution was that the standard of living for the general population in the Western world began to escalate constantly for the first time in history (Industrial Revolution 2020).

In the era between 1760 to 1820 and 1840, the Industrial Revolution was the shift to modern production methods in Europe and the United States. During this transformation, there was a shift from manual production to machinery, advanced chemical manufacturing and processing of iron, improved use of steam and water resources, machine tool creation, and the introduction of a mechanized plant environment. The Digital Revolution has also contributed to a dramatic increase in population growth trends (Industrial Revolution 2020).

During the late 1830s to the early 1840s, the economic crisis accelerated and matured the introduction of the Industrial Revolution's initial innovation, with mechanized spinning and weaving. Late in the century, advances such as the growing usage of locomotives, steamboats, and steam engines; hot blast iron smelters; and emerging inventions such as the electric telegraph, which were generally adopted in the 1840s and 1850s, were inadequate to push fast growth levels. A new generation of developments in the so-called Second Industrial Revolution began to generate fast economic development, since 1870. These advances included modern technologies of steel manufacturing, textile processing, assembly lines, electric grid networks, the widespread use of machine tools, and the usage of more sophisticated equipment for steam power plants (Industrial Revolution 2020).

Then a new generation of developments happened after the implementation of the Third Industrial Revolution, which is considered the beginning of the first computing age. With the end of the Second Industrial Revolution, early machines were very basic, unmanageable, and incredibly huge compared with their processing capacity; however, they laid the groundwork for a future today that is hard to envision without digital technology (The Industrial Revolution from Industry 1.0 to 5.0! – Supply Chain Game Changer™ 2020).

Around 1970, the Third Industrial Revolution included the usage of the development of electronics and information technology (IT). Due to web access, networking, and clean energies, development and automation have improved considerably. Moreover, to execute human functions, Industry 3.0 added more automatic processes on the production line, for instance, utilizing Programmable Logical Controllers (PLCs). Although automated systems were in place, they still relied on human input and intervention. The Fourth Industrial Revolution is indeed a period of intelligent machines, storage, and facilities that can communicate knowledge, activate events, and regulate one another autonomously without any human interference.

The industrial Internet of Things (IIoT) today enables the sharing of data associated with specific key elements such as a cyber-physical system, which is a mechanical device system that is run by computer-based algorithms. The Internet of Things (IoT) is an interconnected network of machine devices and vehicles embedded with computerized sensing, scanning, and monitoring capabilities. Cloud computing uses offsite network hosting and data backup. Cognitive computing is a technological platform that employs artificial intelligence.

Throughout the transition period, the emphasis of Industry 5.0 is on the restoration of human hands, brains, and intuition in the manufacturing sense, which stresses transformation of factories into smart IoT facilities that use semantic processing and interconnect systems via cloud servers. Industry 5.0 has the capability that could reconcile humans and machines and seeks ways to operate together in order to increase manufacturing capacity and performance (The Industrial Revolution from Industry 1.0 to 5.0! – Supply Chain Game Changer™ 2020).

Implementation of a modern technological development is unpredictable, since its possibility of building, and its likelihood of deconstruction, is the product of a specific transition. The Industrial Revolution represents an immense move from the decision maker toward settling the endless needs conditions, such as collective community commitment and willingness, civic influence, market risk reduction, and financial stability.

An industrial revolution induces the replacements and refinements of hand tools to machine and power tools. Through the minds of consumers, quality interest is the perceived benefit of a product or service. This is a crucial term for product creation and capital growth, called a valuable product. If the community could produce a commodity that has great value for consumers at a reasonable price, it will be well marketed. The challenge that is encountered from industries is the individual preferences, for instance color, type, size, etc.; moreover, services, distribution, logistics, and interaction with customers. This requires more technical diversity and support for it to complete a qualified valuable product to customers with almost all preferences to reach customer satisfaction.

The industrial revolution is not based on a single invention, or top-notch group of inventions, but a consistent flow of evolutional inventions. In the 21st century, implementing a new industry, for instance Industry 5.0, is not as easy as it is written theoretically, yet not even practically hard to reach and apply. It is known that the Internet has the ability to cut down physical and temporal distances. This provided interconnected machines associated with smart computers incorporated with artificial intelligence technology that are working in the production processes by using software for simulation, modeling, and calculations and predictions that assist scientists and engineers to have a glimpse of the product outcome and future products before manufacturing.

The interconnection of technological and economic data with customers and suppliers would have an opportunity to create a bar that cannot get underneath them anymore. That is due to the excessive incessant flow of inventions and data from different fields. The main issue of an economic life is how to utilize most efficiently a body of knowledge that cannot be owned or centralized by any authority.

Open access to innovation is the parameter for learning by trial and error that encourages companies to successfully transform according to the stimuli that come from different conditions. The innovation that can sustain greater value and turnover is often the original application of something that has been created and invented in another context and for other purposes; it is a phenomenon that is already observed in the past, but the sustained innovation will show more spread and persistence. The point here is to illustrate that every innovation is based on a previous limitation.

The leading model of corporate cooperation is the public-private partnership that leads to transparency, that more than one country will provide support and benefit from both sides in the public and private sectors. The model must bear in mind, from market and economic viewpoints, that no issues occur with the estimates and the modern industrial development systems in order to boost the strength of the gross domestic product (GDP); this is achieved by raising sample size and consumption levels of the population requirements. For example, the Industry 4.0

revolution could not be obtained without the decisive contribution of the state by giving excess to the necessary "4.0 infrastructures", such as the Internet broadband, develop suitable norms and standards, and grant tax incentives.

The majority of people who resided in the countryside increased because the growth of cities coincided with the growth of the industry; this showed change is hard for the society in different areas to adapt quickly. This is due to the implementation of a new industrial revolution by applying the concept of industrialization to the nearby neighborhood.

Industrialization has a fast urbanization that proceeds to escalate in contemporary times, whereas it influenced the average life expectancy that represented an enormous enhancement in industrial nations. Hence, average incomes have increased as well, which proves that industrialization has improved human's lives in many ways and that from a population perspective as a bulk and not from an individualist perspective per person (The Industrial Revolution from Industry 1.0 to 5.0! – Supply Chain Game Changer™ 2020).

The application of this new industrial revolution implies a great effect from the healthcare perspective, worked on improving poor nutrition, disease, lack of sanitation, and harmful medical care in urban areas that will increase life expectancy. This was harder in the past in the early start of industrialization due to the less employability and people become more dependent on their wealth. Due to the effect of industrialization on income increases, that promoted people from low class to middle class and from middle class to upper class. On the other hand, having a robotic industrialization associated with automated and advanced computational predictions application, people's level of productivity, life expectancy, population status, and wealth might be affected. The employability will surely be changed due to the takeover of automated cobots instead of human beings and to decrease the payroll expenses on the company. The challenge also relies on the ability of mankind to adapt to the changes in industrialization.

In a nutshell, it is known that the implementation of Industry 5.0 definitely will be an added advantage to the individual's status, for instance class level, financial stability, and sustainability; hence, industrial concerns as well. Having a well-organized, packed, and qualified trustworthy product is what everyone seeks for. The improvement of creativity, production, prediction, and credibility will be a strong power for the community's status and independence, hence to induce the ability to think more outside the box, to predict the unpredictable, and to expect the unexpected by dispensing the knowledge that was comprehended into actual practical work, so people can benefit from the power of knowledge.

2.1.1.2 The Differences in Industry 5.0 Compared to Other Industries

As the transformation process moves from Industry 4.0 to Industry 5.0, the result is giving the freedom of style responsibility back to the human. A recent study from White (1983) shows the workspace does not become smaller in terms of producing a cell around the human being; it becomes larger. The employee has a lot of responsibility to finish up with even bigger, lighter surroundings such as the workplace, people around, tools, machine setups, quality control, and assurance that they are safer than the previous one.

In terms of practical application, functions within the cell are becoming more relevant, such as the way the reactant moves from one phase to another until it becomes a product. The manufacturing process, which is more or less machine controlled, enables freedom and flexibility of any process methodology, such as the sequence where the product will be allocated with applied suitable conditions at fixed time, to be figured out with the producer and to help understand the ability to manufacture a product that is more customized, has more content, and is private.

The manufacturing processing methodology is introduced in Industry 5.0 as a production process method. This method alters it into a more efficient and cost-effective way that results in a higher rate of production. This implies that the period of knowledge coming back in from the new technology systems applied is valuable.

If this is taken in advance and the data become true, there would be effortless knowledge among employers, which could ease the manufacturing process and therefore cause a change in the work style. Hence, human employers would leave their production path and let cobots to take over. However, concerns will be on how the cobots will be employed according to specific requirement by employer. This is because there will be many requirements of experiments and trials and errors to gain more data about the new implementation of such a new technology.

Industry 5.0 will offer the industrial countries some flexibility to innovate. Therefore, by pushing the boundaries of physics and geometric measurements on the model styles, this will provide new patterns. However, some restrictions may suppress the new developments that which causes the quantity of information to not be sufficient. This leads to unpredicted circumstances.

For instance, the medical community is moving towards a man-made exocrine gland like the pancreas. It is virtually there, after measuring sugar levels in the blood, that the device transfers information to another device which then produces feedback based on the data collected. The data obtained will be reviewed and feedback will be given to the patients accordingly. The decision of using insulin or glucagon can also be known by referring to the vivid sugar level obtained from the patient's blood.

The virtual exocrine gland device detects humans' glucose level via internal regulatory hormone and could the device could inject insulin or glucagon into the blood vessel accordingly; to retain normal values by returning the values to their original parameters that have been re-checked via a feedback loop to see if the feedback sent was effective or not that based on the feedback there will be an action for either to repeat the process or no to make the process more effective than the previous feedback. It is only one size that fits all; therefore, the skilled medical advisor will perfectly tweak the system for the individual in the corresponding site.

The type-1 diabetes disease device is extremely arduous to regulate due to its different metabolic rates, sizes with different skin thicknesses, behaviors, and lifestyles from patients. The progress to Industry 5.0 means more distinct and sturdy user-friendly devices that are customized for the individual associated with easy-to-use applications that will allow the patient to convey real data to the application that follows their lifestyle and routine on a daily basis. This will help the patient to regulate and manage their blood glucose level within the normal parameter range.

Big data and artificial intelligence (AI) provide business in Industry 4.0 with a large boost due to the utilization of a very narrow limited range of the technology, compared to other industrial revolution periods. The interconnected devices could apply artificial intelligence, machine learning (ML), and Internet of Things (IoT) induced in collaborative robots, which makes Industry 4.0 and the upcoming Industry 5.0 more distinctive and interesting to discover, compared to other industries.

The Industry 5.0 is considered a new era due to the wide range in use of data and sufficient knowledge from the society, compared to other industries. As the digitalized society will apply what they had learned, technology application will produce efficient conceived algorithms by the power of machine learning technology to make their life easier.

Intelligent package solutions are reliable sets of solutions that have the ability to use massive information generated by the amount of trials applied to spot trends and patterns that might be customized to build energy consumption systems. For instance, there are new chemical plants are perpetually adapting to new circumstances and undergoing improvements with no distractions due to the association of the artificial intelligence technology, which could increase the networking level that would help the machine to learn to read between the lines and may result in the invention of new advanced connections in systems, but also solve problems before falling into them that weren't evident or thought of before to the human eye and intuition.

For instance, Siemens provides MindSphere, the cloud-based, open IoT package that will be used to produce link products, plants, systems, and machines. It's one amongst the foremost necessary foundations that agrees on the employment of AI in business. MindSphere performs intensive analyses to form the large amounts of information generated by the Internet of Things (IoT), helpful for improvement, simulation, and decision making.

The digital twin permits virtual testing of a spread of situations and promotes sensible choices in areas like optimizing production processes; within the future, employing a digital illustration of a machine with the associated production methodologies applied in the manufacturing processes. Artificial intelligence is going to be able to acknowledge whether or not the work presently being factory-made meets the quality needs. Moreover, it determines the assembly parameters that require being custom-made to make sure that this remains the case throughout the continuous manufacturing processes. As a result, production is formed that is more reliable, more economical, and even more competitive.

A precondition for each industrial revolution, Industry 4.0 and artificial intelligence could be a progressive and end-to-end IT infrastructure, despite the scale of the corporation because crime is everywhere, simply because it would be easier for hackers to commit cybercrime, which is a prediction to a drawback that might occur in the digital future. However, this should be in the middle of associate degree awareness that occupations in different fields from different sectors and cyber security go hand in hand to be more collaborative in the future to fight against these types of crimes.

The risks are vast while not the correct safeguards in situ. In step with the 2018 World Economic Forum's "Global Risk Report", business losses through crime over a subsequent five years can quantity to $8 trillion dollars. It is an incident that happened in Germany that affected the country's gross domestic product. Comprehensive protection for industrial facilities, as exemplified by the defense comprehensive idea from Siemens, will therefore play a key role within the future. After all, hackers are growing smarter and as the use of new advanced technologies with the accessibility of critical data becomes easier for them to invade and hack large sensitive, corporations must keep ahead of them and updated.

Industry 4.0 faced a problem with cybercrime incidents due to the majority of the population is smart and work in a quiet zone with flexible working hours, which is also labeled as hackers. Investors and implementers have to draw to their attention that there is a big risk of failure from cybercrime. This is why business implementation takes time because risks from different dimensions have to be sensitively calculated before implementation. The society is in a transition state between informative society and digitalized society where both societies are different in one major aspect, which is the application of the knowledge that was learned.

2.1.1.3 The Challenges Faced to Adapt in a New Era

The new paradigm of digitized and connected systems is noted as "Industrial Internet of Things" (IIoT) and the outcome of its work established factories into sensible and autonomous productions.

As the data and communication technologies for dynamic management of advanced business processes imposed, it permits real-time-capable horizontal and vertical Internet-based connectedness of individuals, machines, and objects. Related to this, the new industry is attempting to attain what was restricted and not achieved in Industry 4.0 to form a replacement business that is less restricted and that is Industry 5.0. This aims at overcoming contemporary challenges, like thickening world competition, volatile markets, demands, and required customization, were based on these challenges a decrease in innovation was encountered. Industry 5.0 serves as a helpful and targeted approach to agitate these difficult needs.

Nevertheless, there is still uncertainty and confusion since researchers, consultancies, politicians, and practitioners oftentimes build contradictory statements on Industry 4.0 implications. However, it is common and expected that these will be on the Industry 5.0 aspect to undertake any illegal concepts as much as possible. On the one hand, the policy guarantees to supply manufactures with profitable business models, higher efficiency and quality, and to improve work conditions. As much as the manufacturers and investors are concerned with the application of a new industry that is more optimized, it could benefit the society.

The society's challenges are increasing dramatically in relation to the adaptation ability. Therefore, it is necessary to learn how to survive and to adapt to the changes or else there is no choice but to be the victim. The society is worried about the overwhelming demand of employers for money in assuming that cobots could take over the industrial work. This is because there is still a large group of employers who are categorized with less credibility and level of status. Hence, the replacement of the human workforce to cobots will affect their life expectancy and financial balance. This might cause the segregation between classes, which will show how very obvious the gap is between the classes because only people with high credibility and specificity will be chosen by companies in different majors. After all, their credibility must match the job description and skills required to be able to work and innovate.

Suicide level and theft incidents will escalate due to the immediate gratification concept that is sociological terminology, which emphasizes how the society wants to finish early with regards to studies, as well as to earn high income in return in a short period. People who are poor or normal class, who are called proletarians and middle class, respectively, will continue to look at what the high-ranking people have without seeing what they have, and this will certainly increase their chance of robbery or even extreme slaughtering. This is adding stress on poor families that lets them to go seek knowledge at an old age to avoid society's criticism and labeling. This is the only way for them to gain money. Rich families also find difficulties in getting the acceptance to a certain job title because people are dying due to starvation or no equal opportunity in education, which is given to the next generation. This has the ability of breaking the unity in a country.

From the first side, following up with another example, If the applicant is accepted for a job interview and then rejected, this will cause heavy toxic stress on the applicant due to the enhancement of communication and broad connections between companies, which is called intercommunication. That will surely conceive a stigma on that particular applicant, which will make it even harder to be accepted in another job in another company.

Some companies do prefer human beings over cobots, because cobots can certainly handle their prescribed tasks. However, typical situations are unforeseen to them because cobots can never improve their jobs outside the pre-defined programming algorithm as they simply cannot think for themselves. Cobots are probably not as intelligent as humans; despite AI technology. On top of this, there is a cost of training employees on how to work with cobots, which is uncertain to the company whether it is going to be effective or not.

From the other side, companies would favor cobots over human beings over a long-term point of view, as cobots are much cheaper than human employees and now the cost of cobots is lower. Thus, it is a fact that human capabilities cannot be compared with cobots, but cobots' capabilities are now growing rapidly by the new arising technologies, which makes cobots much more convenient. Cobots are more precise than people; they do not have human hands that tremble or shake. Cobots have smaller and more versatile moving elements that help them perform tasks.

This change in the next upcoming generations is due to the adaptation of the society to the changes induced by the industrial revolution, such as Industry 5.0. The adaptation in gaining knowledge and willingness to gain knowledge is essential during the industrial revolution. This would help the community to fight in solidarity against illiteracy. Another example, one of the new innovations invented by biotechnologists that is helping to reduce worldwide pollution is producing eco-friendly products, following the new green technology concept; also synthetic enzymes that are capable of digesting plastic.

The industrialization process has its advantages and disadvantages, yet there are a lot of hidden patterns to be revealed. Every new door to be opened is a new challenge and a discovery is revealed. The workload will increase, and more and more advantages and disadvantages will be identified after the takeover process of industrialization.

To prove this, there is real-life evidence: to assure that cobots are taking over job position in industries. For instance, according to Ivanov and Webster (2017), "travel, tourism and hospitality companies have started to adopt robots, artificial intelligence and service automation (RAISA) in the form of chatbots, delivery robots, robot-concierge, conveyor restaurants, self-service information/check-in/check-out kiosks, and many others. Despite the huge advancements in social robotics, the research on robots in tourism has been extremely limited".

According to T.L.A. Crenshaw (2013), "cyber-physical systems are a genre of networked real-time systems that monitor and control the physical world. Examples include unmanned aerial vehicles and industrial robotics. The experts who develop these complex systems are retiring much faster than universities are graduating engineering majors. As a result, it is important for undergraduates to gain exposure to these kinds of complex systems. This paper describes UPBOT, a robotics testbed hosted at the University of Portland. The testbed features an extensible robot built from an iRobot Create chassis and a computationally powerful embedded system equipped with a wireless card. In the spring 2012 semester, the testbed was used for a course project designed and assessed in the style of contract learning".

2.1.1.4 The Benefits of Industry 5.0 in Application

Japan defines Industry 5.0 as "Society 5.0", a "human touch" revolution: "A humanitarian society that balances economic advancement with the resolution of social issues by a system that extremely integrates Internet and physical space". The development visualizes an advanced society that is capable of incorporating new, advanced technology.

Science-fiction movies portray the longer term of using automated machines like cobots and the would take over and surpass human being's intelligence. Digitalization would not omit human work in the industry. Instead, it would integrate intelligent automation, devices, and systems at the geographic point to elevate cooperation and collaboration between humans and machines. It would facilitate highly skilled employees to guide robotic machines to work in higher performance with human's interaction; that is called cobots.

Industry 5.0 would solve the requirement for personalization and mass customization of merchandise for patrons. It would stimulate human intelligence and thoughtful ideas into computers, which is a process referred to as psychological feature computing. The cobots of the modern factories would even be smart enough to grasp the human operator's desires, the cobots able to predict the right time to decide to help their employers, and facilitate their work accordingly. Furthermore, it would profit the employers in two ways, such as upskilling and providing added tasks in production. It would conjointly mix intelligent systems to the present workflows to leverage human ability, mental capacity, and improve operational efficiencies.

For instance, there is an argument that is partially valid that nurses can be replaced in Industry 5.0 because machines might customize the merchandise by analyzing historical knowledge and patterns to transfer them in the technologies supported by machine learning (Ml) and artificial intelligence (AI) technologies, whereas feedback can be directly sent to the doctor in charge without the help of nurses. However, technology cannot be a replacement for human intelligence; they might be collaborative due to the emotional role that nurses provide that cobots could not naturally provide. That is considered one of the biggest limitations that cobots have. Emotional care is one of the greatest essentials in healthcare.

Standardization and legalization are one of the essential factors for human rights that will offer assistance to anticipate any genuine issues between innovation, society, and businesses. Within the following mechanical transformation, people are anticipated to include more dedication and sensitivity in manufacturing policies in new industrial revolutions to be in the safe zone.

Particularly, senior individuals of society and partners will discover it much more troublesome to adapt to the modern mechanical revolution easily. Fast and exceedingly effective fabrication due to anticipation may result in an overproduction phenomenon that might result in distrust between the government and the society.

The implementation of straightforwardness and transparency to the society ought to moreover be taken into consideration by considering how independent frameworks can join moral principles of the society's norms. There ought to be logical moral behavior arrangements from independent systems; for instance, the incorporation of ethical behavior in independent frameworks.

2.1.1.5 What Is Bio-manufacturing?

Bio-manufacturing is in contrast to existing methods of chemical manufacturing; bioconversion characteristics such as the capacity to work in mild temperatures and pressures and to achieve a high degree of carbon and energy output for one-unit operations results in more streamlined and less technologically complex processes. This is known as a type of biotechnology manufacturing that uses biological systems to commercially produce vital biomaterials and biomolecules for medicines, food, and beverages (Clomburg, Crumbley, and Gonzalez 2017). Moreover, industrial applications are mostly made up of natural resources such as microbes, animal cells or plant cells, and other resources (North Carolina Association 2006). For instance, this type of manufacturing or biotechnology helps medical researches to develop new drugs and enhance an old drug's efficacy, which will increase the bioavailability to help it effectively penetrate the target required without the influence on the drug or the body.

Bio-manufacturing is also involved in genetically engineered food crops to be more nutritious and valuable, more resistant to pests, and that give it the resilience to be able to grow in stressful conditions. Furthermore, this revolution helps environmental researchers to manufacture organisms that can decrease the amount of solid waste in landfills. Apart from these, the bio-manufacturing can be applied in various industries, such as the new introduction of industries that work on the production of vaccines by animal scientists to enhance the health of livestock and improve milk and meat quality in production. Bio-manufacturing industries use living cells to be able to produce products, seeking to duplicate or alter the function of a living cell to make capable enough to work in a more efficient way (Rossi 2020).

2.1.1.6 Integration of Bio-manufacturing with New Industry Era 5.0

The history of the industrial revolution started in 1970 and the automation was labeled as Industry 3.0 where the use of electronics and computers escalated and represented a change in the production rate. In 1980, globalization of Industry 3.5 formed an economic perspective where they planned on offshoring and depleting the product cost to make it more accessible to consumers. In the 21st century, it is called digitalization and labeled as Industry 4.0, with the introduction of connected devices, data analytics, and artificial intelligence technologies in the automation processes in the industries.

The future holds what we are processing in right now as the Fifth Industrial Revolution, where the emphasization is on the cooperation between human and machine. The integration between human intelligence and cobot intelligence will produce a digitalized society that can reveal a new solution that was hidden. Consequently, workers will be upskilled to provide value-added tasks in production, proceeding to mass customization and personalization for customers with high-quality standards and effectiveness (North Carolina Association 2006).

For instance, bio-manufacturing has been incorporated with food safety to prolong the shelf-life, whereas it does not affect the food quality and freshness of food that is due to the short shelf-life of many food products and results in many losses with regards to food and money. The importance of having a digitalized society is that it can reveal new solutions that were hidden by using the new technology. On top of this, employees will be upskilled to provide value-added tasks in production, proceeding to mass customization and personalization for customers with high-quality standards and effectiveness.

The Internet of Things is connecting devices on the plant floor that was introduced by Industry 4.0 and is working coincidently with Industry 5.0 emphasizing the interaction between humans and machines to produce collaborative robots (cobots) that are integrated with artificial intelligence and machine learning. Experts state that still there is a lot of facilities that need to be implemented to reach Industry 5.0, whereas it is already initiated by observing humans work alongside machines. Working under connected smart manufacturing plants through devices integrated with society that know how to use the information had been ascribed and still ascribing to put it into an application.

Industry 5.0 is dependent on reaching valuable big data that could provide trust and authenticity to validate that it can produce promising new solutions. It can be done by the association of cyber-physical systems (CPS), Internet of Things (IoT), Industry 4.0, smart factory, and artificial intelligence (AI) in bio-manufacturing to make it the mainstream line to follow in medicine and life sciences. In relation to this, to Engelberger (1980b) has indicated that there is insufficient usage and data for new industrial applications in medicine and life sciences.

Internet of Things (IoT) and Industry 4.0 will transform the knowledge translation from the medical application of science to real life; in other words, from theoretical to practical application that could impact the society's way of thinking, teaching, and learning that might influence in unprecedented ways (Grosdidier et al. 2007). For instance, medical precision requires advanced interconnected diagnostic systems that are customized in modern factories to be able to predict the patient's accurate condition by analyzing and comparing the patient's medical history scheme and present medical scheme.

The use of these new advanced technologies would provide the production of products that are very useful, sustainable, and eco-friendly to the society. For example, the Second International Congress on Food Safety and Quality in Opatija, Croatia, discussed the novel approaches for food safety management and communication with the application of artificial intelligence (AI) that highlighted the process of application of analytical technologies in the food sector associated with data science (Mohareb et al. 2016). Hence, the virtualization in the supply chain to contribute in product's quality, which is closely related to the human's health, therefore by developing a non-linear time series. Forecasting sales models assures both human and product safety.

Recently, the Cambridge-based company opened a manufacturing facility in Smithfield, Rhode Island, working on a project that is titled Rubius therapeutics. This project utilizes reprogrammed red blood cells to treat conditions like cancer and developing biosynthetic enzymes that might treat rare conditions, such as a patient who cannot produce a particular enzyme in their body naturally, which affects their body's biochemistry.

Bio-manufacturing can also be involved in the treatment of genetic diseases such as homology medicines (blood medicines). Despite being easily resolved by CRISPER, due to its ethical concerns it was stopped. Bio-manufacturing has the ability to produce a new delivery method by using a virus instead of CRISPR. The virus is called adeno-associated virus vector human hematopoietic stem cell (AAVHSCs), that is designed to deliver genetic medicines through a gene therapy, which can tackle a broad range of genetic disorders. This is calibrated and assayed by the help of the new evolution of advanced technology, such as artificial intelligence (AI) associated with machine learning (Ml) to predict the results before the application processes.

The discussed examples in this section are utilized by the application of the new advanced technologies, but in a narrow scale. In Industry 5.0, the application of these new technologies would assumingly be used in a wider range to the extent that it could be the most leading technique that can be used in the future. This might be imaginary because it is intangible in the 21st century, but by the application of 3D printing methodologies that will help us to visualize the future. It would be more sensible to put it into consideration.

2.1.1.7 Job Scope Revolution in Industry 5.0 Era

The industrial revolution would affect some occupational positions that most people already are anticipating. Past mechanical transformations illustrate that the manufacturing frameworks and procedures have been continuously changing towards one main goal, which is the production of products with high efficiency to serve the consumer and make them feel satisfied. While on the other side, employers are almost ignoring and forgetting the responsibility and roles that mankind handles to receive rewards in return. Industry 5.0 would create a large impact on the job scope availability especially for fresh graduate despite of their high qualification and creditability. However, industry 5.0 can contribute positively to business owners due to the advanced technologies in terms of employment.

On the other hand, accepting an industrial revolution requires the selection, standardization, and execution of new advanced technologies, which requires claiming the foundation, infrastructure, and developments that are planned before execution. Industry 5.0 will bring phenomenal challenges within the field of human-machine interaction (HMI), as it will put machines exceptionally near the existence of any human. In spite of the obsession with machines, such as programmable assistive gadgets and cars, they are not considered as form of cobot.

Cobots will be exceptionally distinctive as their organization and presentation will contain human-like functionalities such as grasping, squeezing, and interaction based on purposeful and environmental variables. Moreover, the industrial revolution would offer numerous employments within the field of human-machine interaction (HMI) and human computational factor (HCF) analysis.

Industry 5.0 will revolutionize fabricating frameworks over the globe of taking away dull, dirty, and redundant tasks from human specialization, simply by enabling cobots to take over these tasks instead. Intelligent cobots and systems will transform the fabricating supply chains and manufactured products to an unpredictable level without any complaints from the employer. Cobots will be cost effective because they will be conceived by cheap, highly effective materials incorporated with artificial intelligence to produce exceedingly competitive cobots. These cobots are made up of advanced materials such as carbon fiber and lightweight resolute solid materials, fueled by highly optimized battery packs, cyber-attack hardened, with a more grounded data handling process of forms such as enormous data collections, manufactured insights, and a network of intelligent sensors for environmental interaction.

Industry 5.0 will provide various resources and outcomes unprecedented, such as increasing productivity and operational skills; moreover, becoming more environmentally friendly and reducing both workload and harm on humans beings.

The implementation of cobots could also improve the production time cycle. Industry 5.0 will also provide more employment than it takes away. There might be occupations that would be created within each field's framework that desperately need experts who monitor the cobots in their sub-sector work and check their working ethics, such as artificial intelligence (AI) and robotics programming algorithms. By doing so, the cobots could make preparations, plan, repurpose, and innovate a modern range of cobots for construction. In expansion, redundant tasks will not be required to be performed by a human worker. This could allow us to boost enthusiasm to workers to innovatively use diverse shapes and functions of cobots within their workplace.

The shift from Industry 4.0 to Industry 5.0 emphasizes having a digitalized society that could reduce repetitive tasks and perhaps have more time to utilize and think of other useful matters that lead to innovation and discovery. Having cobots in charge will ease daily tasks for employers. This is because cobots could be helpful for monitoring manufacturing processes and checking product quality every now and then instead of working and monitoring all the time from shift to shift without rest. Teaming up with highly effective cobots and expert humans will undeniably result in unexpected outcomes.

According to a recent study, it is discovered that the Fifth Industrial Revolution requires a new manufacturing role: Chief Robotic Officer (Gesrepair 2021). The role of a CRO is expected to be a robotics expert who specializes in human-machine connectivity, responsible enough to make decisions on suitable type of machines or devices to be implemented in active plants and to optimize the production line; thus an approachable and knowledgeable tutor to be able to share their experience with others.

2.1.2 CONCEPTS AND POSSIBILITIES

2.1.2.1 The Advances in Artificial Intelligence (AI), Machine Learning (ML), and Deep Learning (DL) in Creating New Evolutional Businesses in Different Majors and in Bio-manufacturing

2.1.2.1.1 Artificial Intelligence (AI) Technology

Artificial intelligence (AI) in machines is required to do a specific task that also requires human's intelligence as well for different purposes such as learning, predicting, judging, and problem solving. AI technology can be incorporated with biomanufacturing; for instance this technology might be used in the healthcare sector in two scenarios. Firstly, AI can be incorporated with diagnostic machines to be utilized in the clinic or hospitals for patient care by predicting and diagnosing the type of illness and discovering the most effective prognosis for a treatment that can tackle the illness with very minor side effects.

The association of AI in healthcare's machines works by setting a parameter and, based on the results produced, a decision for treatment can be made. The parameters for neuron depolarization is the impulse transmission mechanism in the neuron to transmit chemical neurotransmitter from one node to another. Usually it is a range between 30–40 millivolts (mV), and if it is less than 30 mV then the patient will follow plan A and treatment A. If the value is in between 30–40 mV, then the patient will be considered as normal and no need for any treatment or further check-ups. If the value is above 40 mV, then the patient will follow plan B and treatment B. The decisions have to be taken cautiously by the physician working on a comparative study between the decision predicted and the patient's medical history, checking whether it is complementary with the patient's medical history or not.

Moreover, AI can also be utilized in the research and development (R&D) sector, specifically on drug discovery. New technologies could be used to find solutions to incurable diseases such as multiple sclerosis, Alzheimer disease, cancer, and many other diseases. By feeding all the data required about a particular disease with the addition of all previous trials, a disease history could be attained which can be used to predict and analyze the best pathway for treatment by identifying potential approaches in order to target the disease and finding a suitable match of the drug and the target or receptor in the body. This produces a solution-dependent interaction, such as to suppress the activity of the disease.

In pharmaceutical industries, AI benefits by changing the drug's structure and design to make it complementary to the therapeutic target where the drug must be delivered to in the body, and also discovering new methods of application to deliver the drug effectively. The prediction of an untested drug on trial and wondering about the function and effect before drug testing, these unpredictable answers are predicted by the power of artificial intelligence due to the advances that it has and various types.

There are four types of artificial intelligence:

- **Reactive Machines**
  AI systems are normally reactive, as they perform their tasks based on the information given, like a catalogue with regards to rules and guidelines, that neither form memories nor use past experiences to inform current decisions. Real-life examples are Deep Blue and a chess-playing supercomputer that determines a chessboard, the character's movements, and predicts the opponent's reply. Based on the data collected, the analysis and feedback will be processed. In bio-manufacturing, it is known that an enzyme like amylase only digests amylose. Amylose is a polysaccharide in starch, hence AI determines the action of the amylase enzyme by knowing its mode of action by how the substrate fits to the active site and the AI system discovers and predicts the outcome before applying it by predicting the conformational change of the enzyme shape and sites of bond breakage or formation. This can conserve and save myriads of biotechnologists' time in discovering new unknown enzymes by synthetically adding enzymes' mode of action to the system with the parameters that must be put into consideration such as substrate concentration, enzyme concentration, pH, temperature, and many other parameters. This type of intelligence acts on the current predicted data.
- **Limited Memory**
  This type of intelligent system is dependent on the past, just like the idea of an automated car or in other words "self-drivers", by conceiving a type of an artificial intelligent system that recalls the limited memory of the past furiously. Based on the little experience from the past and learning from the current human interaction, it self-learns on how to use the car in relevant situations without failing in the same mistake once again.
- **Theory of Mind**
  This type of intelligence system emphasizes the formation and enhancement of machine representations and the way it expresses and reacts with the user. More about the understanding of people, creatures, objects, thoughts, and emotions

that reflects on their behavior and, based on the data, the machine would find the most effective way to consult and advise the respondent in return.

The theory of mind is crucial because without the correct and intelligent way of communicating with each other in society. There would be alot of missed opportunities. Hence the connections will be minimal and weak. Thus, an individual's potential to grow, explore, share thoughts and opinions is not guaranteed. Based on these cobots, understanding the human being's mind is considered one of the most complex organs in the human body that could be analyzed and predicted. Hence this theory would let the cobots adjust their behavior accordingly by applying the machine learning (ML) concept.

- **Self-Awareness**
  This type of intelligence system is considered as a follow-up on the theory of mind concept for the implementation of consciousness in the cobot's decisions to be aware of what they are doing and to study the improvization.

For instance, applying an analyzing algorithm to detect the cause factor that resulted with a particular reaction; predicting the reason behind the well-being anger mood by reconsidering what had happened previously to deserve all of these reactions. The cobot in return finds a way to manage and handle their behavior and reactions. This type of intelligence shows how cobots could be utilized not only in industries, but also in homes.

Machines were evolving at a high pace until there was an incident that is documented as a testimony for cobots' evolution, which is about the intelligent cobot called "Sophia", developed and manufactured by the Hong Kong–based company called Hanson Robotics. According to Chris Weller (2017), as of October 25, 2017, Sophia is the first cobot in history to be a full citizen of a country. Sophia was developed by Hanson Robotics Company, led by an AI developer, David Hanson. Sophia spoke at the Future Investment Initiative conference that was held in the Saudi Arabian capital of Riyadh. "Sophia made her first public appearance at the Southwest Festival in mid-March 2016 in Austin, Texas, United States".

According to Saeed Abdolshah et al. (2017), Sophia copies the exact human signals, facial expressions, and is capable of replying to certain questions by forming a straightforward discussion on predefined themes. Sophia is incorporated with a voice acknowledgment system like speech-to-text innovation from Alphabet Inc. The more the cobot is active, the more intelligent it becomes over time. The cobot speech-synthesis capacity is given by CereProc's text-to-speech motor that conjointly permits Sophia to sing. The AI program investigations extricate information that permits the cobot to make stride reactions within the future.

2.1.2.1.2 Machine Learning (ML)

It is the implementation of artificial intelligence (AI) technology that helps the machine to automatically experience and learn without being programmed. This is achieved by the emphasis on the development of computer programs that can access data to self-learn, which makes people ponder for a while and insinuate whether this could this be applied in the future, hence it would provide accessing resources in a short period with a very high storage capacity. This reflects that cobot's intelligence level would escalate exponentially, simply because learning is inevitable.

The main objective of the machine learning (ML) concept is to induce the trait, personalization, and characteristics of a human being that is embodied in a robotic design with computers that learn automatically without human intervention and action.

Machine learning follows a set of algorithms to complete a specific task that is categorized into the following:

- **Supervised machine learning algorithms**
  Supervised learning is having input variables (x) and an output variable (Y) by utilizing an algorithm to learn the mapping function from the input to the output, so the formula generated would be for instance Y = f(X). Its objective is to manipulate the mapping function; when you have new input data (x), the output variables (Y) for that data can be identified.
  The process of algorithm learning from the training dataset can be thought of as a teacher supervising the learning process, and that is why the process is called supervised learning. The algorithm iteratively makes predictions based on the training data and is corrected by the teacher since most of the answers are already known. Learning lessons will be moved to the next level when the algorithm achieves an acceptable level of performance.
- **Semi-supervised machine learning algorithms**
  This type of machine learning algorithm drops in between supervised and unsupervised learning since the algorithm utilizes both labeled and unlabeled information by preparing regularly a small sum of labeled information and an expansive sum of unlabeled information.
  The frameworks that utilize this strategy could impressively make strides in learning precision. Ordinarily, semi-supervised learning is chosen when the procured labeled information requires talented and significant assets to prepare and learn from it. Usually, this type of algorithm acquires unlabeled information, but it does not require extra assets.
  For instance, unlabeled data consists of data which is either taken from nature or created by humans to explore the scientific patterns behind it. Some examples of unlabeled data might include photos, audio recordings, videos, news articles, tweets, x-rays, etc. The main concept is there is no explanation, label, tag, class, or name for the features in data. Labeled data consists of unlabeled data with a description, label, or name of features in the data. For example, in a labeled image dataset, an image is labeled as it is a cat's photo and it's a dog's photo. This is due to in semi-supervised learning, an algorithm learns from a dataset that includes both labeled and unlabeled data, mostly unlabeled. It focuses on the labeled data and then applies it to unlabeled data to reveal the common data by extracting the similarity and differences between the labeled and unlabeled data.
- **Unsupervised machine learning algorithms**
  This type of machine learning algorithm is utilized when the data represented for training is neither classified nor labeled. Unsupervised learning reflects on how frameworks could induce a function to portray a hidden structure from unlabeled information. The framework does not figure out its proper output,

but investigates the information that can draw deductions from datasets to describe hidden structures from unlabeled information.

2.1.2.1.3 Deep Learning (DL)

Deep learning is the application of the machine learning algorithm learning functions that resembled a portion of a broader family based on artificial neural networks with learning representations. Learning can be directed by either semi-supervised or unsupervised.

Deep learning structures such as deep neural networks, deep belief networks, networks systems, recurrent neural networks, and convolution neural systems have been connected to areas counting computer vision, discourse acknowledgment, normal dialect preparing, sound acknowledgment, social organize sifting, machine interpretation, bioinformatics, sedate plan, therapeutic picture investigation, fabric assessment, and board amusement programs. Hence, algorithms have delivered comparative studies between human and cobot intelligence that represented a few cases that cobots outperformed human master execution.

Deep learning (DL) could be used in architecture, according to Weston et al. (2012), "We show how nonlinear semi-supervised embedding algorithms popular for use with "shallow" learning techniques such as kernel method. Kernel methods are a class of algorithms for pattern analysis, whose best known member is the support vector machine (SVM). Any linear model can be turned into a non-linear model by applying the kernel trick to the model can be easily applied to deep multi-layer architectures, either as a regularize at the output layer, or on each layer of the architecture (Zoppis 2019). Compared to standard supervised backpropagation this can give significant gains. This trick provides a simple alternative to existing approaches to semi-supervised deep learning whilst yielding competitive error rates compared to those methods, and existing shallow semi-supervised techniques".

2.1.2.2 The Advances in the Internet of Things (IoT) in Industry 5.0 Era on Bio-manufacturing Products

The innovation of the Internet of Things (IoT) would provide a more reliable sharing platform for all interconnected devices that have the ability to transmit data from one IP address to others without the human-computer interaction (HCI). This is achieved by connecting devices together with a shared Internet access point to mechanical and digital machines associated with unique identifiers (UIDs).

The increment of smart devices has reached a critical mass point where all mechanical devices became available to interpret chemical interactions. Devices such as thermometers use mercury to identify the temperature in degrees Celsius. By the integration of Internet of Things (IoT) in chemically interaction devices, it becomes safer, easy to understand, and user friendly. This can be utilized due to the science and chemical information that were added as data in a chip that is interconnected by an inference engine, where results with an output based on the input is converted into digital data by a digital converter to a digital output that is almost equivalent and even better than not using the IoT in devices.

Moreover, diabetic patients also could benefit from smart devices. Patients can utilize the device more than twice every day to detect their glucose level in their blood. The glucose detector device is more worthwhile than a dipstick, where the diabetic patient uses their urine as the substrate to test for the blood glucose level instead of their blood sample. The Internet of Things (IoT) would be integrated with the glucose detector devices, which makes the device more user-friendly, high quality, representable, efficient, and cost-effective.

Intelligent devices and networked sensors are technologies that are gathered and compiled in the Industrial Internet of Things (IIoT) to be able to be utilized directly on the manufacturing floor, harvesting data to drive artificial intelligence (AI) technology to work on its predictive analysis to provide hints. According to Soley and Schmid (2018), a chief technologist at Deloitte Digital IoT, stated that in Industrial Internet of Things, sensors are connected to physical assets of data that act like an alert system to detect anything misleading.

By inducing Industry 5.0 industrialization, the manufacturing process could be transformed from a linear manufacturing supply chain with a sequential, restricted, limited, and non-integrated processes into multiple, alternative, and flexible process planning. In other words, this is also called a dynamic manufacturing processing by utilizing interconnected systems such as a digital supply network (DSN) that is incorporated with ecosystem partners to analyze and predict from its surroundings, for instance the environment.

These implementations will change the way the products are manufactured and conveyed, making factories more reliable, assuring a high-level of safety for human operations. Not only improvements from a product evaluation point of view, but also economic and business perspective, by the application of Industry 5.0. It would be expensive on the economy as an initial cost, but on the long term, this would save millions of dollars.

The Internet of Things (IoTs) has a prediction power talent that would very useful from an industrial perspective because it focuses on the lacks in the manufacturing process before it continues and could detect it before moving from one process to other. In other words, IIoT sensors will be considered as an advantage to the industry itself that automatically pinpoints where the problem is occurring based on the issue raised and a service request is initiated. This is a plus point to the Industry 5.0 and one of the perks behind the industrialization theory that it would reduce the failure rate production of products, which is considered in the Industry 4.0 as a burden and a waste of time, effort, money, and electricity that any factory or industry is dependent on.

2.1.2.3 The Advances in Nano, Bio-technology, and 3D Printing in Creating New Evolutional Products in Bio-manufacturing Industries

2.1.2.3.1 Nanotechnology

Although atomic force microscopy (AFM) has viewed many considerable advances in the current years, it could nonetheless be a project to get amazing indicators from these imaging devices, simply by just looking on images. AFM was utilized to image the topography of surfaces, but by modifying the tip it became possible to measure other quantities. For instance, changing the tip leads to new evolutional types of AFM with magnetic and electric properties, friction, chemical potentials, and to perform various types of spectroscopy and analysis. AI can be very beneficial in dealing with these types of signal-related issues.

An AI strategy known as functional recognition imaging (FRI) appears to address the problem of microscopic tip misrecognition via the direct identification of nearby movements from measured spectroscopic reactions. This methodology brings together the use of artificial neural networks (ANNs) with principal component evaluation (PCA), utilized to streamline the enter facts to the neural network.

From a chemical modeling perspective, developments have led to the incorporation of AI and the use of complicated interconnected computers to get to know resolution algorithms. There are myriads sorts of parameters that have to be correlated to generate both a picture and a dynamic depiction of a chemical system. The imaging techniques with AI could have a higher analysis to information that would learn from the past by retaining data with regards for instance to chemical structure modeling to create an extra specific illustration of a new chemical structure under study.

On top of this, AI can minimize the degree of error associated with the geometry or measurement of a device, particle, or design. This is specifically beneficial for studying a nanomaterial as the number of outcomes and phenomena viewed with materials like graphene could regularly be tough to re-create.

The portrayal of the structural characteristics of nanomaterials has additionally been resolved to employ the usage of ANNs. For instance, these algorithms have been used to determine the configuration of carbon nanotube buildings by quantifying the structural traits like the alignments and curvatures of the structure. AI in nanotechnology could help to analyze the nano-sized materials as if they are visible with the naked eye and to figure out solutions that would have not been resolved unless it is fixed from the core.

2.1.2.3.2 Biotechnology

Biotechnology profoundly impacted humanity, economy, business, and industrial products from a healthcare perspective. Scientists are leading in the biotechnology sector for thousands of years, with the inventions such as crop cultivation and therefore the domestication of animals. These biotechnological advancements lead to a healthier life for societies.

The healthcare field has perhaps been the most important beneficiary for the production of breakthrough discoveries in life sciences, and as a result, the fields of oncology, neurology, immunology, infectious diseases, and regenerative medicine are among the drivers of biotech research and development. This thrust has shifted biotechnology industries into a booming business; the evidence is that biotech-developed drugs are accounting for about 21% of the worldwide demand for pharmaceuticals to manufacture and develop vaccines, therapeutics, and other medicines since 2012 (Rue 2019).

More evidence on biotech industries' economic growth, according to Ernst & Young's press release for its 2009 Beyond Borders biotechnology report, more evidence on biotech industries' economic growth observed that "the prolonged and systematic funding drought is placing the business model thatfuelled biotech growth for the past 33 years under unprecedented strain" (Lazonick and Tulum 2011). Yet, according to Ernst & Young, in 2008 the revenues of publicly traded biotech companies grew by 12% over the previous year, reaching $89.7 billion, and taken together these companies showed a profit" (Lazonick and Tulum 2011).

In the last decade, the appearance of biotechnologies, for example, the power to convert any blood type into the universal blood donor group O, 3D printers that are capable of printing human organs, non-invasive devices for monitoring fatal genetic abnormalities, and therefore the now-infamous CRISPR/Cas9 gene-editing technique have drawn attention to a heavy influx of interested investors into biotechnology.

On the other hand, according to Elizabeth, the story of Theranos made the biotech industry a little bit doubtful. This example gives a glimpse on how biotechnology is a successful beneficiary. Theranos is a diagnostic company that focused on (hematology) blood testing to diagnose early diseases in a short period that fell well in need of its promises to produce a technology that was capable of running tests with only some drops of blood, the corporation had valued the company's net worth with a big amount of money; this is all before it even had worked to showcase the prototypes diagnostic results that checks if it is true, reliable, and precise or not. After all of this, the company was dissolved because of the fraud and corruption detected from the company. The company was dependent on the investments by investors and actually did not achieve any of the company's objectives and goals (Adorno and Horkheimer's 'Idiotic Plot' and Representations of Elizabeth Holmes' Fraud – Proquest – The Inventor: Out for Blood in Silicon Valley 2019).

These unprecedented incidents made the investors not confident because of the chaotic incidents, such as the failure of Theranos Company. On top of this, there are moral and ethical concerns on the pair of CRISPR-edited babies that were produced in China. There is still no bar to set on investment opportunities when it involves biotechnology. With the knowledge that is available from scientists around the globe it is a good idea to rely more on AI and ML to assist in data analysis tasks. This could also resolve huge pitfalls in experiments that would quickly denote what is and is not working, which will make the process faster.

One of the biggest issues encountering new biotechnology-driven medical devices is that there is a hardship in getting the acceptance of new iterations into the hands of consumers. This happens often due to the long process required for the approval from technology institutions and organizations. The technology institutions and organizations usually follow a specific policy to check and verify with the ethical, economic, importance, and social concerns on the device before the acceptance, although this could benefit the economy and the organization as a whole.

However, if it is known the new invention could contribute to the medical development, the checking process is still worthwhile because it assures weather the device is convenient or not. This puts an unfortunate limitation on the power to scaffold out new biotech-driven devices to the public, which would make the lives of not only healthcare workers healthier, but also the patient's health.

2.1.2.3.3 3D Printing

3D printing is a specific object that is modeled in three dimensions where the object can be visualized and would help to assume the representation of the object in the real world before printing the object. This could be achieved by the use of Auto-CAD software. The incorporation of artificial intelligence (AI) and machine learning (ML) technologies with modeling softwares would create excellent 3D printable models and that is due to the precise and accurate geometric measurements of the model. Hence, a 3D printing can be used to make unprintable objects be printable by predicting new architectural and designing patterns.

SolidWorks revealed SolidWorksEdgine, which is a fantastic tool for the use of artificial intelligence (AI) and machine learning (ML) technologies, growing an Autodesk DreamCatcher tool that would work on replica designs. Hundreds of designs can be generated in just a few hours by the use of this program. This is an incredible way to boost equipment's efficiency that could realize defects inside the 3D model, which in fact would make it impractical to produce. This would continually be there to improve the additive manufacturing process to get manufacture high-quality parts possible. General Electric's (GE) labs in New York have begun developing computer vision technology that accepts microscopic fractures to be determined in machine parts.

2.1.2.4 The Product's Production Rate in the Industry 5.0 Era on Bio-manufacturing and the Manufactured Product's Quality

The increment of consumption rate of craftsmanship and personalized products is one of the main goals for any company to achieve the targeted sales value. The possibility to produce a personalized product can be very impactful to the end users. For example, the medical devices industry produced an artificial pancreas system. This interconnected system is initiated because of Type 1 diabetic patient's issues, who have to follow a strict treatment guideline. Hence, this device helps patients to constantly maintain their blood sugar levels.

A synthetic pancreas gadget works in the following: a glucose screen draws blood and detects the glucose stage in it, and then talks to another gadget which supplies insulin via a tube connected to the patient's skin. This one-size-fits-all gadget for patients would be challenging to tweak the managed machine for the individual, as exclusive diabetic sufferers have one-of-a-kind metabolic rates and different body parameters.

Moving to Industry 5.0 permits the production of synthetic pancreas structures to supply men and women with a mobile app that follows their special lifestyles and applies advanced AI methods to define how a patient's physique reacts to a particular device. After patterns are defined, the patient's data could be fed into the device to make the synthetic pancreas tailor-made for the individual patient.

Industry 5.0 will be a right choice, as many industrializations are able to handle automation being as a section of the manufacturing process. However, the industry craves the private imprint of human manufacturing blueprint, which produces something exclusive through their dedication and effort. This could be performed by the tight collaboration between people and machines by applying science techniques to collaborate and not to alternate human beings. Therefore, to accelerate cobot's performance, human beings would be more capable to spend more time on strategizing and planning as properly as on other high-value tasks.

To acquire this collaboration in the workspace, Industry 5.0 suggests cobots or collaborative robots. Cobots are utilized to optimize the manufacturing processes and make work safer. It is the use of cobots that have contributed to bringing the human issue and complaints in manufacturing to decrease. As technology advances, the quality rate advances as well to a higher level, in a sense of moving from quality 4.0 to 5.0 is more focused on the use of both autonomic collaborative robotic machines with human reactions that utilizes cyber-physical systems to achieve having a cobot. That would intelligent enough to lower the workload on the human being to help them relax from too much work.

The industrialization of Industry 5.0 would change the societies' behavior pattern and has been observed happened in China and India in two waves. The first wave started from 1996–2010 and the second wave from 2011–2020 periods, which increased the development of technology and economy.

The transformation experienced in China and India is due to the implementation of "Quality 5.0" to the society. Quality 5.0 made the society learn more about technology. This is due to the successful marketing campaigns that urged the society to focus on learning more on these new technologies, which made it a trend that would reach to an extent, for instance, labels the person who has purchased the new technology device as genius, updated, and rich. Therefore, this affected the goods' and services' quality by lifting their levels to compete with the Western ones. The fifth quality wave also affects the digitalization of technology and amplifies to change on the consumers' attitudes, thereby growing the expectations for services.

2.1.2.5 The Employer's Potential Adaptation in Industry 5.0 Era

Ivanov and Webster (2017) drew attention on the interconnection of the trends of geopolitical development, technological revolution, changes in the natural environment, and the globalization of the planet.

Germany is considered to be the world leading country in Industry 4.0 technology. Japan is also shifting towards its vision to induce "Society 5.0". Japan is forced to shift because of its increasing ageing population. The implementation of Society 5.0 would make the use of cutting-edge technology, such as IoT, AI, CPS, big data, and others to be accessible, which would clear the pathway for the society in reaching the fifth stage of civilization. The improved civilizations happened due to the industrializations that had happened ever since Industry 1.0 that moved in the following sequence: after hunters, agricultural, industrial, and information evolutions. In relation to this, Japan made the interpretation of data from users easier by the use of artificial intelligence (AI) technology incorporated in sensors to calibrate information from sensors in objects, for example, machines in the industry, household equipment, cars, and mobile phones.

Artificial intelligence (AI) technology is involved in several things such as tracking locations by the use of GPS, social networks for interests, and credit card companies for commercial activities and economic growth. The ease in accessing these big data by the help of artificial intelligence (AI) technology made it too simple to come up with an automated analyze and conclusion in a very small duration, which would increase customer satisfaction. This is because customers are receiving their needs with high quality, professionalism, less customer work, and application process like filling personal data. Everything became automated so instead of writing, there is a voice-over machine that calibrates the voice, and then interprets the data and converts it to digital data with less time consumed from the customer and the employer.

The 5th Basic Science and Technology Program was implemented by the Japanese government in April 2016. This covers several areas, including the fostering of creativity and internationalization. Nevertheless, one focal point to emphasize is the society's development processes to deviate into a digitalized society, Economy 5.0. The underlying poster (Figure 2.1.1) represents the rapid development of information technology that now enables the real world to combine cyber space information with the physical space. The combination of both is Cyber-Physical Systems (CPS), real-world objects combined together and enhanced with more data. This would bring unprecedented major social change.

The main aim of any industrial revolution that happens is to improve the life expectancy and status level of the societies and also focuses on individuals from the health regulation, movement, education, consumption, recreation, and work. This should also be implemented by correlating and balancing between the falling birth

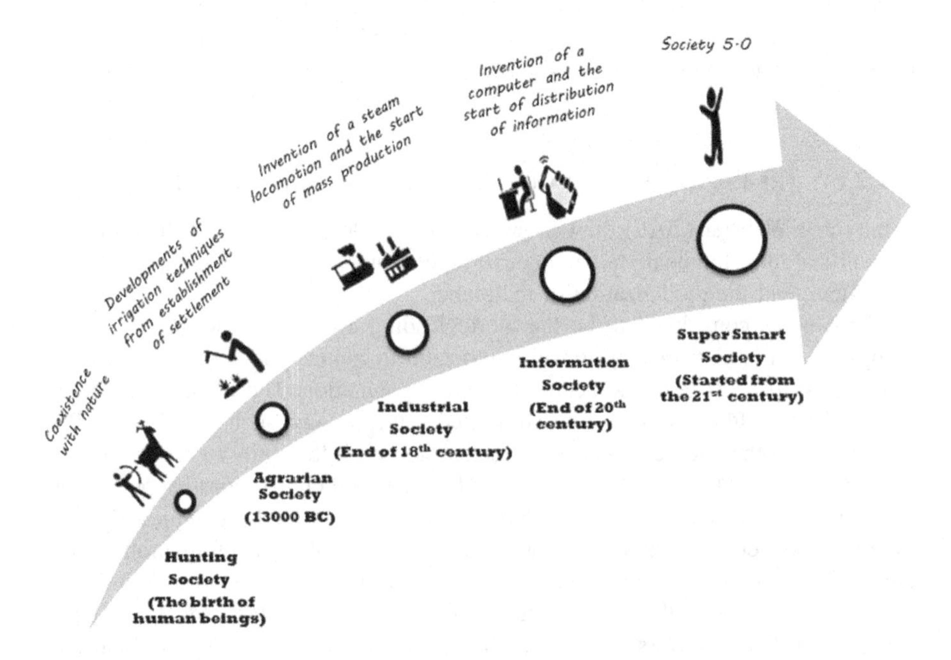

FIGURE 2.1.1 The evolution time-lapse of societies up to Society 5.0.

rate and ageing population, natural disasters, natural environment, and energy. Based on Figure 2.1.1, a new economy and society are conceived by increasing the power of individuals of every person in the society including senior citizens and women. This is because it would increase the probability for them to reside in a secure and safe manner as well as a comfortable and healthy life that could possibly make each individual realize their desired lifestyle.

The rise of new companies is due to the takeover of Industry 5.0, which provided a new set of values because of the improvements in productivity level via the digitization and promotion of revolutionized business models that results with innovation and globalization. The furnishing of new business and service applications is supported and developed by leading companies. Therefore, the solution for social problems such as population depreciation, extravagant ageing society, and natural catastrophe could be achieved by inducing social enterprise businesses.

The possibility of tackling the previously mentioned issues would require a supply of new values and services via recreation and innovation to escalate the momentum of overcoming the national difficulties from the new economy. The use of physical space power from Cyber-Physical Systems (CPS) would provide the economy with benefits due to the factors discussed as follows:

- **Disruptive innovation**
  The disruptive innovation follows the *Blue Ocean Shift* book written by Renée Mauborgne and W. Chan Kim. It illustrates that the production of a new market works on a specific product that consumers are in need to which would be a great success from the business developer. Hence, the product price and quality leads to expand a value network, which could be publicized in a short period. Therefore, this distracts an existing market, which the new pierced market could reach to a level where displacement could be established in the long run. The strategy is simultaneously differentiating and providing a simple golden concept by giving the product fame is much worthwhile than its value. This concept would make the product sell itself and open up a new market space that could help the team conceive a new demand to the society.
- **Invisible manufacturing and innovation based on social problems**
  An invisible manufacturing is a software that is incorporated with artificial intelligence (AI) system and associated with machine learning (ML). The combination could be used for applications such as perform tasks, predict hidden patterns, analyze, and conclude better than the human beings themselves. The identification of the societies' issues in any country and merging them with the industrial strengths by integrating them to invisible manufacturing, disruptive innovation, and innovation based on social problems would create a new strength and various issues would be resolved and reformed.

In general, any innovation has to be practiced for a couple of years before application in order to assure the outcome reliability and accuracy. This gives out a practical experience for first-time users to be familiarized with the innovation. In relation to the feedback obtained, inventors could improvise the challenges faced in a short period of time. The application of a new industry and society such as the

Industry 5.0 and Society 5.0 are labeled as the Digitalized Society. Any new revolution should have sufficient time given to adapt to the new changes that have been implemented. Adaptation of an innovation totally depends on the reach of knowledge to individuals.

2.1.3 PROSPECTS AND CHALLENGES

2.1.3.1 Economic Perspective on Machines' Initial Cost and Maintenance in the Long Run

The National Institute of Standards and Technology (NIST) made an encouraging research effort to advance the efficiency of manufacturing processes, where workers are actively involved in the creation of standards that eventually reduces the costs and losses associated with the maintenance of manufacturing environments.

The research is aimed at the adoption of advanced maintenance techniques and improvization of data analysis. U.S. manufacturers invested $50 billion dollars in maintenance and repair in 2016, making it a significant part of overall operating costs. Maintenance also applies to facilities and other damages including the loss of productivity. There are currently limited estimates on the total cost of production facilities, including equipment maintenance at the national level. This is usually decided after the consent of Census Bureau of Labor Statistics.

The manufacturing environments are constantly changing because of the rapid development of new technologies and standards. Competitive techniques are produced by companies by utilizing their expertise, skills, supply chains, and processes that could manufacture superior products at lower prices. The application of effective maintenance processes in such a competitive environment would distinguish the difference between a successful productive firm and the one that loses sales and money.

The frequency of maintenance can affect the quality of the product, the cost of the capital, labor costs, and even the cost of inventories amounting to production losses for both manufacturer and consumer. These possible drawbacks could influence the investors to invest in potential innovative new maintenance systems. NIST aims to promote the implementation of advanced maintenance techniques, including identifying the most beneficial equilibrium between different types of manufacturing processes. It involves identifying the most desirable equilibrium between reactive, predictive, and preventive manufacturing maintenance.

The world is currently experiencing Industry 4.0 revolution, which emphasizes specific types of maintenance that is based on these types of maintenance. The world is pushing forward to transform Industry 4.0 into Industry 5.0 through the impact of industrialization and globalization associated with the adaptation of society.

The three basic maintenance systems are in the following:

- **Predictive maintenance**
  Predictive maintenance is initiated by predicting the expected process failure that could exist in the machine by utilizing qualitative data, such as capturing the surrounding temperature, noise, and vibration.

- **Preventive maintenance**
  Preventive maintenance follows the manufacturing processes step by step, which has the potential to maintain product quality by spotting any irrelevant process that does not match the correct algorithm, procedure, or sequence. Once the sensors spot the error; it orders the machine to stop working before it continues to other processes. This could conserve the machine's good manufacturing process (GMP) by avoiding the possible damage to the machine and product. Steps are based on a cycle or time that is related to scheduled and well-organized maintenance.
- **Reactive maintenance**
  The implementation of reactive maintenance processes in machines is planned based on predetermined units such as the machine run time or number of operating cycles. A reactive maintenance system in companies operates the equipment until it breaks down or needs repair. Usually, machine repair exists when the machine is broken or halted. The repair system performs by measuring the run-to-failure rates, possible corrective repair, fault-based maintenance, and fail-to-fail maintenance. In relation to the repair costs, it is projected that plant repair costs vary from 15% to 70% of the costs of goods that are manufactured, although some of these are non-maintenance prices, such as capital structure amendments.

2.1.3.2 Business Perspective on Machines' Initial Cost and Maintenance in the Long Run

Manufacturers strive to satisfy the constantly evolving requirements of the market. This leads to evolved calls for an adaptive, smart, and scalable production line to fulfill revised requests from demanders. Such incorporation requires a significant change in industrial processes and strategies. Moreover, the convergence of different facets of a business, including manufacturers, production lines, and consumers could only be accomplished with a solid common ground.

The common ground is the Internet of Things (IoT), which is the main asset of Business 4.0, and is considered as the core multi-faceted application. The transformation from Industry 4.0 to Industry 5.0 applies both Internet of Things (IoT) and inducing artificial intelligence (AI) to enhance the processes system by shifting it from a minor to macro scale. In the area of human-machine interaction (HMI), Industry 5.0 would pose unparalleled difficulties to the society because cobots are almost the same as human beings, and in some circumstance cobots could be even better than human being's natural intelligence. Despite the fact that the societies are fascinated with computers, such as programmable aids and programmable vehicles. The programmed devices are recognized as cobots although they have been created with integrated advanced systems and the community did not complain, yet instead the societies are satisfied and wish for more innovation of technology.

The organization and implementation of cobots would be very specific because they involve human-like features such as pinching, intention-based contact, and environmental factors. Industry 5.0 would generate a large number of jobs in the HMI region. There would be vacancies in technical maintenance department as only technical experts would able to handle the cobots. It is very beneficial back to the society that more young people would be employed into technical department to handle cobots training programs, initial machine costs, machine maintenance, electricity, generators, and unplanned risk management expenses.

The business model produced must be monitored in terms of consumption and production rates to establish recorded parameters. These concerns helps the manufacturers to determine the timeline of a factory to break even, which is quite unpredictable in the beginning due to the inconsistent of equipment fees and the business feeder is not yet to be identified and analyzed. The business feeder is determined based on the success of marketing campaigns to publicize the product's quality and efficiency from revolutionized 5.0 machines associated with cobots. Industry 5.0 would change production processes globally, besides human workers' interaction. Intelligent robotics and devices would make the production chains and factory floors reach an unparalleled level.

The development of more inexpensive and highly capable cobots made of advanced materials such as carbon fibers with light and durable structures, fueled by highly optimized battery packs, intense cyber-assaults with advanced data processing, for example, artificial intelligence (AI) and sensitive sensor networks would make it possible to build a cost-effective suitable cobot (Engelberger 1980a). Industry 5.0 could improve efficiency and productivity, lowering job injuries, shortening manufacturing periods, and reducing pollution by becoming more environmentally friendly. The teamwork of artificial Intelligent (AI) machines, advanced cobots programming, and intelligent maintenance systems would create a significant increase in the number of vacant occupation opportunities. Industrialization time is variable, so it's better to prepare for the unprepared. Since the worker does not have to do repetitive activities, it could improve flexibility throughout the workplace by enabling every worker whether it is in industries or not to use various forms of cobots with different functions at work. In the business outline, bear in mind that intelligent devices, intelligent systems, and intelligent advanced automations are incorporated with the human interaction to reduce manpower. The manufacture and research team has to make sure to relate their goals and objectives towards the theme.

There are concerns in Industry 5.0 that the societies would anticipate for the high expectation of humans to implement high-valued tasks in the production of policies. This would be implemented to resolve any serious issues between technology, society, and business by the application of standardization and legalization. Furthermore, senior members of society and stakeholders could face difficulties in adapting to the new industrial revolution. On top of this, society might experience an overproduction phenomena due to the highly paced production of products in Industry 5.0, which could be resolved by applying transparency and more clarification to the recipient.

Moreover, ethical reviews and principles have to be considered as well because the recipients have to know how autonomous the systems are. Industry 5.0 would provide an essential skill gap such as Chief Robotics Officers (CROs) in the future. The job description of that particular position is monitoring and managing the entire manufacturing systems in brief, where investors have to throw their spotlights on them.

2.1.3.3 Credibility for the Transformation to Industry 5.0

The credibility of the new advances in technologies such as Internet of Things (IoT), Artificial Intelligence (AI), Machine Learning (ML), and Deep Learning (DL) prove outcomes would give a glimpse of a blurry promising vision that might potentially conceive the confidence and trust to the economy. On top of this, it would give investors the encouragement to start to rethink in investing in invisible manufacturing, which could come up with life-changing outcomes.

Over recent years, the science of artificial intelligence (AI) and machine learning (ML) has proved remarkable strides, which is widely available starting from the 21st century to companies of all sizes across channels such as the cloud sector, artificial intelligence (AI), and machine learning (ML). But it does not mean that the technology is approved or used, as a professional industry officer understands that it could end up on the shelf. The Fifth Industrial Revolution would bring people back the incorporation of human intelligence and creativity in combination with work-flows and smart systems which could improve the processes performance. While the main concern of Industry 4.0 is the insufficient data to form cobots, Industry 5.0 would link the collaboration of humans and autonomous machines. The self-employed are receptive and aware of human desire and purpose. The human race would operate with cobots with peace of mind and without terror, realizing that their computer coworkers could comprehend to their instructions without rest, in a well manner, and are capable to work effectively with human beings.

It would contribute to an extremely efficient and cost-effective manufacturing process, thriving to trusted freedom, reduction in waste, and reasonable costs. The expression "robot" is modified by Industry 5.0 to "cobot", which is defined as a collaborative robot. Cobots would not only be programmable computers that always develop specific function, but also intelligent self-learner cobots that act as companions to execute repetitive tasks.

The next industrial revolution would bring about a next generation of cobots that quickly learns and intuits by processing the surroundings and individuals around. The technical data are obtained by the cobot via sensitive sensor devices that have almost an equivalent sensitivity to the human touch. The cobots are aware of the presence of humans; therefore it takes a good care of human's health and any emergency situations, such as a sudden heart attack of a patient at home. The cobot is installed with first-aid principles that would deal with such incidents until the ambulance arrives. One of the features cobots have are the sensation of individual behavior, and it assumes the human's priorities, aspirations, actions, and emotions.

Cobot's trainees stated that cobots obtain human roles by observing their actions to process the advanced automated systems with machine learning (ML) algorithms. Moreover, cobots also predict the type of role, definition, and action could be observed to identify the respondent. The cobots execute their required tasks after they are trained. According to the trainees, it takes only one time to observe what would make the cobot respond based on the action they had observed with processing other relevant actions predicted related to the action. Therefore, operating alongside cobots would make people feel special.

The procedure exists in the following stride, where the worker starts a mission, and the cobot uses a camera that is located on a gadget to track the worker process. The head of the cobot is a camera and the cobot is also attached to an image-capturing machine, which conducts image processing and master-learning to know the patterns. It often studies the human being's actions and tracks the surroundings around the object, and then it processes the data obtained. Hence represents what could the user do operate next by using deep learning (DL) technology to analyze the human purpose of doing a particular action.

These data were obtained by the cobot by using functional near-infrared spectroscopy (fNIRS) over a wireless medium for the retrieval of signals from the human brain. It is a key tool that could be used to understand the human intentions. The functional near-infrared spectroscopy (fNIRS) is an essential function that does not require time-consuming setup, measuring adjustments, or reprogramming. The cobot depends on their data collaborated with advanced predictive technologies to help the human worker in their tasks. This would feel like another entity watching and attempting to support the human worker, which would increase the overall productivity with reduced uncertainties while processing. For instance, the cobot predicts that a certain component or tool in the next phase going to be used by the human operator. Therefore, the cobot gives an order to go and take the tool in advance, thus lends it in the appropriate time to the human worker.

2.1.3.4 Degree of Acceptance in the Implementation of a New Industry

The new technologies that link together physically, technically, and biologically in the world are addressed to societies. These new technologies could affect every profession, culture, and business that would even question the individual's ideologies on the importance of life. These innovations have tremendous potential for continuing to bring billions of users to the web, hence significantly increasing the efficiencies of companies and organizations.

For such tremendous change, the community has to adapt and be ready for it as all the resources are almost ready and big data is out there. This would influence every single person, but it depends on the preparation of an individual to adapt to these upcoming changes. In terms of political, commercial, and social systems of the 21st century, not all adjustments can be made to fulfill the Fifth Industrial Revolution. Despite the fact that these major changes would exist in our societies, weather the economies are prepared or not, there would be some sacrifices.

According to Schwab, who is an author that published a book named *The Fourth Industrial Revolution* stated that "the developments have been so dramatic that there has never been a moment of greater hope or possible danger, from human history. Nevertheless, decision-makers too often find themselves in conventional and non-disruptive mode or distracted by the immediate concerns of politically considering the powers of disruption of creativity that form our future". Figure 2.1.2 below represents the East Asia's Authoritarian Development cycle mind map, which is never meant to be an ideal or permanent political system that the society must follow.

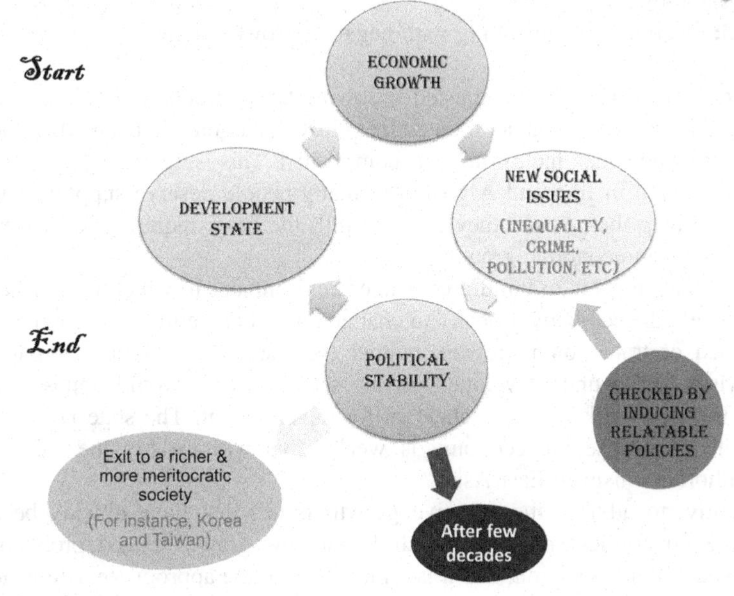

FIGURE 2.1.2 East Asia's authoritarian development mind map.

An application guideline of a new system such as Industry 5.0 is very essential as it has a possibility to promote the economy.

It is a transient and complex comfort system that expresses the purpose of driving the nation from the pit of deprivation towards industrialization. The danger to national unity or health is usually severe internally or externally, whereas this may arise as a consequence of policy fraud or applying irrelevant policy to the new social uprising issue. Then after conforming to the relevant policies related to the new social issue usually lasts a few decades, and it would be a great success to produce a transient developmental state on the economy. By applying the East Asian's Authorial development concept, the country could shift to new systems of higher incomes with more democratic institutions.

Western traditions do not necessarily follow and make political totalitarian developments to achieve an economic growth. That is precisely why East Asian developing countries are criticized as non-democratic by the West, especially by the United States. But many of them have evolved after a few decades into high-income, more competitive economies that are already achieved by Korea and Taiwan in the 21st century.

Figure 2.1.2 represents a summary for the meaning of what a growing authoritarian should take note to avoid an unplanned economic recession that is in the following:

- **Task 1:** Developing a competitive market-based economy if one of the social conditions is not fulfilled, the country's development process is jeopardized

- **Task 2:** Maintaining and handling economic, global incorporation, and political stability
- **Task 3:** Dealing and preventing with negative growth factors

The factors of growth need to be adjusted following the particular conditions, but the statement also serves as a general guideline. Growth can only happen when the political stability and social inclusion are accomplished. This is the prerequisite for all aspects. Although in Iraq and Afghanistan many people deserve support, it is very difficult to help them, since they do not fulfill the basic requirements to undertake to achieve an economic growth.

One of the challenges is to build a consumer environment in which it does not function to enable the economy globally to change into a competitive environment. In a developed or transitioning region, neither the market nor competition immediately arises. In an underdeveloped private sector, people would oppose the ideology of the free market as a mechanism for development. The state needs to assume the lead because the economy is weak. This was exactly the role of structural authoritarianism in East Asia.

Consequently, to address the negative growth issues that have already been addressed, the government must be mindful that new growth-related problems contribute to economic recession, and it is a must to take the appropriate actions to reduce them. The development cycle would break down until new policies are implemented. With policies implementation by government, cooperate economists leaders especially in East Asian countries could succeed in achieving an economic growth. If neither of these functions is applied, it would create a catastrophic mistake that could drive them off the road of economic growth.

This would create an opposition from labor unions and policymakers, as there will be pressure to improve wages rises, with the gains of Industry 4.0 achievements. Nevertheless, the advancement of process improvement through the adoption of advanced technology does not imply that the society or economy have to stay on the back foot. Industry 5.0 would be discussed as the approach that could be accomplished by applying the new developments to the improvement of process efficiency. Industry 5.0 would be discussed as the approach to pursue once the end of reverse drives.

2.1.3.5 Employability in Industry 5.0 Era

The drastic changes that the world would face in Industry 5.0 are enormous and that is due to the excessive selective job vacancies, which proves that Industry 5.0 could escalate the employability rate. Yet, this would require from applicants the ability to critically predict the context and tasks given within allocated time and envision future potentials and hidden challenges. In the Fifth Industrial Revolution, guaranteeing a job is doable, but the candidate has to be competitive as the society transfers from one industrial revolution to other. A new set of rules and guidelines are required and only smart people would be accepted. One of the main characteristics of a smart candidate is having great leadership skills, competitiveness, and the capability of achieving and renewing their aims and objectives in their projects.

However, the concern in applying Industry 5.0 by big companies will be the inconsistency of efficiency. This is due to the demand in new roles that the current system has to adapt. According to Enrico Moretti (Boffo and Fedeli 2018), it is recommended to have a cultured civilized critical education level. In a sense of almost reaching to the same competition level of the opponent candidates, which requires preparedness. Innovation has an immense importance for high-, medium-, and low-skilled employers to focus on the growth of skills is an educational level to become an important competitor in society.

In the past, a career was found right after university and until retirement. In this modern age, people are more interested in finding new careers to gain new experiences. However, some of the more modern strategies are becoming less common. People do not want to see their dream jobs mostly in the newspaper any more. Job seekers became more innovative by using online platforms to hunt candidates. The secret in finding a new occupation is by following these helpful bits of advice, which have shown a great outcome.

2.1.3.5.1 Networking

Networking would take a long time to locate employment opportunities, and there is a possibility that the job seeker could not meet someone who has direct requests for non-working applicants for offering job opportunities. In-person and online networking could be achieved through professional associations, attending graduation activities, or links to professionals working in the same field. There are also many online resources such as LinkedIn, which enable you to network and communicate about potential job opportunities with professionals from different or relevant experiences. It could be possible to meet other experts through social networking platforms such as Facebook or Twitter.

2.1.3.5.2 Referrals

Opportunities are also provided by close connections, but this way you may apply for a role without looking for a new job by just referring the job seeker to guarantee a position in a workplace. Many employers offer their workers opportunities to recommend a good applicant to their organization, which is a win-win opportunity for all.

2.1.3.5.3 Job Boards and Career Websites

Traditionally, the job boards are advertised openings for employments. While some of these boards remain, other boards have migrated to become online. For instance, federal and state governments must also provide job boards and employments in banking for instance to jobs seekers. Job seekers could also use job search engines on the Internet and many specialized pages, including Monster.com or CareerBuilder.com or company websites could also locate workstations.

2.1.3.5.4 Job Fairs

Job fairs are usually aimed to particular companies; typically the fair provides fliers or advertisements, including a list of organizations or companies present at the fair. The fair provides a range of opportunities such as CV writings, reviewing, and checking. Moreover, seminars on what the human resource (HR) would expect from the applicant by illustrating conversations with recruiters as mini-interviews that could help the job seeker to understand what happens in a real interview and what are the selection processes to differentiate applicants from each other and to try to avoid them.

The employability in the Fifth Industrial Revolution is high and open publicly, yet it is very peaky due to the knowledge required is greater and more advanced than the previous industrializations, so the candidate has to work on themselves from now and on, simply because you never know what the future holds. It's better to expect the unexpected and predict the unpredicted before the present comes into action. Always prepare for worst-case scenarios.

A Greek philosopher, Heraclitus, stated that "change is the only constant", for every industrialization there are new doors to open. Every new innovation has its opportunities and challenges associated with optimized rules and guidelines. To guarantee a job opportunity, it would be challenging since the knowledge required will be greater than the previous industrializations. However, the revolution of an industry has to take place as the world is evolving fast, regardless of the consequences.

REFERENCES

Abdolshah, Saeed, Damiano Zanotto, Giulio Rosati, and Sunil Agrawal, "Performance Evaluation of a New Design of Cable-Suspended Camera System," *In 2017 IEEE International Conference on Robotics and Automation (ICRA)*, pp. 3728–3733, 2017.

"Adorno and Horkheimer's 'Idiotic Plot' and Representations of Elizabeth Holmes' Fraud – Proquest – The Inventor: Out for Blood in Silicon Valley." 2019. search.proquest.com. https://search.proquest.com/openview/d57b397ec8f166f3f537d4bca8543fcd/1?pq-origsite=gscholar&cbl=2043477.

Boffo, Vanna, and Monica Fedeli. 2018. "Employability & Competences: Innovative Curricula For New Professions." *Google Books*. https://books.google.com.my/books?id=i65TDwAAQBAJ&pg=PA448&lpg=PA448&dq=industry+5.0+%22employability%22&source=bl&ots=o7iLPCvP-N&sig=ACfU3U1kMuaC7u7z9qcvSnL4zW0vAdrZZA&hl=en&sa=X&ved=2ahUKEwjg5prw_oroAhWMH7cAHdMVBNcQ6AEwAHoECAoQAQ#v=onepage&q&f=false.

Clomburg, James M., Anna M. Crumbley, and Ramon Gonzalez. 2017. "Industrial bio-manufacturing: The future of chemical production." *Science*, 355 (6320): aag0804.

Crenshaw, T.L.A., "Using robots and contract learning to teach cyber-physical systems to undergraduates," in *IEEE Transactions on Education*, vol. 56, no. 1, pp. 116–120, February 2013.

Engelberger, Joseph F. 1980a. "Robotics in Practice: Management and Applications of Industrial Robots." *Google Books*. https://books.google.com.my/books?hl=en&lr=&id=r1Z-BgAAQBAJ&oi=fnd&pg=PT9&dq=cost+effective+robots+in+the+future&ots=9vcaFLyoLv&sig=S0MrE552cJtE27rqKBMhIgIwH3E&redir_esc=y#v=onepage&q&f=false.

Engelberger, Joseph F. 1980b. *Robotics in Practice Management and Applications of Industrial Robots*. Springer. https://www.springer.com/gp/book/9780850386691.

Gesrepair. 2021. What Is Industry 5.0—and How Will It Affect Manufacturers?" 2021. https://gesrepair.com/industry-5-0-will-affect-manufacturers/.

Grosdidier, Aurélien, VincentZoete, & Olivier Michielin. 2007. "EADock: Docking of Small Molecules into Protein Active Sites with a Multiobjective Evolutionary Optimization."

Proteins: Structure, Function, and Bioinformatics 67 (4): 1010–1025. https://doi.org/10.1002/prot.21367

"Industrial Revolution." *Wikipedia*. Wikimedia Foundation, March 5, 2020. https://en.wikipedia.org/wiki/Industrial_Revolution.

Ivanov, Stanislav Hristov, and Craig Webster. 2017. "Adoption of Robots, Artificial Intelligence and Service Automation by Travel, Tourism and Hospitality Companies – A Cost-Benefit Analysis". Prepared for the International Scientific Conference "Contemporary Tourism – Traditions and Innovations," Sofia University, 19–21 October 2017. Available at SSRN:https://ssrn.com/abstract=3007577.

Lazonick, William, and Öner Tulum. 2011. "US biopharmaceutical finance and the sustainability of the biotech business model." *Research Policy* 40 (9): 1170–1187. doi:10.1016/j.respol.2011.05.021.

Leknes, Stefan, & Jørgen Modalsli. 2019. "Who Benefited from Industrialization? The Local Effects of Hydropower Technology Adoption in Norway." *Journal of Economic History*. https://doi.org/10.1017/S0022050719000743.

Mohareb, Fady, Olga Papadopoulou, Efstathios Panagou, George-John Nychas, & Conrad Bessant. 2016. "Ensemble-Based Support Vector Machine Classifiers as an Efficient Tool for Quality Assessment of Beef Fillets from Electronic Nose Data." *Analytical Methods* 8 (18): 3711–3721. https://doi.org/10.1039/C6AY00147E.

North Carolina Association. "Mapping Your Future Careers in Biomanufacturing." Biogen Idec Foundation, North Carolina Biotechnology Center, 2006. http://www.ncabr.org/downloads/curricula/mapping-your-future.pdf.

"Quality 5.0." Forum SIQ. Accessed March 9, 2020. https://forum.siq.se/den-femte-kvalitetsvagen/.

Rossi, Ben. "Industry 5.0: What Is It and What Will It Do for Manufacturing?" Raconteur Media Ltd., February 7, 2020. https://www.raconteur.net/technology/manufacturing-gets-personal-industry-5-0.

Rue, Noah. "Recent Developments in Biotechnology." Medium. *Becoming Human: Artificial Intelligence Magazine*, August 29, 2019. https://becominghuman.ai/recent-developments-in-biotechnology-77b10ed54927.

Soley, Richard, & Robert Schmid. 2018. "Industrial IoT: How Connected Things Are Changing Manufacturing." *WIRED*. https://www.wired.com/wiredinsider/2018/07/industrial-iot-how-connected-things-are-changing-manufacturing/.

"The Industrial Revolution from Industry 1.0 to 5.0! – Supply Chain Game Changer™." 2020. Supply Chain Game Changer™. https://supplychaingamechanger.com/the-industrial-revolution-from-industry-1-0-to-industry-5-0/.

Weller, Chris. 2017. "Meet the First-Ever Robot Citizen—A Humanoid Named Sophia That Once Said It Would 'Destroy Humans'". Jewishcamp.Org. https://jewishcamp.org/wp-content/uploads/2018/05/Sophia-Article-Golem.pdf.

Weston, Jason, Frédéric Ratle, Hossein Mobahi, and Ronan Collobert. 2012. "Deep learning via semi-supervised embedding." *Lecture Notes in Computer Science*, 639–655. doi:10.1007/978-3-642-35289-8_34.

White, Otis. 1983. "How Computers Are Changing the Way We Work: Across America, Inexpensive Technology Is Igniting a New Industrial Revolution; What Started in Factories Is Spreading to Offices [and Other Business Enterprises]." *Florida Trend* 26 (September): 51–55. https://search.proquest.com/scholarly-journals/how-computers-are-changing-way-we-work-across/docview/59297106/se-2?accountid=135175.

"Why Is Industrialization & Industrial Development Important?." 2020. EM Founders Group. http://eaglemountainutah.com/why-is-industrial-development-important/.

Zoppis, Italo. 2019. "Kernel Method – An Overview." Sciencedirect Topics. Sciencedirect.com. https://www.sciencedirect.com/topics/biochemistry-genetics-and-molecular-biology/kernel-method.

2.2 Significance of Industry 5.0

Yoong Kit Leong, Jian Hong Tan,
Kit Wayne Chew, and Pau Loke Show

CONTENTS

2.2.1 IMPORTANCE OF INDUSTRIAL REVOLUTION

The British brought the world into its First Industrial Revolution with a myriad of discoveries. A new source of energy was found in Britain which was coal. Its energy was harvested by burning it in the newly invented steam engines, which brought the trains alive and moved them onto railroad network that travel across the country (Clark 2008). The rise of mechanical invention started the transformation of manual labor to mechanized mass production which boosted industrial productivity. It sparked the transition of Great Britain from an agrarian society into an industrial society with textile industry dominating (Crafts 2005). The First Industrial Revolution marks a major turning point in history and brought change to all aspects of the world from growing the economy, transforming industries as well as improving living standards and rising population growth through healthier nutrition (Mohajan 2019).

Subsequently, the Second Industrial Revolution (Industry 2.0) pioneered in the United States with electricity and crude oil as new source of energy. Telephone was the new form of communication, and automobiles being the new form of transportation started filling up the streets. Industry 2.0 also improved public health and sanitation through public health initiatives and improvement in the health and pharmaceutical industry with better medicine and medical instruments (Mohajan 2020). The second wave of technology revolution opened up an exponential rise in international trade for the world. For example, export rates of Belgium increased from 1.1% to 1.5% per annum (Huberman, Meissner, and Oosterlinck 2017). Although there was a delay of technological diffusion, the second industrial revolution still led the world into a new economy of electricity. It resulted in higher growth in productivity, improving the living standards of people (Atkeson and Kehoe 2001).

From the 1960s onwards, rapid technological progress significantly lowered the prices of computers and equipment, which correlates to 60% of economic growth around 1974 (Greenwood 1997). The third wave of the industrial revolution, which is also known as the digital revolution, led us from an industrial society into an information society (Karvonen 2001). Transistors, integrated circuit chips and microcomputers were the examples of inventions that made the digital revolution possible. Computers and its networks have opened up opportunities for everyone and anyone to share their knowledge through the Internet. This age of information has driven innovation and productivity to new heights, influencing the economy and creating an economy of digital information (Brynjolfsson and McAfee 2011). This was when companies like Intel and IBM were developing computer chips and systems which shaped the digital reality of today.

Industry 4.0 was first announced at the Hannover Fair in 2011 with public awareness reaching a peak at the 2016 Davos World Economic Forum. The motivation behind the Fourth Industrial Revolution lies in Smart Manufacturing and Smart Factory (Demir and Cicibas 2017). To achieve smart production, new and advanced technologies such as Cyber-Physical systems, cloud computing, IoT, AI robotics and Big Data are required (Bahrin et al. 2016). Other technologies such as targeted gene editing, advanced bionics, synthetic biology and biomanufacturing are examples of biological technologies that will bring changes to the world of Industry 4.0 (Schwab 2017).

A summary of the main characteristics of all industrial revolutions is shown in Table 2.2.1. In all the industrial revolution, they share technical advancements of mainly three areas:

1. Communication Technologies: Improve communication more efficiently and effectively
2. Source of Energy: Provide effective and efficient power that drives our economies
3. Modes of Mobility: Allows effective and efficient locomotion

When three technologies of each area synergize, it creates a new general-purpose technology platform, a new infrastructure that changes the way society behaves,

TABLE 2.2.1
Main Characteristics of Industrial Revolutions

Industrial Revolution (Period)	Periods for Transition	Source of Energy	Mode of Mobility	Mode of Communication	Technological Advancement	Identifying Characteristic
First (1760–1820)	1860–1900	Coal, Steam	Trains, Steamships	Newspaper, Telegraph	Steam engine, Mechanical loom	Mechanization
Second (1760–1820)	1940–1960	Fossil fuel, Electricity	Trains, Cars	Telegraph, Telephone, Television, Radio	Internal combustion engine	Mass production
Third (1960–2000)	1980–2000	Fossil fuel, Electricity, Nuclear	Cars, Airplanes	Mobile phones, Instant text messaging, E-mails	Computers, Robots	Automation
Fourth (2010–Present)	2000–2010	Green Renewable Energy	Electric cars, Ultra-fast trains	E-mails, Internet messaging, Online video calls	Internet, 3D printer, Genetic engineering	Cyber-physical systems

Source: Created based on Peterson (2008), Prisecaru (2016) and Demir, Döven, and Sezen (2019).

how governments operate and how the economy flows. In the subsequent revolutions, we can see important technological advancements that shape our lives today. And the Fifth Industrial Revolution will be no different.

2.2.1.1 Importance of Industry 5.0

Industry 5.0 is coming soon in the near future, and what are the expectations that are set for the Fifth Industrial Revolution? The fifth industry has been predicted to utilize the full potential of collaborations between AI machines and humans, where human-machine interaction will be more frequent and publicly implemented into society. Technologies other than AI and machine learning (ML), such as 3D printing, autonomous vehicles are innovations from Industry 4.0 (Skobelev and Borovik 2017). These technologies would be massively implemented into society, moving us forward to Industry 5.0. The visions and themes of Industry 5.0 predicted by the futurists are presented in Figure 2.2.1.

All of the technology developed in Industry 4.0 will be integrated horizontally and vertically, applying on our everyday lives on an enormous scale (Bahrin et al. 2016). This revolution will bring in the usage of machines to purely automate production on a super large scale, with only machine-machine interaction and human assistance. As for human workers, they will be tasked to be creative, innovate and personalize products for clients, businesses and society. This will allow the society to cater needs on a personal level, thus bringing forth the usage of personalization in products. This is why Industry 5.0 will be known as the "personalization revolution" (Özdemir and Hekim 2018). However, as the industry begins to have more personalization in their products, the complexity of the industry will skyrocket and workers on the frontline might not be able to cope. Hence, Industry 5.0 is likely to cause smart automation partially taking over human jobs and some jobs will be highly collaborative with robots (Nahavandi 2019).

This is where human-robot collaboration comes in. Even though the future customers will flock to the idea and concept of personalization in every industry that

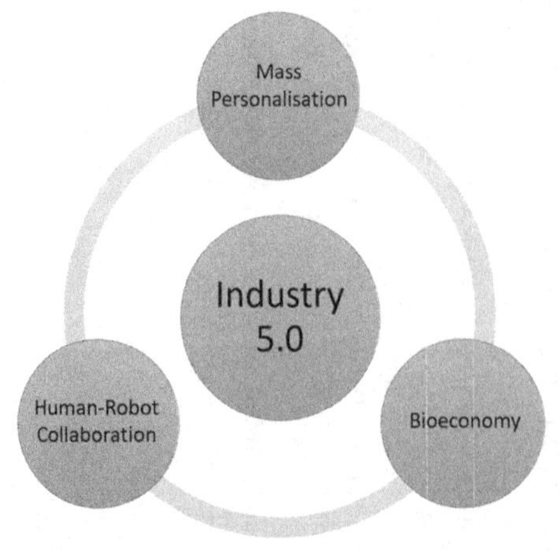

FIGURE 2.2.1 The principle of Industry 5.0. Created based on Demir, Döven, and Sezen (2019), Pathak et al. (2019) and European Commission (2018).

we can think of, but the personalization would not be possible without the creativity and empathy of humans. Humanities are what connects all humans as a society, understanding the needs and wants of each other through empathy. Therefore, although the present jobs will be taken over by AI and industrial robots in the future, new jobs that require vocational skills, human's creativity and empathy will emerge. Helping civilizations to adapt and accept the introduction of AI will be a crucial part in the transformation of Industry 5.0 and will require step-by-step and gradual introduction. Many variables will affect this, such as culture, age and physical environment will all come into play with how a person and the community accept the transformation. A critical factor in the acceptance of AI will be fairness and equality, and several measures have to be put in place to ensure AI can achieve this (Demir, Döven, and Sezen 2019). Nonetheless, the collaboration between a human being and a robot symbolizes a new reality and we need to define the boundaries, ethics, and the rules between human and machine interaction. We could see in an impressive example during Google I/O 2018 presented by Sundar Pichai, CEO of Google, where a voice assistant called to make an appointment and the woman answering the call didn't realize that she was speaking to a robot. The implementation of AI will likely not be the binary selection of the stepping stone to a "Utopian" or "Dystopian", but this doesn't mean that the inevitable upcoming revolution should not be handled carefully (Makridakis 2017).

Aside from robots and personalization, the main focus of Industry 5.0 also includes sustainability. With the United Nations' 17 Sustainable Development Goals (SDGs) in mind, we can achieve this through bioeconomy and biologization of the industries, which reconciles nature, ecology, society and economy (Schütte 2018). Solving the critical global issues such as energy crisis, climate change, poverty and global food insecurity will never be an easy task. The human economy needed to be reformed to move away from fossil fuel resources and shift toward bio-based resources. Encouraging non-bio-based industries to embrace renewable resources like biofuels will help to reduce the emission of greenhouse gases and mitigate climate change (Staffas, Gustavsson, and McCormick 2013). The success of the bioeconomy requires continuous discussion on how our society chooses to integrate sustainability into economic growth in Industry 5.0. This requires adaptations of societies, continuous development of policies and strategies and finally cooperation from every single human on this planet.

2.2.2 HEALTHCARE, MEDICINE AND PHARMACEUTICALS

Healthcare is one of the paramount industries in the present society, which consist of medicines and pharmaceuticals among many other things such as healthcare professionals and infrastructure. Healthcare demands a lot of manpower, with both paper and digital networks utilized to process patient's data into database. This is very tedious and time-consuming and more often not, there is possibility of human errors in patients' medical records (Thomas 2009). The enormous hassle of processing electronic health records and clinical notes can be much easier with the use of AI. AI can help to automate these processes and tasks, allowing nurses and doctors to focus more on patient care, saving valuable time.

In the society of Industry 5.0, personalization is greatly emphasized within healthcare. By incorporating IoT and AI technologies, it would revolutionize how we treat patients and save lives (Sheth et al. 2017). Medical centers will be able to utilize biosensors and genetic sequencing to disclose a person's genotype and learn about the person's pre-existing health conditions, thus predicting how they may react to the medicine. Moreover, AI can improve and aid in patient diagnosis which allow early detection of diseases. It can also aid in matching patient treatments, clinical decision support, improve clinical workflows and check symptoms for diagnosis. Thus, patient care and experience would be enhanced through the capabilities of AI-human interface and AI applications (Schork 2019).

In modern times, patient care can be enhanced by opportunities in innovation with the usage of IoT. Along with 5G data networks and IoT, test results can be sent to doctors and nurses in real time. Eventually, this technology can reduce the time taken to run diagnoses on patients, making it easier, especially for elderly patients (Thomas 2009). To make things even more interesting, augmented reality (AR) has also been adopted in surgery. Medical fields such as laparoscopic, oral and maxillofacial, and even plastic surgeries have been trying to adopt AR into their practice (Khor et al. 2016; Sayadi et al. 2019).

The pharmaceutical industry will also be revolutionized by Industry 5.0 mostly, in drug design and discovery through AI and machine learning. Currently, the medical and pharmaceutical practices drug design and development from scratch, which has multiple cumbersome stages. Pharmaceutical drugs are commonly used at a standard, where the mechanism of action along with possible side-effects differ for different persons. Also, there is difference in the dosage of drug, which is dependent on the individual patient's circumstances and requirements. There are a lot of variables when it comes to the efficacy of drugs and medicines as they can be affected by an individual's health and fitness, lifestyle choices, genetic makeup and even sex. Medicine that is effective for one person may be less effective for another highlights the importance of personalized medicine (Fröhlich et al. 2018). The pharmaceutical industry would be so much safer with AI-supported pharmacovigilance, which has less human errors to overlook drug developments (λ).

2.2.3 FOOD SUPPLY

Food security has been a major topic and issue in recent years, particularly due to our rising populations of 7.8 billion. With the climate change affecting supplies of food, unbalance in nature can lead to negative impacts in food production. For example, the 1988 U.S. Midwest drought led to a 30% corn production drop in the United States (Rosenzweig et al. 2001; Porter et al. 2014). All living beings can't live without food and the global food supply is in jeopardy, but here's where AI can intervene and help us. When food is freshly harvested, the harvest is sorted by its size and quality according to a set of standard. Sorting produce is one of the most tedious and time-consuming processes, however, incorporating AI and IoT with infrared detectors can help to differentiate healthy harvest or diseased produce as well as determine its quality and nutrition (Elakkiya, Karthikeyan, and Ravi 2018).

To manage the harvest and make sure it reaches every table in each home, it is important to manage the supply chain. The logistics of food transportation has to be highly efficient in the distribution process to ensure a stable food supply, and this can be achieved by utilizing AI monitoring. AI in food production can help predict the demand for food, hence deciding transportation mode and provide better pricing. Monitoring and managing inventory, tracking of food origins and deliveries with AI can ensure transparency as well as earning the customer's trust and reducing food waste (Luthra et al. 2018).

By using blockchain technology, farmers can now manage their land and property in a safer and more transparent way, thus, improving their rights and preventing fraud or corruption (Naudé 2019). The high level of safety through fault tolerance and transparency enable blockchain technology to be applied to every level of the food supply chain. Blockchain technology can provide information from the amount of fertilizers and pesticide applied to the processing methods of the produce, and even the shipping details (Kamilaris, Fonts, and Prenafeta-Boldú 2019).

The current food supply system is highly inefficient as there is great amount of food wastage. In the United States of America, it is estimated that there is 54% of edible food is wasted, which adds to around 70 million metric tons of food wastage every year (Morone et al. 2019). Food wastage can be significantly reduced through AI applications. Starting from restaurants, grocery stores and malls, AI can help to analyze the market demand, their customer's preferences and habits to predict the demand and decide on the amount of food to be produced. By implementing online websites or a service system that could recommend and advertise specific foods that are in abundance, this helps to cut down fresh produce going to waste (Morone et al. 2019). The range of ideas is wide, such as supermarkets can install voice-enabled shopping software and devices that will suggest the customers what to order and even automatically order a complete supply of food or household goods through the habits and needs of customers. The same idea can be applied to restaurants and cafes. AI-assisted food tracking enables us to buy and sell food and reduce the amount that go to waste. Additionally, these technologies enable food producers to connect with the communities, making food supply more effective and efficient.

2.2.4 FUELS AND BIOFUELS

Currently, societies around the world are focusing on many issues revolving around fuel, such depletion of fossil fuel reserve, the damage of these fossil fuel cause to our plants and climate change due to carbon emissions (Höök and Tang 2013). Therefore, bio-based fuels were created in hopes to replace fossil fuels (Patermann and Aguilar 2018). The first and second generation of biofuels were made from plants such as food crops and agricultural waste (Naik et al. 2010). However, the first-generation biofuels sparked a backlash for using food crops as a fuel source, jeopardizing global food security. As for the second-generation biofuels, they have questionable benefits of reducing greenhouse gas emissions due to excessive land use.

Under Industry 5.0, white biotechnology and synthetic biology will be the major tool to re-engineer and improve the sustainability of biofuel production. The combination of technologies will create new ways of producing biofuels with higher efficiency (Sachsenmeier 2016). Examples include microalgae-based biofuel which doesn't require expansive land use, thus avoiding excessive land use and maintain the current forestry (Shuba and Kifle 2018). Through synthetic biotechnology, *Porphyridium cruentum*, *Tetraselmis suecica* and other algae are examples of algae strains that were found to be highly potential as biofuel source (Sachsenmeier 2016; Jagadevan et al. 2018). This changes the way in which sources of biofuels can be created that are renewable and sustainable, which fits the bioeconomy vision of Industry 5.0.

2.2.5 FINE CHEMICALS AND BIOPOLYMERS

Common chemicals, fine chemicals and biopolymers largely revolve around modern human life. They can be found in a vast array of applications from automobiles, medicines, to aerospace and even more. Fine chemicals are important to pharmaceutical drugs and the manufacturing industry because they are largely used to make specialty chemicals which include agrochemicals, paints, polymers and food additives (Straathof, Panke, and Schmid 2002). With the recent global environmental awareness of plastic pollution and climate change, sustainability has become the center of attention. The use of biopolymers, such as bio-based biodegradable plastics has been on the rise (Mohanty, Misra, and Drzal 2002). The use of synthetic biology, evolutionary algorithms and biotechnology will be the highlight of Industry 5.0 for the chemicals industry.

In Industry 5.0, synthetic biology and biotechnology can bring sustainable solutions for the productions of biodegradable materials. It can also help design and develop sustainable industrial processes that can be found in nature (Merk et al. 2018). With the help of AI and biotechnology, microorganisms could be re-engineered to biomanufacture biopolymer at higher rates (Clomburg, Crumbley, and Gonzalez 2017). During the production process, IoT along with AR/VR technology can help specialists to monitor bioreactors in real time or make any last-minute tweaks and changes, thus allowing customization (Wang et al. 2020). Down the production line, robots will autonomously work on intelligent packaging, control and assure the quality through sensors. When 3D-printing technology comes into play, 3D-printed biopolymers can be easily done at home, for any purposes, such as biodegradable bags or toys (Liu et al. 2019).

2.2.6 MANUFACTURING

The world and its economy have been relying on manufacturing to complete productions ranging from small to large scale. Once powered by steam and water, machines are now connected with smart robots that autonomously complete the manufacturing process (Mohajan 2019). As AI and industrial IoT come into play, humans will work alongside robots via device connections. In Industry 5.0, there will be more human-AI machine interactions and interfaces, which encourages improved integration, allowing faster, better automation paired with the power of human brains (Pathak et al. 2019).

Instead of AI fully "taking over the world", humans will work together with AI machines and robots to improve the manufacturing process and overall productivity. Industrial robots will be a critical component of the Fifth Industrial Revolution (Nahavandi, 2019). While much of what defines Industry 5.0 involves a human's ability to customize and personalize a product at a mass scale, this is only possible with advanced robotic capabilities. By fully and efficiently automating the entire production process, humans are left free to create and innovate without having to worry about production constraints (Doyle-Kent and Kopacek 2019). Unlike in Industry 4.0 where robotic capabilities take center stage, industrial robots will take a backseat to human intelligence in Industry 5.0. They will remain a critical component, especially when industrial IoT will be adapted into manufacturing allowing large amounts of data to be collected into Industrial Big Data. This allows the industry to analyze customers and clients or analyze the factory and its equipment, enabling entirely new production methods (Mourtzis, Vlachou, and Milas 2016).

Virtual Manufacturing and Maintenance are examples of what Industry 5.0 can change in the industry. Imagine an engineer that wears a VR headset or an AR device to perform maintenance of aircraft remotely from the comfort of his own home (Palmarini et al. 2018). Then, somewhere far away in a shipyard, the ship is built with that design by an industrial robot supported by AI, machine learning and industrial IoT. This would mean that engineers and specialists will no longer need to work inside a manufacturing environment, even for maintenance, where they can access the working site through 5G speed and secure connection off-site. Thus, it increases efficiency and reduces workplace injuries and fatigues. On top of that, AI and IoT can support the specialist with predictive maintenance which would help to monitor the conditions and track performance of equipment or parts. This could be applied in all manufacturing industries to help engineers predict and detect the defects before a failure happens.

It is likely that in the coming years, housewares, hardware and accessories could be manufactured from home under Industry 5.0. People will be able to fully customize clothes or trinkets as 3-D printing will allow for custom prints for customers' requested item. 3-D printing allow for very intricate designs to be easily made where previously have to be created with a very unique mold or production method, this will significantly increase the ease of production, customizability and creative possibilities for myriads of purposes.

2.2.7 IT AND COMMUNICATIONS

With the upcoming integration of AI into civilization, it is important that if the integration is to be as efficient and accepted as possible that humans will be able to communicate at least basic instructions to the AI. AI is a crucial part of the upcoming Industry 5.0 in terms of economy, business and social impact and there is great pressure to make the digital transformation as smooth as possible. Robots are utilized through coding and are usually unable to communicate with humans through speech or gestures, and will only change the work they do if they are given instructions via control panels or changes in coding (Pandey and Gelin 2018).

However, there have been some robots developed that have heightened levels of communication through utilization of speech recognition, sensors and IoT technology, a good example being the wheel-based humanoid robot developed in Japan known as "Pepper". Pepper has shown to be incredibly advanced in terms of communicative intelligence, it has the capability to understand different languages, acknowledge a person's tone of voice and gestures to recognize a person's emotion and react accordingly. The robot can be utilized in many settings as a method of cognitive support, information relay and societal-based needs support with a high level of safety due to the many sensors and bumpers around the chassis. Pepper has already been successfully employed in hospitals, care homes, restaurants, railways stations and will soon see applications in other sectors of business (Pandey and Gelin 2018). Between humans, meetings and all other forms of communication would utilize 5G and projector technology such as VR/AR calls could be performed.

2.2.8 SUPPLY CHAIN AND LOGISTICS

In Industry 5.0, the supply chain will become a much more efficient and simple process; soon enough there will be self-driving delivery vehicles. Self-driving vehicles can keep on working without rests or breaks, unlike man-manned vehicle where the only time they need to stop is when the vehicles are picking up or dropping off deliveries, refueling or for maintenance. Thus, it would help the manufacturers and suppliers to save time and money in terms of efficiency.

The next addition is predicted to be one of the most disruptive new technologies so far to the supply chain, as most supply chain "improvements" over the past decade have been seen as incremental, this hyped technology is known as "augmented reality, AR". Augmented reality can affect the supply chain heavily; for instance, with AR "smart glasses", workers could get an onscreen display of their upcoming jobs, how to perform them and what to do next (Merlino and Sproģe 2017). They could also be remotely contacted through IoT, which would reduce downtime of workers waiting for a manager's help or waiting to know their next action. For example, a warehouse picker will have the next item needed to be picked up displayed on his field of view. This will allow him to access the item much quicker rather than having to ask a manager or look down at papers or a device. Keeping the users' eyes up which would increase safety in a warehouse environment with vehicles and machines. The device would also provide a constant up-to-date tutorial on how to perform actions, which would mean workers no longer have to have extensive training or extra training to learn how to perform a new task which would heavily speed up the full training of new employees. Another benefit is this device could provide relevant health and safety in regard to the task, which would heavily reduce the amount of injury and time off due to injury, even people who are up to date with health and safety would benefit, as with repetitive work sometimes all a person would need is a reminder to stay safe (Grabowski, Rowen, and Rancy 2018).

5G technology is expected to be around 20 times faster and more reliable than 4G. Using this immensely increased speed, networks will be able to transmit data at a much higher rate and with less latency (AlMousa and AlShahwan 2015). The usage of 5G will allow for the supply chain to utilize technologies that require higher data such as self-driving delivery vehicles. The usage of 5G will also allow for any issues or maintenance requisites to be communicated much faster, which will lessen any time loss on these issues. This works in synergy with the increasing usage of IoT devices and blockchain technology. This allows a further increase of collection time and analysis of data while maintaining cyber-safety. 5G will even make warehouse workers' lives easier, 5G networks would allow for easier access to monitor data, easier communications amongst the workers, and better access to logistics.

2.2.9 SUSTAINABLE ECONOMY

In the period of the First Industrial Revolution, there are exponential economic growth for both European countries and America (Komlos 1998). Major shifts were observed in the industrial sector as the institutional framework modernized. However, people of the late 18th century started to have decreased height and weight (Komlos 1998). This was caused by the change of diet from protein-rich food to carbohydrate-rich food due to a rise in food prices. All in all, Industry 1.0 grew the economy but it also affected the physical stature of the people, which can heavily reflect how a person's health and development is affected by change of culture and industry (Komlos 1998). During the Second Industrial Revolution, the economy and productivity grew with the existence of electricity and other technologies. However, the economic growth took time of almost 20 years, from 1899 to 1919, for the electricity to be implemented into 50% of the industry in the United States (Atkeson and Kehoe 2001). Coming into Industry 3.0, where the information age digitalization had boosted economic growth in the United States by 60% (Greenwood 1997). Just entering into Industry 4.0, the economy has become an open and connected world economy, where zero marginal cost is coming closer and factories work automatically (Schwab 2017). However, Schwab (2017), Morrar, Arman, and Mousa (2017) and Kergroach (2017) have all expressed concerns of inequalities and social cleavage that would arise from emerging technological changes. Therefore, Industry 5.0 envisioned a sustainable economy for all, through the bioeconomy vision (Demir and Cicibas 2017; European Commission 2018).

Bioeconomy stresses the need to have sustainability and circularity that covers all sectors, industry and systems. Few countries have started to explore bioeconomy, which includes EU, USA, Canada, Germany and few other countries (Staffas, Gustavsson, and McCormick 2013). In Germany, the value of bioeconomy has seen its rise from 115 billion euros to 140 billion euros, which translates to a growth rate of 22% from the year 2002 to 2010 (Schütte 2018). Bioeconomy aims to build a nature-based circular economy, which emphasizes on encouraging industries such as sustainable agriculture and fishery, aquaculture, forestry, biorefinery, food, renewable energy and biotechnology (Patermann and Aguilar 2018), thus creating more jobs and enhancing economies through diverse and sustainable industries (Staffas, Gustavsson, and McCormick 2013; Schütte 2018). Under the extensive collaboration between human-and-robots of Industry 5.0, it is inevitable that there is a possibility of robots being a part of the human economy. As robots can perform exchange and consumption of services and goods with humans and/or robots, it creates its own value and growth (Ivanov 2017), thus creating a robot economy also known as robonomics, which aims to create an economy of robots in order for humans to exchange products with robots (Lonshakov et al. 2018). Through blockchain and IoT technology, the simple framework of robot economics could allow payments with its own digital currency between humans and robots (Arduengo and Sentis 2018).

2.2.10 BUSINESS

AI and Machine Learning are currently employed as a business tool where it covers everything from employee screening, responding to customers queries and targeted marketing with the help of intelligent robots. Throughout the production line, warehouse management and customer deliveries, artificial intelligence is supporting or replacing human expertise in many domains with improved efficiency and lower cost (Finlay 2017). Examples include AI deciding on insurance premiums, aiding the HR department on deciding who to hire or fire and automatically identifying customers as they walk into your store which would help them decide what to buy. Something similar would happen to how businesses market themselves. AI could offer precision and effective marketing strategies (Wirth 2018). Through Big Data and algorithms, potential customers could be easily tracked and identified. Moreover, this technology could be used to identify specific problems which the business is facing, and then personalize solutions for these problems. Predictive analysis could be applied to all clients, customers and business partners to better understand them and provide the right solutions while reducing uncertainty. In the future of Industry 5.0, businesses will have their own personalized predictive model to make business decisions in a smoother, efficient and effective manner (Finlay 2017).

Small and medium enterprises (SMEs) are a vital part of the economy and is essentially the crux of societies. Following the accelerated development of SMEs, the economy grows exponentially as well. In Industry 4.0, SMEs have been transforming into digitally capable businesses that are more diverse and technologically advanced. As SMEs use AI and other technologies such as cloud computing, robotics and material sciences, it allows these high-tech SMEs to flourish by increasing the productivity while lowering the cost of setting up the business (Antoniuk et al. 2017). Therefore, the same will happen in Industry 5.0, where big data analytics and business intelligence (BI) will help our society create new innovations and foster a new generation of entrepreneurs (Sun, Sun, and Strang 2018).

2.2.11 JOB AND LABOR MARKET

As Industry 5.0 progresses, it is predicted that the worker productivity will rise, not through humans but robots. Robots will be used along assembly lines to provide work for mundane, repetitive and heavy tasks. Therefore, people will be left with unique tasks that utilize our humanity, leaving their brain open for creativity and innovation (Nahavandi 2019). Another predicted productivity boost is that workers will be injured at a much lesser rate and will have more energy due to the cumbersome jobs being performed by machines.

Due to the mass digitization of industries, great change happened within the labor market. With the increased speed of technological advancement and complexity, labor markets will require manpower equipped with vocational skills instead of pure academics. This includes all corporate companies, industrial entities, policymakers and even universities around the world are looking for skilled workers. Countries like the UK, Germany and Denmark have been running vocational programs and systems to train more people to fit skill-intensive jobs, such as. This is crucial because the change in demand of the workforce affects and changes the education system, such as pressuring universities to shift into developing vocational programs and complex equipment skills (Madsen, Bilberg, and Hansen 2016).

In a working environment, managing an organization and its workers is no easy feat. Hence, AI systems have been tested out on managing employees, whether it be monitoring, coordinating their employees. The AI system of employee management is very effective and efficient in organizations. However, improvements and optimization still needed to be done in terms of fairness and equality. As an example, it was found that the AI-powered recruitment engine in Amazon has a gender-bias towards males (Robert et al. 2020). Job and income opportunities will be massively influenced by Industry 5.0 and its future labor market. It is undeniable that a lot of jobs will be lost to AI and robots. However, new jobs will appear based on skills needed to accommodate technological advancement, such as cyber-insurance providers. And some jobs will remain with a new set of required skills (Eberhard et al. 2017).

2.2.12 TRANSPORTATION

Currently, vehicles are innovated to become more digitalized; through digitization of vehicles, the addition of smart sensors and allowing the vehicle to connect to wireless network allowing vehicles to integrate with IoT. IoT technology brings many benefits for transportation sector due to its fast and precise data collection and information relay to the user. Transportation and logistics companies see promising opportunities in IoT, the technology when properly utilized can perform accurate analysis of all steps of shipping and accurately monitors the delivery status. It is important that there is a heavy amount of monitoring when it comes to shipping vehicles as variables such as temperature, movement of items, humidity and light conditions can affect the product and thus affect the revenue and profitability (Manoj Kumar and Dash 2017). Companies can also use IoT to predict the maintenance required before a problem arises by using collected data on the IoT sensors (Kong et al. 2017), which reduces downtime of the vehicle used and will lead to increased revenue. Fuel costs are another factor that comes into play when accounting for the cost of shipping and logistics. However, IoT can predict the most fuel-efficient shipping route by avoiding traffic jam, road blocks, bad weather and others (Manoj Kumar and Dash 2017).

2.2.13 HUMAN WELFARE AND EQUALITIES

It is without a doubt that in the early years of Industry 5.0, many jobs will be nullified by automation. Jobs that are repetitive and mundane, such as production, administration and others will be replaced by computers and robots with majority are of low skill and low wages. While automation largely benefits the employers by reducing operation and production cost, the over-reliance on computers and robots will heavily affect the income inequality caused by economic growth and technological advancement (Degryse 2016).

As technology improves, the demand for high-skill workers trained specifically for the related sector increases, often accompanied by high pay grades. Another factor that cause income equality is productivity, as technology improves high-skilled jobs, but low-skilled jobs will have remained the same due to the lack of difference in their work performance, and the work they typically perform are generally repetitive in nature with little room for innovation. With AI and robots spearheading the progress and growth of our economy in Industry 5.0, inequalities within the economy will be the greatest concern for the world. As some countries yet to caught up to the current technological advancement, poverty and economic disparity might worsen if technological advancement continues to leave these countries out (Prisecaru 2016).

The effect that automation have in regards to income equality has been examined by Hong and Shell (2018) in relation to the "Gini coefficient". The Gini coefficient is a scale that measures the equality of distribution of income across the population and workers of all occupation with the scale of zero to one. For example, Gini coefficient measure of 1 would mean that the income distributed to the population is the least equal, while a measure of 0 would mean that the income distributions are completely equal. They calculated the probability of an occupation being taken over by automation and applied three different variables. The first variable is where the workers of post automation become unemployed and earn zero income, the second variable is where the workers earn the minimum wage, and the third variable is where the workers take a 20% pay cut on their income. All of these scenarios lead to a conclusion that increased Gini coefficient causes a greater income inequality, with the first scenario being the most impactful (Hong and Shell 2018).

There is no doubt that Industry 5.0 will affect the welfare at work. While the jobs performed by factory workers during Industry 5.0 will be easier and less strenuous, the increase in working alongside the robots will undoubtedly have psychological effects on some. Humans are social creatures and have the drive to socialize, yet their co-workers most likely are machines. In the future of Industry 5.0, employees will want to work in tight-knitted groups with valuable interactions due to high interactions with AI and robots (Welfare et al. 2019). A key part in the addition to AI and robotics to the workplace is to guarantee that the AI is completely fair and equal to all workers and to manage the instances of unfairness. If businesses decided to try and add social features to the robots, some people may find easier to work alongside them. However, some may see the uncanny aspect of a machine with a social aspect and may become aversive or uncomfortable to work around them (Robert et al. 2020).

2.2.14 ENVIRONMENT AND CLIMATE CHANGE

Currently, our world still utilizes coal and fossil fuels as primary energy source with 80% of global energy consumption are derived from them. Majority of carbon dioxide emissions come from transportation and factories which burn coal and fossil fuels to power their engines, leading to massive carbon dioxide emissions and heavy smoke-related air pollution, leading to environmental issues and health complications (Berhe, Alemayehu, and Fortuin 2014). Water bodies such as rivers and ocean are polluted by companies and factories dumping their industrial waste resulting in the destruction of aquatic wildlife and habitat, such as the River Thames of London (Andrews 1984). The situation worsens as chemical pollution such as mercury was found in fishes and waters of Mithi River of Mumbai and Pearl River Delta. It contaminated the food web, thus jeopardizing global food security (Wong 2017; Bhave and Shrestha 2018). The growing urbanization also leads to more people using cars as mode of transport, which is one of the biggest contributors to the climate change (Wuebbles and Jain 2001).

In the future of Industry 5.0, green technologies will be utilized with the aims to achieve sustainability by protecting and preserving nature (Pathak et al. 2019). Through the bioeconomy vision of Industry 5.0, the societies will switch from fossil fuel to green renewable energy including biomass, biofuels, solar energy, wind energy and more (Patermann and Aguilar 2018; European Commission 2018). Bioeconomy would be a circular economy that integrates environmental preservation and climate change mitigation. The system mainly consists of policies and strategies that promote the use of renewable energy to power facilities. For sectors in agriculture, forestry and other bio-based sectors, policies that pressures companies and factories to opt for operations and processes with greater reduction of GHG emissions. The bioeconomy empowers the future generations to protect and preserve nature while co-existing with our technologically advanced societies.

The human economy will be significantly digitalized through the mass robotification of industries. Studies have shown that digitization can help in the reduction of greenhouse gases (GHG) emissions through lifestyle changes, including reduction in the use of paper minimize deforestation (Al-Khouri 2013; Bieser and Hilty 2018). However, under Industry 5.0, the increased usage of electrical and electronic equipment such as computers, cell phones and refrigerators would also create waste of electrical and electronic equipment (WEEE). Currently, the main treatment strategies for WEEEs are reutilization, recovery/recycling, recovery for energy generation and finally landfill or incineration. Under Industry 5.0, the WEEEs could be efficiently disassembled with human-robots collaboration for processing and recycling (Renteria and Alvarez-de-los-Mozos 2019). Waste management through robots and AI would be more efficient and effective.

2.2.15 CONCLUSION

By all counts, it is likely that Industry 5.0 will be an incremental but necessary shift in the industry, society will see the adoption of AI into the majority of organizations and companies where some labor force will be replaced by AI. IoT will have a greater impact on people's lives as most of their devices will become digitalized and connected worldwide. Alongside these human- and society-based benefits provided by Industry 5.0, nature and Earth will be complemented by the replacement of GHG emitting fossil fuels with renewable energy such as wind and solar power or greener energies such as biofuels. While all the current knowledge of Industry 5.0 is based on the theory of future technologies and we can't be sure exactly how these technologies will be put in place, but we can be certain that we will be able to reap the benefits of them.

REFERENCES

Al-Khouri, A.M. 2013. "Environment sustainability in the age of digital revolution: A review of the field." *American Journal of Humanities and Social Sciences* 1 (4): 202–211.

AlMousa, E., and AlShahwan, F. 2015. "Performance enhancement in 5G mobile network Processing." *Lecture Notes on Information Theory* 3 (1).

Andrews, M.J. 1984. "Thames Estuary: Pollution and Recovery." In *Effects of Pollutants at the Ecosystem Level*, Wiley & Sons, 1984, 195–228.

Antoniuk, L., Gernego, I., Dyba, V., Polishchuk, Y., and Sybirianska, Y. 2017. "Barriers and opportunities for hi-tech innovative small and medium enterprises development in the 4th industrial revolution era." *Problems and Perspectives in Management* 15 (4): 100–113.

Arduengo, M., and L. Sentis. 2018. "Robot Economy: Ready or Not, Here It Comes." arXiv preprint arXiv:1812.01755.

Atkeson, A., and Kehoe, P.J. 2001. *The Transition to a New Economy after the Second Industrial Revolution*(No. w8676). National Bureau of Economic Research.

Bahrin, M.A.K., Othman, M.F., Azli, N.N., and Talib, M.F. 2016. "Industry 4.0: A review on industrial automation and robotic." *Jurnal Teknologi* 78 (6–13): 137–143.

Berhe, A., Alemayehu, T., and Fortuin, K.J.P. 2014. "Environmental impact study of cement factory using a multi-criteria analysis: Evidence from Messebo Cement Factory, Ethiopia." *Developing Country Studies* 4 (24): 151–161.

Bhave, P., and Shrestha, R. 2018. "Total mercury status in an urban water body, Mithi River, Mumbai and analysis of the relation between total mercury and other pollution parameters." *Environmental Monitoring and Assessment* 190 (12): 711.

Bieser, J.C., and Hilty, L.M. 2018. "An Approach to Assess Indirect Environmental Effects of Digitalization Based on a Time-use Perspective." In *Advances and New Trends in Environmental Informatics* (pp. 67–78). Springer: Cham.

Brynjolfsson, E., and McAfee, A. 2011. *Race against the Machine: How the Digital Revolution Is Accelerating Innovation, Driving Productivity, and Irreversibly Transforming Employment and the Economy*. Brynjolfsson and McAfee.

Clark, G. 2008. *A Farewell to Alms: A Brief Economic History of the World* (Vol. 25). Princeton University Press.

Clomburg, J.M., Crumbley, A.M., and Gonzalez, R. 2017. "Industrial biomanufacturing: The future of chemical production." *Science* 355 (6320): aag0804.

Crafts, N. 2005. "The first industrial revolution: Resolving the slow growth/rapid industrialization paradox." *Journal of the European Economic Association* 3 (2–3): 525–534.

Degryse, C. 2016. "Digitalisation of the Economy and Its Impact on Labour Markets." ETUI Research Paper – Working Paper.

Demir, K.A., and Cicibas, H. 2017. "Industry 5.0 and a Critique of Industry 4.0." In *4th International Management Information Systems Conference*, Istanbul, Turkey (pp. 17–20).

Demir, K.A., Döven, G., and Sezen, B. 2019. "Industry 5.0 and human-robot co-working." *Procedia Computer Science* 158, 688–695.

Doyle-Kent, M., and Kopacek, P. 2019. "Industry 5.0: Is the Manufacturing Industry on the Cusp of a New Revolution?" In *Proceedings of the International Symposium for Production Research 2019* (pp. 432–441). Springer, Cham.

Eberhard, B., Podio, M., Alonso, A.P., Radovica, E., Avotina, L., Peiseniece, L., Caamaño Sendon, M., Gonzales Lozano, A. and Solé-Pla, J. 2017. "Smart work: The transformation of the labour market due to the fourth industrial revolution (I4. 0)." *International Journal of Business & Economic Sciences Applied Research* 10 (3).

Elakkiya, N., Karthikeyan, S., and Ravi, T. 2018, March. Survey of Grading Process for Agricultural Foods by Using Artificial Intelligence Technique. In *2018 Second International Conference on Electronics, Communication and Aerospace Technology (ICECA)* (pp. 1834–1838). IEEE.

European Commission. 2018. *A Sustainable Bioeconomy for Europe: Strengthening the Connection between Economy, Society and the Environment.*

Finlay, S. 2017. *Artificial Intelligence and Machine Learning for Business: A No-Nonsense Guide to Data Driven Technologies.* Relativistic, Great Britain.

Fröhlich, H., Balling, R., Beerenwinkel, N., Kohlbacher, O., Kumar, S., Lengauer, T., Maathuis, M.H., Moreau, Y., Murphy, S.A., Przytycka, T.M. and Rebhan, M. 2018. "From hype to reality: Data science enabling personalized medicine." *BMC Medicine* 16 (1): 150.

Grabowski, M., Rowen, A., and Rancy, J.P. 2018. "Evaluation of wearable immersive augmented reality technology in safety-critical systems." *Safety Science* 103, 23–32.

Greenwood, J. 1997. *The Third Industrial Revolution: Technology, Productivity, and Income Inequality* (No. 435). American Enterprise Institute.

Hong, S., and Shell, H. 2018. "The impact of automation on inequality." *Economic Synopses,* (29): 1–2.

Höök, M., and Tang, X. 2013. "Depletion of fossil fuels and anthropogenic climate change—A review." *Energy Policy* 52, 797–809.

Huberman, M., Meissner, C.M., and Oosterlinck, K. 2017. "Technology and geography in the second industrial revolution: New evidence from the margins of trade." *The Journal of Economic History* 77 (1): 39–89.

Ivanov, S.H. 2017. *Robonomics – Principles, Benefits, Challenges, Solutions.* https://www.academia.edu/33711776/Robonomics_principles_benefits_challenges_solutions. PowerPoint Presentation.

Jagadevan, S., Banerjee, A., Banerjee, C., Guria, C., Tiwari, R., Baweja, M., and Shukla, P. 2018. "Recent developments in synthetic biology and metabolic engineering in microalgae towards biofuel production." *Biotechnology for Biofuels* 11 (1): 185.

Kamilaris, A., Fonts, A., and Prenafeta-Boldú, F.X. 2019. "The rise of blockchain technology in agriculture and food supply chains." *Trends in Food Science & Technology* 91, 640–652.

Karvonen, E. 2001. *Informational Societies: Understanding the Third Industrial Revolution.* Tampere University Press.

Kergroach, S. 2017. Industry 4.0: New challenges and opportunities for the labour market. *Форсайт (Foresight and STI Governance)* 11 (4 (eng)): 6–8.

Khor, W.S., Baker, B., Amin, K., Chan, A., Patel, K., and Wong, J. 2016. "Augmented and virtual reality in surgery—The digital surgical environment: Applications, limitations and legal pitfalls." *Annals of Translational Medicine* 4 (23): 454.

Komlos, J. 1998. "Shrinking in a growing economy? The mystery of physical stature during the industrial revolution." *The Journal of Economic History* 58 (3): 779–802.

Kong, L., Khan, M.K., Wu, F., Chen, G., and Zeng, P. 2017. "Millimeter-wave wireless communications for IoT-cloud supported autonomous vehicles: Overview, design, and challenges." *IEEE Communications Magazine* 55 (1): 62–68.

Liu, J., Sun, L., Xu, W., Wang, Q., Yu, S., and Sun, J. 2019. "Current advances and future perspectives of 3D printing natural-derived biopolymers." *Carbohydrate Polymers* 207, 297–316.

Lonshakov, S., A. Krupenkin, A. Kapitonov, E. Radchenko, A. Khassanov, and A. Starostin. 2018. *Robonomics: Platform for Integration of Cyber Physical Systems into Human Economy. White Paper.*

Lu, Y., and Da Xu, L. 2018. "Internet of things (IoT) cybersecurity research: A review of current research topics." *IEEE Internet of Things Journal* 6 (2): 2103–2115.

Luthra, S., Mangla, S.K., Garg, D., and Kumar, A. 2018. "Internet of Things (IoT) in Agriculture Supply Chain Management: A Developing Country Perspective." In *Emerging Markets from a Multidisciplinary Perspective* (pp. 209–220). Springer, Cham.

Madsen, E.S., Bilberg, A., and Hansen, D.G. 2016. "Industry 4.0 and Digitalization Call for Vocational Skills, Applied Industrial Engineering, and Less for Pure Academics." In *Proceedings of the 5th P&OM World Conference on Production and Operations Management (P&OM).*

Makridakis, S. 2017. "The forthcoming Artificial Intelligence (AI) revolution: Its impact on society and firms." *Futures* 90, 46–60.

Manoj Kumar, N., and Dash, A. 2017, November. "Internet of Things: An Opportunity for Transportation and Logistics." In *Proceedings of the International Conference on Inventive Computing and Informatics (ICICI 2017)* (pp. 194–197).

Merk, D., Friedrich, L., Grisoni, F., and Schneider, G. 2018. "De novo design of bioactive small molecules by artificial intelligence." *Molecular Informatics* 37 (1–2): 1700153.

Merlino, M., and Sproģe, I. 2017. "The augmented supply chain." *Procedia Engineering* 178, 308–318.

Mohajan, H. 2019. "The first industrial revolution: Creation of a new global human era." *Journal of Social Sciences and Humanities* 5 (4) 377–387.

Mohajan, H. 2020. "The second industrial revolution has brought modern social and economic developments." *Journal of Social Sciences and Humanities* 6 (1), 1–14

Mohanty, A.K., Misra, M., and Drzal, L.T. 2002. "Sustainable bio-composites from renewable resources: Opportunities and challenges in the green materials world." *Journal of Polymers and the Environment* 10 (1–2): 19–26.

Morone, P., Koutinas, A., Gathergood, N., Arshadi, M., and Matharu, A. 2019. "Food waste: Challenges and opportunities for enhancing the emerging bio-economy." *Journal of Cleaner Production* 221, 10–16.

Morrar, R., Arman, H., and Mousa, S. 2017. "The fourth industrial revolution (Industry 4.0): A social innovation perspective." *Technology Innovation Management Review* 7 (11): 12–20.

Mourtzis, D., Vlachou, E., and Milas, N.J.P.C. 2016. "Industrial Big Data as a result of IoT adoption in manufacturing." *Procedia CIRP* 55, 290–295.

Nahavandi, S. 2019. "Industry 5.0—A human-centric solution." *Sustainability* 11 (16): 4371.

Naik, S.N., Goud, V.V., Rout, P.K., and Dalai, A.K. 2010. "Production of first and second generation biofuels: A comprehensive review." *Renewable and Sustainable Energy Reviews* 14 (2): 578–597.

Naudé, W. 2019. *New Technology, Entrepreneurship and the Revival of Manufacturing in Africa: Opportunities for Youth and Women?* (No. idrcdpru4ir).

Özdemir, V., and Hekim, N. 2018. "Birth of industry 5.0: Making sense of big data with artificial intelligence, 'the internet of things' and next-generation technology policy." *Omics: A Journal of Integrative Biology* 22 (1): 65–76.

Palmarini, R., Erkoyuncu, J.A., Roy, R., and Torabmostaedi, H. 2018. "A systematic review of augmented reality applications in maintenance." *Robotics and Computer-Integrated Manufacturing* 49, 215–228.

Pandey, Amit Kumar, and Rodolphe Gelin. 2018. "A mass-produced sociable humanoid robot: pepper: The first machine of its kind." *IEEE Robotics & Automation Magazine* 25 (3): 40–48.

Patermann, C., and Aguilar, A. 2018. "The origins of the bioeconomy in the European Union." *New Biotechnology* 40, 20–24.

Pathak, P., Pal, P.R., Shrivastava, M., and Ora, P. 2019. "Fifth revolution: Applied AI & human intelligence with cyber physical systems." *International Journal of Engineering and Advanced Technology* 8 (3): 23–27.

Peterson, M.J. 2008. *Roots of Interconnection: Communications, Transportation and Phases of the Industrial Revolution.*

Porter, J.R., L. Xie, A.J. Challinor, K. Cochrane, S.M. Howden, M.M. Iqbal, D.B. Lobell, and M.I. Travasso. 2014. Food security and food production systems. In *Climate Change 2014: Impacts, Adaptation, and Vulnerability. Part A: Global and Sectoral Aspects. Contribution of Working Group II to the Fifth Assessment Report of the Intergovernmental Panel on Climate Change* [Field, C.B., V.R. Barros, D.J. Dokken, K.J. Mach, M.D. Mastrandrea, T.E. Bilir, M. Chatterjee, K.L. Ebi, Y.O. Estrada, R.C. Genova, B. Girma, E.S. Kissel, A.N. Levy, S. MacCracken, P.R. Mastrandrea, and L.L. White (eds.)]. Cambridge University Press, Cambridge, United Kingdom and New York, NY, USA, pp. 485–533.

Prisecaru, P. 2016. "Challenges of the fourth industrial revolution." *Knowledge Horizons – Economics* 8 (1): 57.

Renteria, A., and Alvarez-de-los-Mozos, E. 2019. "Human-Robot Collaboration as a new paradigm in circular economy for WEEE management." *Procedia Manufacturing* 38, 375–382.

Robert, L.P., Pierce, C., Marquis, L., Kim, S., and Alahmad, R. 2020. Designing fair AI for managing employees in organizations: A review, critique, and design agenda." *Human–Computer Interaction* 35, 545–575.

Rosenzweig, C., Iglesius, A., Yang, X.B., Epstein, P.R., and Chivian, E. 2001. Climate change and extreme weather events; Implications for food production, plant diseases, and pests. *Global Change and Human Health* 2, 90–104.

Sachsenmeier, P. 2016. "Industry 5.0—The relevance and implications of bionics and synthetic biology." *Engineering* 2 (2): 225–229.

Sayadi, L.R., Naides, A., Eng, M., Fijany, A., Chopan, M., Sayadi, J.J., Jamasb J. Sayadi, Ashkaun Shaterian, Derek A. Banyard, Gregory R.D. Evans, Raj Vyas, and Widgerow, A.D. 2019. "The new frontier: A review of augmented reality and virtual reality in plastic surgery." *Aesthetic Surgery Journal* 39 (9): 1007–1016.

Schmider, J., Kumar, K., LaForest, C., Swankoski, B., Naim, K., and Caubel, P.M. 2019. "Innovation in pharmacovigilance: Use of artificial intelligence in adverse event case processing." *Clinical Pharmacology & Therapeutics* 105 (4): 954–961.

Schork, N.J. 2019. "Artificial Intelligence and Personalized Medicine." In *Precision Medicine in Cancer Therapy* (pp. 265–283). Springer, Cham.

Schütte, G. 2018. "What kind of innovation policy does the bioeconomy need?" *New Biotechnology* 40, 82–86.

Schwab, K. 2017. *The Fourth Industrial Revolution.* Currency.

Sheth, A., Jaimini, U., Thirunarayan, K., and Banerjee, T. 2017, September. "Augmented Personalized Health: How Smart Data with IoTs and AI Is about to Change Healthcare." In *2017 IEEE 3rd International Forum on Research and Technologies for Society and Industry (RTSI)* (pp. 1–6). IEEE.

Shuba, E.S., and Kifle, D. 2018. "Microalgae to biofuels: 'Promising' alternative and renewable energy, review." *Renewable and Sustainable Energy Reviews* 81, 743–755.

Skobelev, P.O., and Borovik, S.Y. 2017. "On the way from Industry 4.0 to Industry 5.0: From digital manufacturing to digital society." *Industry 4.0* 2 (6): 307–311.

Staffas, L., Gustavsson, M., and McCormick, K. 2013. "Strategies and policies for the bioeconomy and bio-based economy: An analysis of official national approaches." *Sustainability* 5 (6): 2751–2769.

Straathof, A.J., Panke, S., and Schmid, A. 2002. "The production of fine chemicals by biotransformations." *Current Opinion in Biotechnology* 13 (6): 548–556.

Sun, Z., Sun, L., and Strang, K. 2018. "Big data analytics services for enhancing business intelligence." *Journal of Computer Information Systems* 58 (2): 162–169.

Thomas, J. 2009. "Medical records and issues in negligence." *Indian Journal of Urology: Journal of the Urological Society of India* 25 (3): 384.

Wang, B., Wang, Z., Chen, T., and Zhao, X. 2020. "Development of novel bioreactor control systems based on smart sensors and actuators." *Frontiers in Bioengineering and Biotechnology* 8, 7.

Welfare, K.S., Hallowell, M.R., Shah, J.A., and Riek, L.D. 2019. "Consider the Human Work Experience When Integrating Robotics in the Workplace." In *2019 14th ACM/IEEE International Conference on Human-Robot Interaction (HRI)* (pp. 75–84). IEEE.

Wirth, N. 2018. "Hello marketing, what can artificial intelligence help you with?" *International Journal of Market Research* 60 (5): 435–438.

Wong, M.H. 2017. "Chemical pollution and seafood safety, with a focus on mercury: The case of Pearl River Delta, South China." *Environmental Technology & Innovation* 7, 63–76.

Wuebbles, D.J., and Jain, A.K. 2001. "Concerns about climate change and the role of fossil fuel use." *Fuel Processing Technology* 71 (1–3): 99–119.

2.3 Transition of Bio-manufacturing Industry from 4.0 to 5.0

Advances and Challenges

Zahid Majeed, Muhammad Mubashir, and Meng-Choung Chiong

CONTENTS

2.3.1 INTRODUCTION

Bio-manufacturing is economic and sustainable processes of utilization of biological systems such as living organisms, cells and enzymes to produce nature-inspired and newly engineered and intelligent biomolecules for industrial innovation and societal applications. History of bio-manufacturing could be classified into the five generations of revolutions including, bio-manufacturing 1.0, 2.0, 3.0, 4.0 and 5.0. Table 2.3.1 shows the classification of bio-manufacturing revolution and representative products.

Referring to the Table 2.3.1, bio-manufacturing 1.0 revolution focuses on the manufacturing of primary metabolites and bio-manufacturing 2.0 focuses on the production of secondary metabolites. Meanwhile, manufacturing of large-size biomolecules such as enzymes is categorized in bio-manufacturing 3.0.

Bio-manufacturing 4.0 is another classification that focuses on human tissues, artificial starch synthesized by *in-vitro* bio-systems, iso-butanol production using metabolic engineering and synthesis of biology driven organisms. Bio-manufacturing 4.0 revolution could address most important challenges including, food safety, energy production and sustainability, water supply issues and environmental changes (Zhang, Sun, and Ma 2017). Furthermore, adaptation of digital technologies and AI has become prerequisite and competitive in the bio-manufacturing field. Therefore, many bio-manufacturing industries are transforming from human reliance to robots. However, complete implementation and realization of robots is still far (Nahavandi 2019).

In recent years, the bio-manufacturing industry is dependent on the evolution of the Internet of things (IoT) technologies. The concepts of industry have changed into society where things work in networks based on data-driven information. Industry 4.0 encompasses the bio-manufacturing world, which is characterized by use of cyber-physical-based systems. Digital transformation, cloud technology and big data drive massively revolutionized Industry 4.0 which has reshaped our daily life. There are four designs which include, interoperability, information transparency, technical help and decentralized decision. Interoperability is the unification of machines, tools and vehicles through the IoT framework. Subsequently, information transparency is to produce virtual replicas of real-world things. Meanwhile, technical assistance is artificial intelligence to perform a physical activity. On the other hand, decentralized decisions are the stand-alone systems which independently act and complete tasks with high

TABLE 2.3.1
Arrangement of Bio-manufacturing Revolutionary History

Bio-manufacturing Revolutions	Starting Time	Products
Bio-manufacturing 1.0	1910s	Acetone, n-butanol, glycerol, amino acids
Bio-manufacturing 2.0	1940s	Penicillin, tetracycline, streptomycin
Bio-manufacturing 3.0	1980s	Insulin, growth of hormone, enzymes, amylase, cellulose
Bio-manufacturing 4.0	2000s	New food, artificial starch, hydrogen production

accuracy. However, Industry 4.0 revolution has a serious issue which is machine-to-machine communication and thus, it reduces the performance and stability (https://gesrepair.com/industry-4-and-5/). In order to avoid these issues, industrial revolution from 4.0 to 5.0 is needed in the field of bio-manufacturing.

Industry 5.0 pays attention to the human role and IoT-based technologies. In the Industry 5.0 revolution, man and machine work as a team to find solutions together to improve bio-manufacturing industries. In this transient revolution, it is predicted interaction of human intelligence and cognitive computation would be advanced which benefit humans with ease in tasking of bio-manufacturing. Subsequently, Industry 5.0 is more centric to human socialization, integrity and association with nature. In the realm of advancement, a more practical approach is required. The synthetic biology has a central role in reshaping the bio-manufacturing as it uses the principles of biology and engineering.

Overall, transition of the bio-manufacturing industry is complicated and challenging, which needs to be reviewed critically prior to the complete transformation from Industry 4.0 to 5.0. Therefore, in the present book chapter, bio-manufacturing transformation from Industry 4.0 to 5.0 has been critically reviewed. Subsequently, progression methods for bio-manufacturing transformation are highlighted. Furthermore, recent advancement and challenges on bio-manufacturing transformation from 4.0 to 5.0 are deeply analyzed. Besides, various applications of transition bio-manufacturing industries are highlighted in this book chapter.

2.3.2 BIO-MANUFACTURING TRANSFORMATION FROM 4.0 TO 5.0

Industrial transformation from 4.0 to 5.0 is anticipated with more electronic pollution, which obviously needs more smart solutions to address these problems. Transition to Industry 5.0 seems more sustainable, which makes humans more responsible while relying on machines for sustainability, creativity and innovation using man-made intelligent systems. Of course, this synergy will help to fill in the gap of Industry 4.0 in bio-manufacturing processes for process efficiency and sustainability. Industry 4.0 automation will be partially replaced with humans and self-sufficient and machine intelligence. Autonomous workforce will have enhanced human-informed capability to make decisions in Industry 5.0.

Humans teaming up with robots has been seen in the Hotel of Japan for taking orders and serving food; hospitals of China specially deliver food to persons infected with COVID-19 in China. Therefore, it is believed humans working alongside robots will be exceptionally efficient, value-added production processes, reduce waste and running expenses under a regime of trust autonomy. In Industry 5.0 a robot is a programmable machine and can perform repetitive tasks with intelligence as humans do with greater capacity to know and learn through experience.

How bio-manufacturing is done in Industry 5.0 and where robots and humans can work in collaboration. This is important to understand before we take in length different bio-manufacturing under current scenario. Human working is mimicked by a robot. A camera on the robot recorded the activity and sent it to the computer in the form of an image and processed information. This pattern information is retained in memory of robots. Functional near-infrared spectroscopy receives signals via wireless communication channels from the human brain. Robots make predictions, and once confident, it executes function and hence will increase the process efficiency. The improved presentation of current technologies may have transformed machine data and their potential for arraying to cloud computing. This will increase the accessibility to more data-driven services for bio-manufacturing systems. Extensive data sharing across companies and countries is required in production-related sectors in Industry 4.0. Big data collection from wide-range sources and inclusive analysis supports product and quality optimization, making real-time decisions and improving services (Bahrin et al. 2016).

The development of industrial transformation will provide strategic theory support for future industrial development and research direction. It was then applied to explore the higher level of function emerged in the next industrial revolution. The Fifth Industrial Revolution can be triggered by machines with learning functions that will continuously emerge to lead Industry 5.0. Miehe and his co-workers (2020) reported the characterization of bio-manufacturing transformation using systematic knowledge about the biological sciences in order to increase the biotechnology information using machine and industrial learning processes (Miehe et al. 2020). The process of bio-manufacturing transformation can be classified into three modes as shown in Figure 2.3.1 (Miehe et al. 2020). First mode is the inspiration which confirms translation of biological mechanisms into technical value formation systems, functionalities and organizational solutions. Subsequently, the second mode is the information of bio-manufacturing applications which can be used in biological systems to enhance the production system. Meanwhile, the third mode is the development of relation between information and biological systems to produce the new technology which is known as bio-intelligent manufacturing systems.

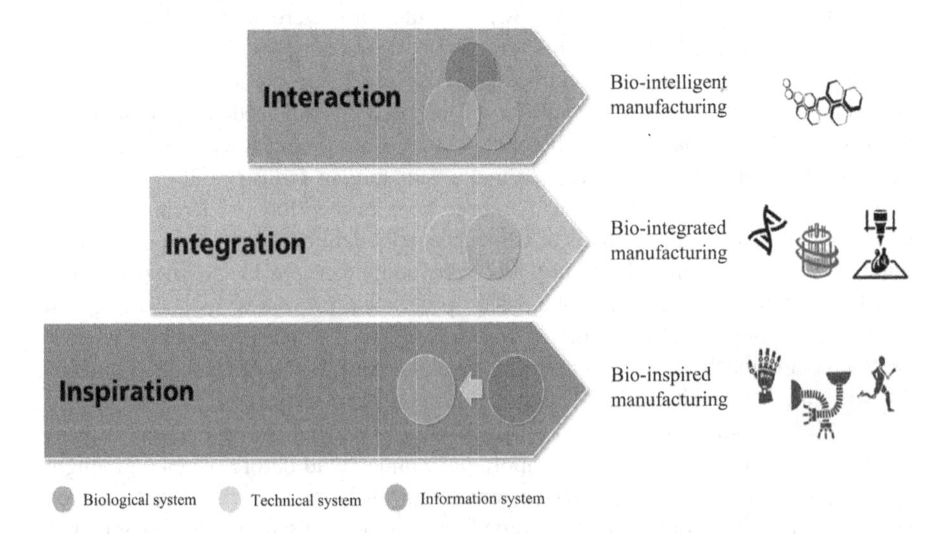

FIGURE 2.3.1 Different modes of bio-manufacturing transformation (Miehe et al. 2018, 2020).

2.3.3 BIO-MANUFACTURING TRANSFORMATION DRIVERS IN INDUSTRY 5.0

Artificial intelligence (AI), synthetic biology, bioengineering and biotechnology are the bio-manufacturing drivers in the industrial transformation to 5.0. AI and synthetic biology are interconnected through natural-like intelligence wherein applying biochemistry to the artificial modelling and recreation of natural intelligence for bio-manufacturing of novel molecules. Biologically inspired artificial systems (biological-like robots) are programmatic transitions from "software" to "hardware models" of natural cognitive processes surely represents for AI a significant embodiment-oriented novelty.

Emerging techniques of chemical synthesis and assembly, applied to biological processes, parts and systems make synthetic biology capable of modifying extant biological cells but more interestingly building synthetic cells, synthetic genome transplantation (Strychalski et al. 2016) and/or through the construction of chemical models (Luisi, Ferri, and Stano 2006). Synthetic biology succeeds in incorporating in these systems self-regulating mechanisms of biological self-organization and self-production with interest for AI (Damiano and Stano 2018). Figure 2.3.2 shows the computer engineered-inspired hierarchy for synthetic

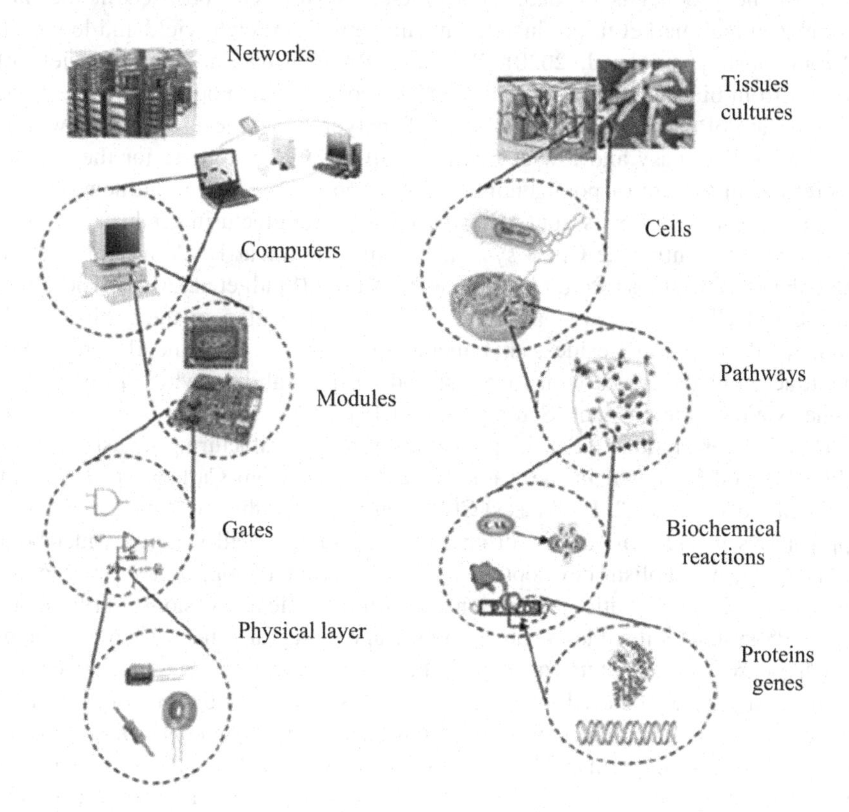

FIGURE 2.3.2 Depiction of computer engineered-inspired hierarchy for synthetic biology (Andrianantoandro et al. 2006).

biology (Andrianantoandro et al. 2006). Referring to Figure 2.3.2, a synthetic biology starting point is to consider biological organisms as systems composed by interconnected parts, in analogy with electronic systems composed by individual components (Andrianantoandro et al. 2006). Furthermore, application of new models of biological materials is very much linked with driving inter-sectorial, interdisciplinary connection, materials science, associated science and AI technology sectors are the significant issues to apply the materials from biological point (Le Feuvre and Scrutton 2018).

On the other hand, cell-free protein synthesis (CFPS) in biotechnology and synthetic biology has significant approaches in *in-vivo* systems by using AI (robotic behaviour) to enhance their abilities for sensing and production using different commands. These potential abilities can be achieved using nanorobotics which have been designed through the dynamic nanomaterials, which can produce the cycling motion. However, to understand the robotic behavior in bio-manufacturing industries still need further research (Ayoubi-Joshaghani et al. 2020).

Development of appropriate systems which have potential to increase production capacity, to make a simple bio-manufacturing system and enhance the yield of the product is needed. This efficient system can be used in the biopharmaceutical market to produce the medicine with efficient yield and low cost. (Ayoubi-Joshaghani et al. 2020). Subsequently, fabrication of higher yield of protein from bio-manufacturing plants at low cost became noticeable through the introduction of pioneer protein synthesis. This type of synthesis of protein will be rapid as well as easy and low cost which will be very beneficial for the human. Therefore, in the era of post-genomic, CFPS approach has been attracted by the various researchers for its application in the bio-manufacturing industry (Chong 2014). Subsequently, the CFPS system contains the linear DNA system to eliminate the cloning steps of old plasmid methods used (Seidi et al. 2018). Therefore, LET-based CFPS method is a potential for its application in the evaluation of engineered proteins. Besides, this method can be used in the different bio-manufacturing industries with low cost and higher stability, which provides the higher yield of the product (Schinn et al. 2016).

Detailed descriptions on each application in bio-manufacturing industries using CFPS method is shown in the Table 2.3.2, adopted from Carlson et al. (2012). Referring to Table 2.3.2, LET-based CFPS could provide the novel platforms for its applications in the bio-manufacturing industries such as cell synthesis, metabolic engineering, metabolism development, novel experimentation, protein production, gene synthesis, therapeutics production and virus particle expressions. Furthermore, the CFPS system is flexible in nature and it can be integrated into different systems which improves its monitoring capabilities to intricate the protein engineering. Besides, this system can reduce the complexity as well as multi components which reduces the cost and time constraints steps in the *in-vivo* engineering platforms (Rosenblum and Cooperman 2014). On the other hand, CFPS can be used in the cell system to control its properties. Even this system can be used to control the obstacles of living organisms by providing different functions in genetic engineering (Shimizu et al. 2006).

TABLE 2.3.2
CFPS System Applications in Biotechnology and Biology Reported in Literature (Ayoubi-Joshaghani et al. 2020)

Specific Potential(s)	Examples	
Production-screening	The rapid and scalable characterizing CRISPR technology, including	
Production and self-assembly of macromolecules	Co-expression and assembly of Virus Like Particles (VLPs) composed of the cytotoxic A2 protein and the coat protein of the bacteriophage Qβ	
Production-folding	Production of membrane	
Production	Immunoglobulin G	
Pathway/network prototyping	UDP-N-acetylglucosamine and UDP-GlcNAc pathway	Zhou et al. (2018)
Bio-sensing	Cheomogenic detection of estrogenic endocrine disruptors (hERb)) in human blood and urine	Seidi et al. (2018)
Glyco-engineering	Site-specific controlled glycosylation of proteins (glycoproteins) using *E. coli* extracts enriched for oligosaccharyltransferases (OSTs) and lipid-linked oligosaccharides (LLOs)	
Synthesis-purification	DNA-modified agarose microbeads and nickel ion-modified agarose for production of EGFP (144.3 μg/ml, 10.1 μg per batch)	
Genetic switches (biosensor)	Programmable, point of care (POC) diagnostics actuated by tiny-molecule (glucose) and RNA (strain-specific Ebola virus) on paper	
Production and labeling (protein engineering)	RNA immobilized magnetic beads coupled with the quasi-continuous transfer of RNA templates to enable automated CFPS for production of the cytotoxic protein Pierisin with simultaneous incorporation of non-canonical amino acid for fluorescence labeling	
Transcription activation-repression (genetic networks)	Two-component oscillator with an activator (sigma factor 28)–repressor (C protein) motif and delayed negative feedback as monitored by deGFP reporter signal	

2.3.4 PROGRESSION METHODS

The progression methods in bio-manufacturing are classified into three categories which includes, cell-based bio-manufacturing, cell-free bio-manufacturing and digital bio-manufacturing, as shown in Figure 2.3.3. Detailed descriptions of each method are given below.

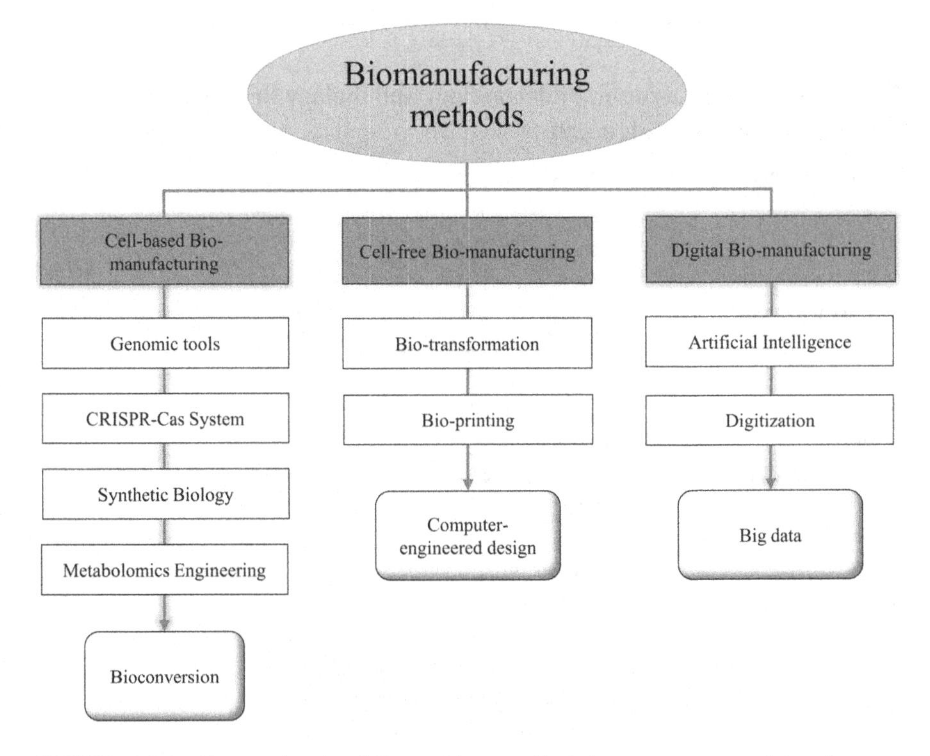

FIGURE 2.3.3 Progression in different bio-manufacturing processes evolving for next generation industrial revolution 5.0.

2.3.4.1 Cell-Based Bio-manufacturing Methods

Cell-based bio-manufacturing methods include genomics tools, clustered regularly interspaced short palindromic repeats (CRISPR) attached with protein scheme and synthetic biology. Genome engineering possesses significant potential, which can affect the scientific knowledge, bio-manufacturing industry, medicines and genetic engineering such as improvement of DNA fabrication. However, the genome possesses the significant disadvantages of weak coordination and integration between the large team which is a very challenging task and thus, it needs to be addressed effectively (Bartley et al. 2020). Subsequently, large delivery of DNA assembly in genomes using efficient methodology is complicated and challenging.

Meanwhile, the CRISPR-Cas system is an RNA-guided next-generation strategy for genetic modifications. This RNA system has been used as a power method for genome editing and heterologous hosts (Komor, Badran, and Liu 2017) for the bio-manufacturing industry. Therefore, application of CRISPR–Cas systems in evaluation and selection of different organisms have reduced the time requirements which is very beneficial at the industrial scale level (Clomburg, Crumbley, and Gonzalez 2017). Furthermore, manufacturing of the CRISPR-Cas system for genetic engineering is necessary for its improvement towards the industrial-scale applications (Westbrook, Moo-Young, and Chou 2016). The CRISPR system uses an alternative endonucleases approach with different recognition technologies along with CRISPR-RNA mechanisms (Ungerer and Pakrasi 2016; Yan et al. 2016).

Synthetic biology is another cell-based bio-manufacturing method that is used in the multidisciplinary area for fabrication of biological components. Synthetic biology refers to the transformation of ability in redesigning biological systems, mainly for industrial application. Synthetic biology plays an important role in helping to turn bioprocessing into industrial production as the challenges of sustainability intensify (Clarke and Kitney 2020). Therefore, the manufacturing of automated design technology is challenging and further research is needed (Gendrault et al. 2014).

2.3.4.2 Cell-Free Bio-manufacturing Methods

Cell-free bio-manufacturing methods can be classified into two categories which includes bio-transformation and bio-printing. Biotransformation can be defined as modification of a defined compound to produce a product with structural similarity by using biological catalysts (Lilly 1994). There are two types of bio-transformation according to the bio-catalysts, which includes microbial and cell-free systems.

On the other hand, bio-materials, printing of cells and extracellular matrix, are called bio-printing (Poh et al. 2016). Bio-printing is complicated, which is limited to synthesis of paradigms which possess small proportions. Therefore, various researchers reported the bio-printing and found innovative designs such as bioreactors that are capable of printing large constructs which can maintain the nutrients and transportation of waste through the cell during the fabrication processes.

2.3.4.3 Digital Bio-manufacturing Method

Digital bio-manufacturing methods have two types, which include AI technologies and digitization methods. AI technologies are based on machine learning in which algorithms are trained on data to extract knowledge driven patterns in systems metabolic engineering (Presnell and Alper 2019). AIs historical success combined with the rise in the data size used to build models and upgrade hardware. The creation of novel chemical descriptors such as topological descriptors (Gozalbes, Doucet, and Derouin 2002) and molecular fingerprints (Willett 2006; McGregor and Muskal 1999) facilitated artificial intelligence in drug discovery, increasing the size/descriptor categories determined from training sets dramatically. Hence, interest in applying artificial intelligence techniques to drug discovery has grown (Vamathevan et al. 2019). Artificial neural networks reflect a form of computing based on how the human brain carries out computations (Beale, Demuth, and Hagan 1996).

On the other hand, digitization is the process of converting information into a digital format. Digitalization has been identified as key strategic activities for the next few years to face these challenges. Bio-manufacturing revolution 4.0 is currently transforming through the addition of digitalization and changing of fundamentals of industries. Besides, the production rate of the product in the bio-manufacturing industry is also enhanced through the application of digitalization in the industrial revolution of 4.0 (Beier et al. 2017). Digitization connects equipment, materials and people. Bio-manufacturers can stand to benefit from process efficiencies, optimized process design, real-time monitoring of supply chain, product quality assurance and ultimately achieve real-time product release.

2.3.5 CHALLENGES AND ISSUES WITH INDUSTRY 4.0–5.0 TRANSFORMATION

Bio-manufacturing transformation from 4.0 to 5.0 is facing challenges and issues that need to be addressed prior to the transformation. These challenges and issues include manpower requirements, optimization of process parameters and production of materials. Detailed descriptions on each parameter are provided in the following subsections.

2.3.5.1 Manpower Requirement

The rapid transformation of the bio-manufacturing industry from 4.0 to 5.0 requires significant manpower to establish the system within industry. Therefore, this issue should be addressed prior to the transformation. This issue can be solved by training programmes which can be divided into two categories: namely university-based education courses and industrial training on bio-manufacturing orientated modules.

2.3.5.2 Optimization of Process Parameters

Optimization of process parameters such as temperature, pressure, feed composition, flow rate and feed ratio are another challenging issue which need to be addressed prior to the transformation. Process parameters in the bio-manufacturing interact with each other, which subsequently affect the performance of industry. Therefore, its optimization is a serious issue during the transformation. Outlook of the world's growing industries, transition from 4.0 to 5.0 is still inadequately understood and hardly anticipated in strategic plans (Sachsenmeier 2016). These process parameters can be optimized via application of different software such as central composite design coupled with response surface methodology.

2.3.5.3 Production of Bio-intelligent Materials

Highly efficient bio-manufacturing may result in overproduction phenomenon and could affect the demand and supply. Implementation transparency can be considered prior to the transformation of industry in order to control the production. Subsequently, the ethical principles should be applied in an autonomous system. Change from 4.0 to 5.0 is anticipated to include high-value assignments in bio-manufacturing approaches. Standardization and legalization will offer assistance to avoid any genuine issues between innovation, culture and businesses (Nahavandi 2019). The robots are interconnected with the human brain and work as partners to monitor development (Nahavandi 2019).

2.3.5.4 *In-vitro* Metabolic Engineering

Simulating and guiding the design of *in-vitro* metabolic engineering is a promising method, especially with the rapid and higher performance of biological measurements of experimental data (Iniesta, Stahl, and McGuffin 2016). However, simulation and design of the *in-vitro* metabolic engineering is challenging and complicated, which needs to be addressed prior to its application. Currently, data-driven models are widely used and one of the bottlenecks is the limitation of high-quality and well-curated data (Mitchell, Michalski, and Carbonell 2013). Numerous *in-vitro* metabolic designing considers have been executed and distributed, there's no database that standardizes these considers, which hinders the creation of data-driven calculations. Building such a database requires both time and effort. Be that as it may, the advancement of a gigantic database, containing thousands of datasets in three to five days is still attainable (Guo, Sheng, and Feng 2017).

2.3.6 BIO-MANUFACTURING INDUSTRY TRANSFORMATION FROM SYNTHETIC TO BIO-INTELLIGENT SYNTHETIC SYSTEMS

In the past few years, bio-manufacturing industries are in the transition state to transform from synthetic products into bio intelligent biosynthetic production systems essential for entering into Industry 5.0. Figure 2.3.4 shows the different transitions in the bio-manufacturing industry in bio-hybrid electronic devices. Electronic to bio-hybrid electronic devices, petroleum-based plastics to bio-plastics, non-living sensor to bio-sensors, tissue transplant to tissue engineering, synthetic raw material to highly functional, efficient and environmental friendly biomass system, reactor to bioreactors, unnatural design to biomimetic designs and computer to soft robotics as shown in Figure 2.3.4. Detailed descriptions on each application are provided below (Guvendiren et al. 2016).

2.3.6.1 Bio-hybrid Electronic Devices

Additive manufacturing bio-hybrid materials and electronic components are of highest relevance for the biological transformation for bio-manufacturing in the next-generation industry. Recent work findings indicate progress in producing these devices, in which, for example, semiconductors made from plant extracts or gelatine insulators can be printed with additive processes on biodegradable circuit boards (e.g., compostable plastic). Later work appears advanced within the innovation required to empower 3D printing with frequently profoundly variable and inhomogeneous biomaterials (Guvendiren et al. 2016). The creation of high-performance skin-like terminals is called for by developing electronic skins with applications in on-body detecting and human-machine interfacing. Profoundly tough, straightforward and breathable epidermal cathode made up of a scaffold-reinforced conductive nanonetwork (SRCN) jam the contacts between the silver (Ag) nanowires by undertaking the lion's share of the stacked push (Fan et al. 2018).

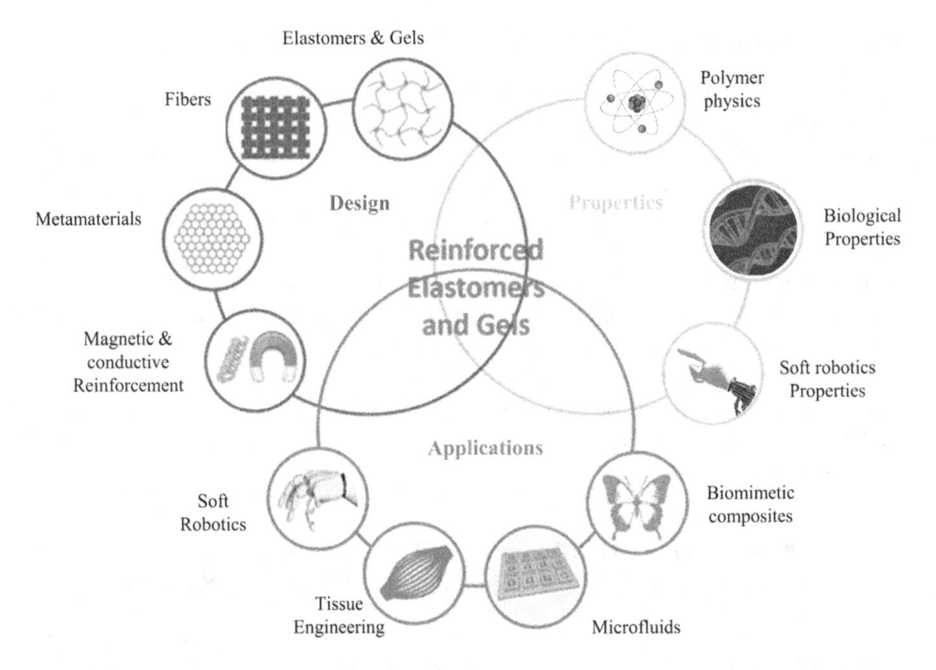

FIGURE 2.3.4 Application of transition industry in bio-hybrid electronic devices (Zhalmuratova and Chung 2020).

2.3.6.2 Bioplastic

A large variety of bio-based plastic materials are available today. Most are biodegradable but there are also long-lasting, reusable and recyclable forms available (Kabasci 2020). 3D printing and fiber composite technology have been applied to produce bio-plastics such as 3D printing and fiber composite technology (Wegst and Ashby 2004). In 2019, plastics fabrication, injection and molding manufacturing industries were in the transition state. The plastic toy bricks have hardly changed their composition in Denmark in the last 50 years. Likewise, other businesses like LEGO enter the sustainable plastics bandwagon by setting the target of making their toys from recycled plant materials by 2030 (de Lorenzo et al. 2018). Bio-based handling of ethylene glycol starts with bioethanol, taken after by lack of hydration to ethylene, oxidation to ethylene oxide and in the long-run hydration to ethylene glycol. The Coca-Cola Company actualized this prepared conspire for their Plant-Bottle development made from partially bio-based polyethylene terephthalate. In addition, direct fermentation of microorganisms with hemicellulose-accessible xylose substrates is under progress (Kabasci 2020). This decision represents one of the shifts with modern bio-manufacturing processes, techniques and products to come in the plastics industry (Romeo 2019). Polyhydroxyalkanoates and other bio-polymers with diverse structures within the shapes of homo-polymers, arbitrary copolymers and piece copolymers are also developed utilizing nano-robots within the bio-industry (de Lorenzo et al. 2018).

2.3.6.3 Biosensors

A biosensor is composed of a component of organic acknowledgment and a physical sensor (transducer), in coordinate touch. A biosensor can be utilized to identify an organic test, and after that create a physical flag (Hellinga and Looger 2017). Key applications of these sensors are man-machine interfacing, which are progressively critical in prosthetics, virtual reality and future fabricating situations among others. In this sense, by connecting human nerve cells with technological components, neurorobotics will dramatically contribute to an advancement of the current technologies.

Biosensor has versatility features, rapid response, high robustness, excellent durability (>10,000 tests), design cut ability and no energy consumption (Liao et al. 2020). Current biosensors often make use of a variety of physical mechanisms linked to electrons to achieve high sensitivity and low detection power. All things considered, these sensors are still particular from the ion-related natural forms of the material sensation of people, and subsequently absent from the reason of bionic applications. Bio-sensors combine the benefits of simple manufacturing processes, ionic-type detection mechanisms and ion injection processes that demonstrate practically possible applications for future wearable electronic and bio-electronic devices (Ding et al. 2020).

2.3.6.4 Novel Pharmaceuticals

Industrial bio-processes have been advanced to produce the medicines and drugs. The use of recent techniques and automation have played an important role at industrial production of medicines (Jullesson et al. 2015). Artificial intelligence methods have moved towards the advances. However, it is necessary to be transparent about these methods to be used to produce the advanced medicines (Walters and Murcko 2020). Subsequently, artificial intelligence is also used for the proper use of medicines at healthcare centers. Predictive analytics for drug-related information are already used in different industries (Zhavoronkov, Vanhaelen, and Oprea 2020).

Some of the pharmaceutical industry's greatest problems are drug research and production that can take years and cost hundreds of millions of dollars. Therefore, these issues can be solved by using different AI and transition of industrial revolution (Zhavoronkov, Vanhaelen, and Oprea 2020). For example, deep learning methods which have recently been used to extend antibiotic arsenal by discovering structurally distinct antibacterial molecules. Halicin – predictions from ZINC15 database compiled by 107 million molecules. Hilacin shows bactericidal movement against a huge extend of pathogens counting mycobacterium tuberculosis and carbapenem-resistant (Stokes et al. 2020)

2.3.6.5 Biomimetic and Soft Robotics

Robots are an intelligent, automated computer designed and developed by humans. These robots are modified with keen computer programs to oversee human-given multi-tasks. The rise of mechanical autonomy has made the bio-producing segments more profitable by sparing time and squandering the coming about items (Kumar and Srinivas 2019). Biomimetic and delicate mechanical technology work, impacted by numerous natural species, has centered on composites of delicate components being fortified by organized hardened components. In specific, structures determined from develop material innovation and recently developing bio-producing methods are fruitful in deterministically accomplishing complex biomimetic structures (Zhalmuratova and Chung 2020).

Soft robotics points to fabricate robots made of adaptable components that allow numerous valuable capabilities, such as shape distortion, control of sensitive objects, encompassing adaptation and development totally different situations within the bio-producing businesses (Martinez et al. 2013). Soft robotics are the potential innovations that will obscure the boundaries between people, robots and the physical labor conveyance (Whitesides 2018). Therefore, it has been widely proposed in the different bio-manufacturing industries. However, application of soft robotics in different bio-manufacturing industries could cause the issues related to the human job recession (Manti, Cacucciolo, and Cianchetti 2016).

2.3.6.6 Tissue Engineering

Design of different materials and their development to interact with the biological systems is called tissue engineering. In recent years, tissue engineering has been modified and modernized using robotics and artificial intelligence at bio-industries. A number of biomaterials have been designed and produced to date for medical treatment such as cancer therapy, ligament and tendon repair, orthopaedic applications, ophthalmic applications for contact lenses design, wound healing, nerve generation reproduction therapy, breast implants and the manufacture of various surgical devices (Biswal, BadJena, and Pradhan 2020). As of late, three-dimensional (3D) and four-dimensional (4D) printing is promising bio-manufacturing advances in biomedical applications for the improvement of custom bone prostheses and useful scaffoldings. The shape memory impact is utilized in materials with current 3D printing methods to form energetic 3D-printed structures beneath the impact of different boosts (Dong et al. 2020) as shown in Figure 2.3.4.

Tissue building ensures the repair or substitution of tissues that are debilitated or unhealthy. Complications in organ transplants tend to be autologous methodologies in bio-manufacturing industries. 3D bioprinting promises to produce entire organs in single setup in the field of bio-manufacturing industries (Hickerson et al. 2020). In addition, mechanical advancements of tissue building of regenerative pharmaceuticals have made a difference researchers get muscle tissue from a parcel of living cell culture tests, clearing the way for *in-vitro* meat generation (Arshad et al. 2017).

2.3.6.7 Biomass-Based Green Energy Systems

The generation and storage of bio-based energy is an integral prerequisite of industrial bio-manufacturing. Both the importance of sustainable bio-based energy systems is substantially growing in the sense of an imminent decarbonization of energy production. A prominent example are the bio-refineries, which are mostly self-sufficient energy units that obtain the necessary energy directly from the processed biomaterial. Robotics and AI in the bio-refinery is increasing which contributes to improve the bio-refinery process as well as products (Amarasekara, Tanzim, and Asmatulu 2017; Zhen et al. 2017). Therefore, an integrated bio-refinery is turning into a promising solution which could produce the efficient biofuel, bioactive compounds and biomaterials (Cervantes, Torres, and Ortega 2020).

2.3.6.8 Bioreactors

Manufacturing of bioreactors is critical for large-scale production of refined chemicals on sustainable energy conserved processes. Bioreactors could conclusively contribute to enhance the production rate of the products in the bio-manufacturing. Therefore, bioreactors are significantly applied for the production of phototrophic organisms which includes micro-algae and bacteria or solar energy sources in the bio-manufacturing industry (Pulz 2001).

Recently, AI and IoT are rapidly entering into the process and bio-manufacturing industry and it will be beneficial to the bioprocess industry. Bio-manufacturing at industrial scale uses advanced analytical tools to analyze the data and enhance the operation performance. Besides, these tools can also be used to scale-up the methodology for the production at industrial scale. Therefore, quantity as well as quality of data obtained from the tools in the bio-manufacturing industry for biofuels and bio-based chemicals are not known as "Big Data". Hence, it reduced the opportunities of process enhancement by data mining (Cuellar and Straathof 2020).

2.3.7 CONCLUSIONS

In the present chapter, contemporary challenges and current trends have been highlighted to open a new perspective for the transition of the bio-manufacturing industry from 4.0 to 5.0. Challenges for the transformation of the bio-manufacturing industry include big-data storage, curation, access, standardization and societal and organization issues are challenges to handle. Furthermore, manpower, which is able to be worked as a workforce for this revolution, is limited and training is needed. Based on the reported literature, it has been found that the innovation in the industrial process is a continuation process of transformation driven by emerging tools of automation to AI. Subsequently, transformation of bio-manufacturing is based on synthetic biology, metabolic engineering and soft material. Furthermore, AI methods such as neural networks have been used to increase the human intelligence in robots that could be used to produce the next generation industrial revolution 5.0.

ACKNOWLEDGMENTS

Authors duly acknowledged the University of Azad Jammu & Kashmir, Pakistan, Asia Pacific University of Technology and Innovation, Malaysia and University of Nottingham Malaysia for the technical support.

REFERENCES

Amarasekara, Asanga, Fairus Sakib Tanzim, and Eylem Asmatulu. 2017. "Briquetting and carbonization of naturally grown algae biomass for low-cost fuel and activated carbon production." *Fuel* 208: 612–617.

Andrianantoandro, Ernesto, Subhayu Basu, David K. Karig, and Ron Weiss. 2006. "Synthetic biology: New engineering rules for an emerging discipline." *Molecular Systems Biology* 2 (1).

Arshad, Muhammad Sajid, Miral Javed, Muhammad Sohaib, Farhan Saeed, Ali Imran, and Zaid Amjad. 2017. "Tissue engineering approaches to develop cultured meat from cells: A mini review." *Cogent Food & Agriculture* 3 (1): 1320814.

Ayoubi-Joshaghani, Mohammad H., Hassan Dianat-Moghadam, Khaled Seidi, Ali Jahanban-Esfahalan, Peyman Zare, and Rana Jahanban-Esfahlan. 2020. "Cell-free protein synthesis: The transition from batch reactions to minimal cells and microfluidic devices." *Biotechnology and Bioengineering* 117 (4): 1204–1229.

Bahrin, Mohd Aiman Kamarul, Mohd Fauzi Othman, N.H. Nor Azli, and Muhamad Farihin Talib. 2016. "Industry 4.0: A review on industrial automation and robotic." *Jurnal Teknologi* 78 (6–13): 137–143.

Bartley, Bryan A., Jacob Beal, Jonathan R. Karr, and Elizabeth A. Strychalski. 2020. "Organizing genome engineering for the gigabase scale." *Nature Communications* 11 (1): 1–9.

Beale, Hagan Demuth, Howard B. Demuth, and M.T. Hagan. 1996. "*Neural Network Design*." PWS, Boston.

Beier, Grischa, Silke Niehoff, Tilla Ziems, and Bing Xue. 2017. "Sustainability aspects of a digitalized industry – A comparative study from China and Germany." *International Journal of Precision Engineering and Manufacturing – Green Technology* 4 (2): 227–234.

Biswal, Trinath, Sushant Kumar BadJena, and Debabrata Pradhan. 2020. "Sustainable biomaterials and their applications: A short review." *Materials Today: Proceedings*, 30, 274–282.

Carlson, Erik D., Rui Gan, C. Eric Hodgman, and Michael C. Jewett. 2012. "Cell-free protein synthesis: Applications come of age." *Biotechnology Advances* 30 (5): 1185–1194.

Cervantes, Gemma, Luis G. Torres, and Mariana Ortega. 2020. "Valorization of Agricultural Wastes and Biorefineries: A Way of Heading to Circular Economy." In *Industrial Symbiosis for the Circular Economy*, 181–194. Springer.

Chong, Shaorong. 2014. "Overview of cell-free protein synthesis: Historic landmarks, commercial systems, and expanding applications." *Current Protocols in Molecular Biology* 108 (1): 16.30.1–16.30.11.

Clarke, Lionel, and Richard Kitney. 2020. "Developing synthetic biology for industrial biotechnology applications." *Biochemical Society Transactions* 48 (1): 113–122.

Clomburg, James M., Anna M. Crumbley, and Ramon Gonzalez. 2017. "Industrial biomanufacturing: The future of chemical production." *Science* 355 (6320): aag0804.

Cuellar, Maria C., and Adrie J.J. Straathof. 2020. "Downstream of the bioreactor: Advancements in recovering fuels and commodity chemicals." *Current Opinion in Biotechnology* 62: 189–195.

Damiano, Luisa, and Pasquale Stano. 2018. "Synthetic biology and artificial intelligence. Grounding a cross-disciplinary approach to the synthetic exploration of (embodied) cognition." *Complex Systems* 27: 199–228.

de Lorenzo, Víctor, Kristala L.J. Prather, Guo-Qiang Chen, Elizabeth O'Day, Conrad von Kameke, Diego A. Oyarzún, Leticia Hosta-Rigau, Habiba Alsafar, Cong Cao, and Weizhi Ji. 2018. "The power of synthetic biology for bioproduction, remediation and pollution control." *EMBO Reports* 19 (4), e45658.

Ding, Hanyuan, Zeqin Xin, Yueyang Yang, Yufeng Luo, Kailun Xia, Bolun Wang, Yufei Sun, Jiaping Wang, Yingying Zhang, and Hui Wu. 2020. "Ultrasensitive, low-voltage operational, and asymmetric ionic sensing hydrogel for multipurpose applications." *Advanced Functional Materials*, 30, 1909616.

Dong, Guirong, Yichen Hu, Yige Huyan, Weiming Zhang, Chenyang Yang, and Longchao Da. 2020. "3D-Printing of Scaffold Within Bionic Vascular Network Applicable to Tissue Engineering." In *Proceedings of the Seventh Asia International Symposium on Mechatronics*.

Fan, You Jun, Xin Li, Shuang Yang Kuang, Lei Zhang, Yang Hui Chen, Lu Liu, Ke Zhang, Si Wei Ma, Fei Liang, and Tao Wu. 2018. "Highly robust, transparent, and breathable epidermal electrode." *ACS Nano* 12 (9): 9326–9332.

Gendrault, Yves, Morgan Madec, Martin Lemaire, Christophe Lallement, and Jacques Haiech. 2014. Automated design of artificial biological functions based on fuzzy logic. In *Proceedings of 2014 IEEE Biomedical Circuits and Systems Conference (BioCAS)*.

Gozalbes, R., J.P. Doucet, and F. Derouin. 2002. "Application of topological descriptors in QSAR and drug design: History and new trends." *Current Drug Targets – Infectious Disorders* 2 (1): 93–102.

Guo, Weihua, Jiayuan Sheng, and Xueyang Feng. 2017. "Mini-review: *In-vitro* metabolic engineering for biomanufacturing of high-value products." *Computational and Structural Biotechnology Journal* 15: 161–167.

Guvendiren, Murat, Joseph Molde, Rosane M.D. Soares, and Joachim Kohn. 2016. "Designing biomaterials for 3D printing." *ACS Biomaterials Science & Engineering* 2 (10): 1679–1693.

Hellinga, Homme W., and Loren L. Looger. 2017. Biosensor. Google Patents.

Hickerson, Darren, Sita Somara, Almudena Martinez-Fernandez, Chi Lo, Todd Meinecke, Cynthia Wilkins-Port, and Julie G. Allickson. 2020. "Chapter 9 – The Next Wave: Tissue Replacement and Organ Replacement." In *Second Generation Cell and Gene-based Therapies*, edited by Alain A. Vertès, Devyn M. Smith, Nasib Qureshi and Nathan J. Dowden, 243–268. Academic Press.

Iniesta, R., D. Stahl, and P. McGuffin. 2016. "Machine learning, statistical learning and the future of biological research in psychiatry." *Psychological Medicine* 46 (12): 2455–2465.

Jullesson, David, Florian David, Brian Pfleger, and Jens Nielsen. 2015. "Impact of synthetic biology and metabolic engineering on industrial production of fine chemicals." *Biotechnology Advances* 33 (7): 1395–1402.

Kabasci, Stephan. 2020. "Chapter 4 – Biobased Plastics." In *Plastic Waste and Recycling*, edited by Trevor M. Letcher, 67–96. Academic Press.

Komor, Alexis C., Ahmed H. Badran, and David R. Liu. 2017. "CRISPR-based technologies for the manipulation of eukaryotic genomes." *Cell* 168 (1–2): 20–36.

Kumar, J.K. Ajay, and G. Srinivas. 2019. Recent trends in robots smart material and its application in aeronautical and aerospace industries. *Journal of Physics: Conference Series*, 1172, 012035.

Le Feuvre, Rosalind A., and Nigel S. Scrutton. 2018. "A living foundry for synthetic biological materials: A synthetic biology roadmap to new advanced materials." *Synthetic and Systems Biotechnology* 3 (2): 105–112.

Liao, Xinqin, Weitao Song, Xiangyu Zhang, Chaoqun Yan, Tianliang Li, Hongliang Ren, Cunzhi Liu, Yongtian Wang, and Yuanjin Zheng. 2020. "A bioinspired analogous nerve towards artificial intelligence." *Nature Communications* 11 (1): 1–9.

Luisi, Pier Luigi, Francesca Ferri, and Pasquale Stano. 2006. "Approaches to semi-synthetic minimal cells: A review." *Naturwissenschaften* 93 (1): 1–13.

Manti, Mariangela, Vito Cacucciolo, and Matteo Cianchetti. 2016. "Stiffening in soft robotics: A review of the state of the art." *IEEE Robotics & Automation Magazine* 23 (3): 93–106.

Martinez, Ramses V., Jamie L. Branch, Carina R. Fish, Lihua Jin, Robert F. Shepherd, Rui M.D. Nunes, Zhigang Suo, and George M. Whitesides. 2013. "Robotic tentacles with three-dimensional mobility based on flexible elastomers." *Advanced Materials* 25 (2): 205–212.

McGregor, Malcolm J., and Steven M. Muskal. 1999. "Pharmacophore fingerprinting. 1. Application to QSAR and focused library design." *Journal of Chemical Information and Computer Sciences* 39 (3): 569–574.

Miehe, R., T. Bauernhansl, M. Beckett, C. Brecher, A. Demmer, W.-G. Drossel, P. Elfert, J. Full, A. Hellmich, and J. Hinxlage. 2020. "The biological transformation of industrial manufacturing – Technologies, status and scenarios for a sustainable future of the German manufacturing industry." *Journal of Manufacturing Systems* 54: 50–61.

Miehe, Robert, Thomas Bauernhansl, Oliver Schwarz, Andrea Traube, Anselm Lorenzoni, Lara Waltersmann, Johannes Full, Jessica Horbelt, and Alexander Sauer. 2018. "The biological transformation of the manufacturing industry – Envisioning biointelligent value adding." *Procedia CIRP* 72: 739–743.

Mitchell, R.S., J.G. Michalski, and T.M. Carbonell. 2013. *An Artificial Intelligence Approach*: Springer.

Nahavandi, Saeid. 2019. "Industry 5.0—A human-centric solution." *Sustainability* 11 (16): 4371.

Poh, Patrina S.P., Mohit P. Chhaya, Felix M. Wunner, Elena M. De-Juan-Pardo, Arndt F. Schilling, Jan-Thorsten Schantz, Martijn van Griensven, and Dietmar W. Hutmacher. 2016. "Polylactides in additive biomanufacturing." *Advanced Drug Delivery Reviews* 107: 228–246. https://doi.org/10.1016/j.addr.2016.07.006.

Presnell, Kristin V., and Hal S. Alper. 2019. "Systems metabolic engineering meets machine learning: A new era for data-driven metabolic engineering." *Biotechnology Journal* 14 (9): 1800416.

Pulz, Otto. 2001. "Photobioreactors: Production systems for phototrophic microorganisms." *Applied Microbiology and Biotechnology* 57 (3): 287–293.

Romeo, Jim. 2019. "Plastics Engineering in 2019: The Technological Runway Ahead: Trends for the coming year include encouraging sustainability, closing the circular economy, and developing viable bioplastics, among others." *Plastics Engineering* 75 (1): 42–47.

Rosenblum, Gabriel, and Barry S. Cooperman. 2014. "Engine out of the chassis: Cell-free protein synthesis and its uses." *FEBS Letters* 588 (2): 261–268.

Sachsenmeier, Peter. 2016. "Industry 5.0—The relevance and implications of bionics and synthetic biology." *Engineering* 2 (2): 225–229.

Schinn, Song-Min, Andrew Broadbent, William T. Bradley, and Bradley C. Bundy. 2016. "Protein synthesis directly from PCR: Progress and applications of cell-free protein synthesis with linear DNA." *New Biotechnology* 33 (4): 480–487.

Seidi, Khaled, Rana Jahanban-Esfahlan, Hassan Monhemi, Peyman Zare, Babak Minofar, Amir Daei Farshchi Adli, Davoud Farajzadeh, Ramezan Behzadi, Mehran Mesgari Abbasi, and Heidi A Neubauer. 2018. "NGR (Asn-Gly-Arg)-targeted delivery of coagulase to tumor vasculature arrests cancer cell growth." *Oncogene* 37 (29): 3967–3980.

Shimizu, Yoshihiro, Yutetsu Kuruma, Bei-Wen Ying, So Umekage, and Takuya Ueda. 2006. "Cell-free translation systems for protein engineering." *The FEBS Journal* 273 (18): 4133–4140.

Stokes, Jonathan M., Kevin Yang, Kyle Swanson, Wengong Jin, Andres Cubillos-Ruiz, Nina M. Donghia, Craig R. MacNair, Shawn French, Lindsey A. Carfrae, and Zohar Bloom-Ackerman. 2020. "A deep learning approach to antibiotic discovery." *Cell* 180 (4): 688–702.e13.

Strychalski, Elizabeth A., Clyde A. Hutchinson III, Ray-Yuan Chuang, Vladimir Noskov, Nacyra Assad-Garcia, Tom J. Deerinck, Mark H. Ellisman, John Gill, Krishna Kannan, and Bogumil J. Karas. 2016. "Design and synthesis of a minimal bacterial genome." *Science* 351 (Science).

Ungerer, Justin, and Himadri B. Pakrasi. 2016. "Cpf1 is a versatile tool for CRISPR genome editing across diverse species of cyanobacteria." *Scientific Reports* 6 (1): 1–9.

Vamathevan, Jessica, Dominic Clark, Paul Czodrowski, Ian Dunham, Edgardo Ferran, George Lee, Bin Li, Anant Madabhushi, Parantu Shah, and Michaela Spitzer. 2019. "Applications of machine learning in drug discovery and development." *Nature Reviews Drug Discovery* 18 (6): 463–477.

Walters, W. Patrick, and Mark Murcko. 2020. "Assessing the impact of generative AI on medicinal chemistry." *Nature Biotechnology* 38 (2): 143–145.

Wegst, U.G.K., and M.F. Ashby. 2004. "The mechanical efficiency of natural materials." *Philosophical Magazine* 84 (21): 2167–2186.

Westbrook, Adam W., Murray Moo-Young, and C. Perry Chou. 2016. "Development of a CRISPR-Cas9 tool kit for comprehensive engineering of *Bacillus subtilis*." *Applied and Environmental Microbiology* 82 (16): 4876–4895.

Whitesides, George M. 2018. "Soft robotics." *Angewandte Chemie International Edition* 57 (16): 4258–4273.

Willett, Peter. 2006. "Similarity-based virtual screening using 2D fingerprints." *Drug Discovery Today* 11 (23–24): 1046–1053.

Yan, Xin, Frances Chu, Aaron W. Puri, Yanfen Fu, and Mary E. Lidstrom. 2016. "Electroporation-based genetic manipulation in type I methanotrophs." *Applied and Environmental Microbiology* 82 (7): 2062–2069.

Zhalmuratova, Dinara, and Hyun-Joong Chung. 2020. "Reinforced gels and elastomers for biomedical and soft robotics applications." *ACS Applied Polymer Materials* 2 (3): 1073–1091.

Zhang, Yi-Heng Percival, Jibin Sun, and Yanhe Ma. 2017. "Biomanufacturing: History and perspective." *Journal of Industrial Microbiology & Biotechnology* 44 (4–5): 773–784.

Zhavoronkov, Alex, Quentin Vanhaelen, and Tudor I. Oprea. 2020. "Will artificial intelligence for drug discovery impact clinical pharmacology?" *Clinical Pharmacology & Therapeutics*, 107, 780–785.

Zhen, Guangyin, Xueqin Lu, Gopalakrishnan Kumar, Péter Bakonyi, Kaiqin Xu, and Youcai Zhao. 2017. "Microbial electrolysis cell platform for simultaneous waste biorefinery and clean electrofuels generation: Current situation, challenges and future perspectives." *Progress in Energy and Combustion Science* 63: 119–145.

Zhou X., Wu H., Cui M., Lai S.N. and Zheng B. 2018. "Long-lived protein expression in hydrogel particles: Towards artificial cells." *Chemical Science* 9 (18): 4275–4279.

3.1 Medicine and Pharmaceuticals Biomanufacturing – Industry 5.0

Zahra Nashath, Doris Ying Ying Tang, Kit Wayne Chew, and Pau Loke Show

CONTENTS

3.1.1 INTRODUCTION

The pharmaceutical industry is often described as a licensed commercial firm to experiment, discover, manufacture, market and distribute the end products (drugs) to those in need of said medication. However, nowadays, changes in consumer behavior, high R&D costs and patient empowerment have impacted the pharmaceutical industry significantly. Additionally, the entire biomanufacturing process with respect to the pharmaceutical industry also faces several challenges, particularly in collecting and processing the large datasets, such as the data from preclinical studies and following phases of clinical trials. Therefore, the coming of Industry 5.0 with the concept of human-machine collaboration with the aid of artificial intelligence (AI) techniques, machine learning (ML), digital apps, 3D printers and other systems will be able to positively revolutionize the pharmaceutical healthcare industry. In other words, the Fifth Industrial Revolution will focus on man-machine collaboration whereby human intelligence operates in conjunction with cognitive computing, resulting in mass customization, automation and personalization in accordance to the needs of each consumer. It is expected to have a dramatic impact on the consumers, pharmaceutical companies, healthcare providers and the world as a whole. To some extent, this paradigm shift is already in motion with the invention of wearable technologies in the healthcare sector, such as small, robust and discrete smart watches that are equipped with advanced sensors. The smart watch is able to monitor all of the body's vital signs, such as heart rate, calories burned and sleep. The data will then be documented and can analyzed by medical practitioners.

Furthermore, due to the large-scale of searchable digital information in a single file, a central healthcare database, known as electronic health records (EHRs), is created to store large quantities of clinical or medical records (Sarkar 2017, 133–51). The deluge of data from several channels or platforms creates the need for a quick and efficient method to analyze this big data for decision making or predictive purposes. The analysis of large datasets by AI is a staple of Industry 5.0 whereby AI is developed to imitate advanced human cognition in order to analyze complicated and large amounts of medical data using algorithms and software. AI technology has evolved to a state where it is able to make good healthcare predictions based on the large datasets available, as proved by the use of the AI Clinician in the treatment of sepsis. The importance of AI in medical diagnostics has also been realized with the development of Lunit, a medical AI software company, that provides AI analysis for chest X-ray, mammography and tissue slides with an accuracy rate of 97%–99% thereby providing appropriate treatment for each patient (Lunit Inc. 2020). Hence, it is essential to ensure that the data produced for analysis is as "clean data" with high-quality standards that requires a standard data structuring system across all platforms and cooperation between the system developers.

Moreover, the use AI in healthcare systems also provides integral opportunities for data collection through doctor-patient interactions. The digitalization of clinical trial data collection allows real-time monitoring without excess expenditure and can also be used in preliminary drug conception stages for drug approval. Moving further down the production line, Industry 5.0 concepts can be applied in the manufacturing stage to identify the variances in batch production and ensure the parameters in all equipment and environmental settings are controlled, thus reducing the chances of equipment or process failure. The demand for personalization has fueled the development of agile manufacturing processes where customized, small-scale batches of medications are produced on demand for each patient based on their medical conditions. In addition, robotic surgery or robot-assisted surgery, a prime example of the possibility of doctor-machine collaborations, has now become commonplace in operating theaters and allows doctors to perform complex surgical procedures with high precision.

Despite the impact and benefits of Industry 5.0 to the pharmaceutical industry, this evolution brings with it several challenges, primarily ethical issues, as technology becomes more intertwined with human lives. Additionally, the use of AI technology in data processing requires further development into synchronized storage systems, data security and automated data scrubbing systems. In short, while there are several challenges and issues still to be resolved before the transition to Industry 5.0, it is clear that it will lead to the advancement of the medical and pharmaceutical industry, particularly in the manufacturing stages, bringing more benefits to humans through machine interactions and AI and in the creation of optimized production lines.

3.1.2 PROGRESSION AND DEVELOPMENTS

The process of drug discovery and development is time (10–17 years or much longer) and cost (approximately $2.558 billion) intensive. Despite the high R&D cost, the success rate of drug approval for marketing is extremely low, usually less than 10% (Wang et al. 2019, 1–10). Catalyzed by an exciting range of cutting-edge technologies in Industry 5.0, all stages of pharmaceutical manufacturing are revolutionized, automated and reshaped, starting from drug synthesis to tabletting or liquefaction to prescription and finally consumption. The greatest asset of the coming Industry 5.0 to the medical industry lies in the cooperation of man (human intelligence) and machine (cognitive computing) to improve the means and efficiency of production. An example is the use of AI to process big data generated through the drug discovery process from multiple users. This can reduce the high production costs and imminent threat from market competition to make the drug discovery process less resource consuming and bring the biomanufacturing process to a new level of speed and quality. Table 3.1.1 indicates the expected changes in the fundamental aspects of the pharmaceutical industry by the Fifth Industrial Revolution.

3.1.3 ADVANCES IN TECHNOLOGY

3.1.3.1 Digitalization of Clinical Trials

A clinical trial is an experiment conducted on a group of volunteer patients to test the efficacy and safety of a new drug, treatment or medical device. It is a critical process in the drug development cycle. Clinical trials are divided into four phases, wherein different phases involve different numbers of participants. For instance, recruitment of 20–80 participants for phase 1; phase 2 involves 100–300 participants; 1,000–3,000 participants for phase 3 and phase 4 involves more than 1,000 participants. Therefore, there is an issue of data collection from these large numbers of participants from multiple regions and countries, especially in long-term follow-up data collection, such as in cancer clinical trials, as most clinical trials still rely on outdated paper-based data collection (Deloitte Luxembourg 2019, 28). Moreover, there are also difficulties in sourcing participants from narrow subsections of society and minority populations. Participation in clinical trials is time-consuming due to the slow enrolment process and requires participants to make regular visits to study sites, normally set in hospitals or

TABLE 3.1.1
The Potential Impacts of Industry 5.0 in the Pharmaceutical Sectors

Impacts	Examples
Advances in technology	• 3D bioprinting (3D-printed organs and living cells) • Human bionics (artificial organs, bionic implants, bionic body part, prosthesis, assistive devices) • Predictive analysis (big data analysis and digitalization of clinical trials) • Cryptopharmaceuticals
Manufacturing process	• Advances on the factory floor (floor monitoring, continuous process verification and identification of nonconformance) • On-demand agile manufacturing and personalization (3D printing of drug and polypill formulations)
Digital therapeutics	• Behavioral programs • Virtual reality (VR) treatment

research centers (Oh et al. 2015, 3–4). The associated inefficiencies and logistical challenges, from the recruitment of participants, data collection and finally study adherence in the early stages of clinical trials, have resulted in eligible participants being reluctant to participate in clinical trials (Deloitte Luxembourg 2019, 28). In fact, less than 10% of eligible individuals are willing to join the clinical trials (Murthy, Krumholz, and Gross 2004, 2722–23) with high dropout rates frequently experienced.

For these reasons, digitalization of clinical trials, also known as virtual or "site less" trials, is slowly gaining traction as a viable option. In this system, clinical trials are conducted outside the study site or in the participant's home (Coravos 2018). Through the digitalization of clinical data collection, participants only need to answer the questionnaire that has been prepared by the investigators through personalized apps installed in their electronic devices, such as wearable technology or smartphones. The data can be obtained constantly and remotely by the investigators for further analysis. The user-friendly mobile apps can notify participants to answer the questionnaire on time and monitor the participants for observational, behavioral or physiological data. Additionally, they allow for direct contact between investigators and participants from other regions or countries and thus allow for timely modifications of the study. The digitalization of clinical trials will also provide data on the daily activities of participants which may affect the findings of the trials to ensure the reliability of the data collected and provide an accurate reflection of the reality and nature of participants' lives (Brucher et al. 2018, 3–4). Instead of going to the clinical center where the trials are conducted in an artificial ecosystem that is set up at the clinical site, the effects of a tested drug can be monitored by the investigators from digital devices worn by participants, providing a whole new clinical trial environment in which more accurate data can be obtained (Edetek 2018). To access patient data, permission can be requested through smartphone apps and users can choose whether to accept or reject access.

The benefits of digitalization of clinical trials are their ability to save time, costs and remove travel obligations of the participants to the testing center. This increases the success of data collection through participants and makes longer monitoring times possible. For example, if a participant visits the clinical sites multiple times a month, the investigator can only gather about 50 hours of data on said participant. However, if the data can be collected passively at home, nearly 4,000 hours of data can be obtained, up to 75 times more as compared to on-site data collection (Coravos 2018). Digitalization of clinical trials enables the integration of data, metadata, systems, standards, processes and resources in one environment (Edetek 2018). Digitalization not only allows for the automated generation of periodic reports, but it also allows for faster generation of ad-hoc reports for timely decision making. This process can increase the engagement and participation of people from all walks of life and thus facilitate the diversification of the population studied to represent the demographic diversity that the new drugs need to cover.

The most concerning issues that arise from the digitalization of clinical trials are missing data and processing of large datasets during the clinical trials which can affect the accuracy of a study. Hence, AI is required to solve this problem and interpret the big data generated. The algorithms are designed to be able to constantly correlate, contextualize and filter the massive raw data in real-time from the sensors without the need for storage. This concept is visualized in Figure 3.1.1 where the sensor in a wearable device measures and collects the data. At the same point, the mobile AI processor analyses the data collected. The results can be saved locally or uploaded to the cloud for storage. Moreover, to process the big data coming from several channels, GNS Healthcare developed the Reverse Engineering, Forward Simulation (REFS) machine learning patterns to analyze the combined clinical trial data for better understanding of the patient's response to certain drugs, predict success rate in the candidate and understand how the drug works in real life. Combined with clinical history, patient treatment and outcome data, REFS can also be used to determine the subpopulations that have positive treatment responses (GNS Healthcare 2020).

Through the digitalization of data collection, data can not only be collected through a centralized healthcare system but also on a patient level through smartphone health apps and wearable sensors. Research into wearable sensors has already

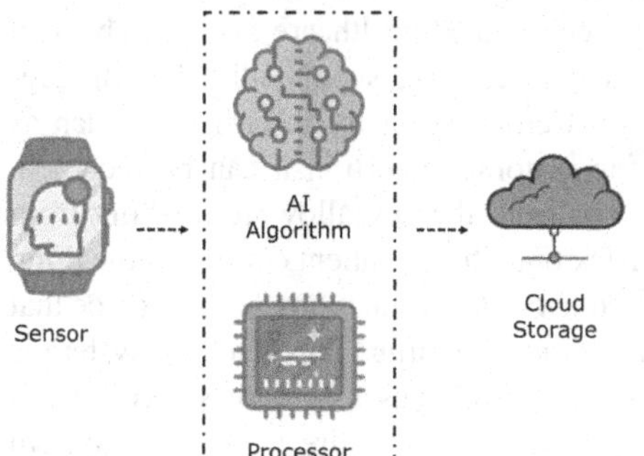

FIGURE 3.1.1 The collection of data and analyzing system through wearable technology.

evolved to a state where sensors are able to track a patient's respiration and emotional state through emotion-related bodily characteristics. A recent review detailed the possibility of detection of continuous temperature mapping through the sensors and stretchable material such as artificial electronic skins (Kumar et al. 2017, 97; Li et al. 2017). Contactless sensing is another monitoring method that forgoes the need for direct skin contact with the use of electrodes and applies the concept of near field coherent sensing (NCS). In this system, microchip tags are incorporated into clothing, for instance near the chest, to monitor vital signs such as heartbeat and blood pressure (Hui and Kan 2018, 74–78). Similar to radar systems, the microchip tags emit radio waves to measure and detect mechanical movement in the organs. The tags are fitted with electromagnetic energy stored in a reader to eradicate the problem of low-battery power supply.

In short, the key to the success of clinical trials is sufficient, appropriate, precise and accurate data for analysis purposes. Since clinical trials are time-consuming as well as requiring constant and continuous monitoring of many participants, the digitalization of clinical data collection will greatly enhance the process, reduce human errors and further the realization of virtual trials.

3.1.3.2 Cryptopharmaceuticals

The increasing demand for drugs puts forward the possibility of drug abuse, raising the need for a method to monitor drug consumption and ensure accountability. The opioid crisis occurring in USA, described by some as "the worst addiction epidemic in American history" (Nachtwey 2019), further cements the necessity for a safeguard system before the widespread use of on-demand drug printing. The sharp increase in medication prices and the resulting financial strain on society is reaching an unsustainable and unacceptable level. Therefore, a strategy must be adopted to reduce costs and while ensuring accountability by rethinking the principles of product design, associated production methods and distribution models. This will ensure all consumers have equal access to medication and maintaining standards for the safety and effectiveness of pharmaceutical products (Nørfeldt et al. 2019, 2838–41).

Therefore, in 2019, a relatively novel concept of cryptopharmaceuticals was introduced through the installation of prototype software in mobile devices such as smartphones. It is a concept that incorporates a blockchain or database of all manufactured and consumed medications into a centralized healthcare system. This can help to monitor and track a drug from its manufacture, supply, distribution, prescription and finally to patient consumption. Certain specialty information, such as changes in temperature during manufacturing, storage and transit can be recorded. Every dose of a medication needs to be serialized, thereby allowing tracking from check in after the manufacturing stage to check out when a patient consumes the drug. The patients will also be able to scan a QR code on the product box for assurance that it is a genuine product and not a generic or counterfeit drug. This tracking system is aided by sensors in wearable technology or smartphones that allows information about the pharmaceutical products to be connected to an entire health care system through the Internet of Things (IoT), a system in which computing devices, mechanical and digital machines are interconnected as displayed in Figure 3.1.2.

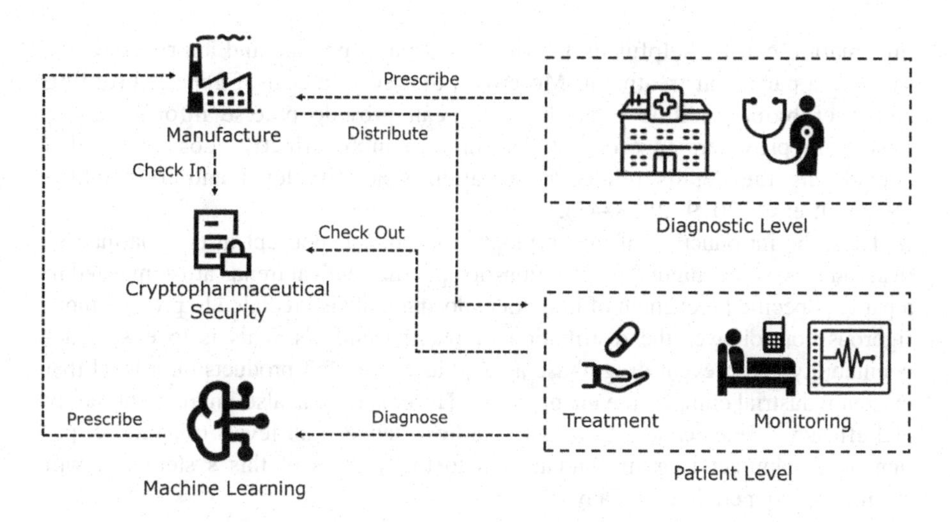

FIGURE 3.1.2 A healthcare system model for Industry 5.0 incorporating IoT.

This system also prevents the production of counterfeit drugs as each dose has a serialized "hash", similar to the Bitcoin system, which is unique to every patient. A hash is a pseudorandom number given in hexadecimal (base 16) and acts as a checksum by enabling data validation without disclosure (Zhang and Ji 2018, 2–3). A fluorescent 3D QR code produced using nanoparticles in colored ink is printed on drug capsules which can be scanned with a smartphone application to decode the code to prove the authenticity of the drug (You et al. 2016, 10096–104). For safety purposes, the QR code produced should be edible. The low-cost QR codes possess high storage capacities per unit area as compared with existing preventative medical counterfeiting measures. The issue of barcode scanning from a digitalized copy to obtain excess medication through this system is raised, so a solution is needed to prevent the scanning of the code from a screen (Nørfeldt et al. 2019, 2838–41). The close monitoring of actual ingestion is becoming a possibility as "smart pills" are approved for use by the FDA. The smart pill contains a swallowable sensor that can track the drug ingestion process from a patient and relay this information to caregivers for greater accountability (Avery and Liu 2011, 331–32). The sensor on the pill is activated as soon as it comes into contact with acidic gastric juice in the stomach. A patch worn on the body works together with the pill in monitoring heart activity and body temperature to ensure drug compliance and send alerts when adverse reactions are experienced or noticed. The smart pills sensor is manufactured with materials found in food, such as magnesium and copper, to prevent rejection or allergic reactions and does not require antennas or batteries.

Additionally, by allowing access to data collected for monitoring purposes, the patient can engage in personalized care and be updated of new dose windows for medication. A growing number of electronic devices are in a position to monitor and report behavioral patterns through installed mobile apps. This information can be helpful in determining a more precise and appropriate dosage for a particular treatment. Moreover, the reduced cost of genetic profiling and microbiota profiling over the years can provide precise information to healthcare providers in order to determine a more effective dosage by also considering the details related to a patient's activity level and food intake (Nørfeldt et al. 2019, 2838–41).

Thus, the introduction of the cryptopharmaceuticals concept in the pharmaceutical industry where unique information-rich pharmaceutical trends are connected in a patient-specific blockchain of individual dosing units is predicted to provide more rigorous control over the distribution of pharmaceuticals. This is to ensure accountability and prevent drug abuse as well as counterfeit products on a level that current industrial climates are unable to do. The concept can also improve the safety and efficacy of medication. Constant data flow between all levels (diagnostic, patient and manufacturing) is fundamental to the success of this system and will require the cooperation of many parties.

3.1.3.3 Human Bionics

Humans bionics is an area which is easy to be visualized as being popularized through Industry 5.0 as it is the actual melding of human and machine. Bionics is a sophisticated technology which can be integrated with various human body parts, where the term "bionic body" originates from. The invention of the bionic eye, an electrical device which helps to restore vision, is an exciting and promising piece of technology. The first bionic implants were tested in 2015 to restore the vision of those diagnosed with retinitis pigmentosa, a rare, hereditary condition in which the light-sensitive retina of the eye progressively degenerates (Humayun, de Juan, and Dagnelie 2016, 89–97). Visual information is obtained from a camera attached to glasses and then transmitted to electrodes connected to the retina to stimulate the retinal cells to direct information to the brain. Patient learning is needed before and after the implantation of bionic eyes. One example of this application can be found in the success of the Argus II Retinal Prosthesis System (retina-based bionic eyes). An analysis of the advances in pixel resolution of the bionic eyes showed an exponential trend similar to Moore's Law, detailing that bionic eyes can reach human eye quality by 2,048 wherein the resolution of bionic eye is predicted to reach 576 megapixels (Bloch, Luo, and da Cruz 2019, 7–8). On the flip side, Argus II Retinal Prosthesis System does not enable the simulation of full controlled color vision or enable the users to perceive colors. Hence, specific parameters for the simulation or generation of color vision needs to be discovered to assist the concept of using electrical stimulation to create color vision (Humayun, de Juan and Dagnelie 2016, 89–97). Future versions of the bionic eye are also expected to have a greater number of smaller electrodes in order to improve the resolution of the observed image (Heiskanen 2019).

In addition to this, there is a system in development that could bypass the retina entirely and relay visual information directly to the brain. This sophisticated bionic eye system is called the Orion Visual Cortical Prosthesis System and has recently gained FDA approval for human clinical trials (Mirochnik and Pezaris 2019, 1–9).

It is a novel visual cortical prosthesis device designed to provide useful artificial vision to people who are blind due to a wide variety of conditions, including glaucoma, diabetic retinopathy, optic nerve damage or eye injury. This system bypasses the retina and optic nerve, the normal visual pathway, and provides stimulation directly to the implants in the occipital lobe of the patient's brain. A transmission coil constantly receives the data wirelessly from external components. The downfall of this system is the necessity of a steep learning curve and lengthy time required for full functionality of the implants because it takes weeks for the electrodes to be individually tuned and requires repetitive calibration exercises. The patient also needs a few months to adapt to the system.

While prosthetic limbs are still the norm worldwide, bionic limbs are slowly gaining popularity due to their increased motor functionality that is comparable to the human limb. Bionic limbs are linked to the neuromuscular system and exploits the residual human nervous system. The electric signals from nerves or muscles above the amputation controls the movement of the limb, allowing the bionic limbs to feel more natural and comfortable to users. To further enhance the experience, sensors are placed along the bionic limb and an algorithm is used to process and deliver the data to the nerve, enabling the user to experience the sensation on their "phantom limb" (Tan et al. 2014, 6–9). Another promising field of human limb bionics is lab printed bones. Currently, scientists are working on the production of ceramic powder that can print artificial bone scaffolds by using a specially configured inkjet printer and CAD software, which can later dissolve as natural bone grows around it (Du, Fu, and Zhu 2018, 4397–412).

Additionally, an exciting development in the field of robotics is the development of robotic hands that are able to "sweat" for thermal management, similar to natural human cooling systems (Mishra et al. 2020, 1–9). This ability allows the soft robot muscle to work for longer periods of time without overheating and the cooling effect is approximately three times more efficient than human systems. When temperatures in the limb exceeds 30 °C, water from the hydrogel is pushed out from micropores on the surface, resulting in water evaporation to cool down the surface by 21 °C in 30 minutes. The micropores are closed once the systems temperature is below 30 °C. The issue of lubrication from the "sweat" which may reduce robotic grip can be addressed by changing the hydrogel's texture to a structure that resembles the wrinkles in human skin. While challenges still lie in the need for a constant water supply which may hinder mobility, it is undoubtably clear this technology will be fundamental to the development of bionic limbs which can imitate human movement mechanisms with added benefits. Moreover, the advancement of bionic technologies in the development of bionic eyes and bionic limbs allows researchers to further explore possibilities beyond the limits of the traditional five senses through the generation of magnetoreception in the future. By 2035, it is predicted that our senses will be upgraded with implants that can detect more signals, for example radio waves and x-rays, through the installation of neuronal implants or small computer chips into the body to interact directly with the nervous systems (Daniel 2012). In short, the advances in bionic technology over the years have helped scientists to develop human bionics, such as bionic arms and bionic legs, to improve our existing abilities and help those with disabilities to live more efficient lives.

3.1.4 MANUFACTURING PROCESS

3.1.4.1 Advances on the Factory Floor

Being the industry that tends to lag behind other industries in technology transition matters, the market dynamics nowadays has generated an urgent need to reform pharmaceutical manufacturing practices. This means all paper-based document management systems will be replaced with electronic document management systems such as Big Data, AI, industrial internet of things (IIOT) and machine-learning. This will have a significant impact on pharmaceutical manufacturing to enhance processes and quality (Brooks 2020). The application of AI can shorten the time needed from the manufacturing process to the final stage of distribution into the market. Every stage of the pharmaceutical manufacture process, from raw material consignment to packaging, provides large quantities of factory data that can be analyzed with AI to reduce manufacturing costs and prevent variances in the production stage. Internet of Things (IoT) sensors can be automated to collect and transfer the factory data within seconds and thus alarm systems can be activated if normal operating conditions are breached. This system is also able to track raw material batch tags, equipment operations, calibration settings and environmental readings such as ambient temperature and pressure (Schmidt 2016). Thus, non-conformance issues can be identified and corrected before the batch is sent for market distribution. Standard procedure in non-conformance cases in pharmaceutical manufacture usually calls for disposing whole batches of drug products and resulting in significant revenue loss and supply problems during epidemic or pandemic periods, for example the coronavirus (COVID-19) pandemic from 2019–2020 and the 2009 flu pandemic. Merck & Co. has developed a system after similar incidents of discarding considerable quantities of vaccines due to non-conformance issues where the data collected by researchers from laboratory testing is processed using software that is able to perform more than 15 million batch-to-batch comparisons in three months, allowing researchers to pinpoint the fermentation stage which may affect the final purification and cause non-conformance (Henschen 2014).

This system can also be used in tandem with continuous process verification (CPV) to ensure consistency and prevent equipment downtimes due to operating failures. In recent years, several regulation authorities, such as the Food and Drug Administration (FDA), require CPV which is the third stage of FDA process validation guidelines to be performed and complied with. If CPV is not carried out by the respective organizations, there is a possibility that the batches of drug products concerned will be withheld from the market. CPV analyses all the aspects of the manufacture process including processing conditions and operating parameters to control the process, prevent batch discards, reduce vulnerabilities in the system, provide continuous improvement and collect a significant quantity of data (Taylor 2019). AI can be used to interpret this big data and identify the areas which require more rigorous control, maintenance or improvement. This further prolongs the lifespan of equipment, minimizes manufacturing downtime and proposes changes to the system based on the monitoring results. After that, a human operator is allowed to take over and implement these actionable changes.

Moreover, the utilization of AI in the biomanufacturing process will revolutionize mass manufacturing, perform repetitive works, reduce human errors and provide high-quality assurance. AI can also create a safe operational environment by reducing the manpower needed to conduct risky and hazardous operations. As a result, the number of workplace accidents will be reduced. Another positive impact is that Internet of Things (IoT) will bring products and services to customers who might not comprehend that they are required. Additionally, IoT can submit in-depth telemetry back to the suppliers and distributors to test quality and identify factors that could lead to failures (Plant Automation Technology 2020). Overall, this proves that many aspects of Industry 5.0 will be applied to the manufacturing process in the pharmaceutical industry to increase overall productivity.

3.1.4.2 On-Demand Agile Manufacturing and Personalization

Agile manufacturing is the new paradigm of pharmaceutical production as conventional methods are gradually losing their efficiency and optimization opportunities. The agile manufacturing concept involves the production of highly customized products while maintaining high standards of quality and, at the same time, controlling the overall production costs. In other words, the manufacturing system should be designed with high flexibility and faster response times to changing customer behaviors, attitudes and demands (Ali, Jahanzaib, and Aziz 2014, 381–86).

In the medical field, personalization is extremely important because different individuals with different medical histories, conditions, genetics, gender, age and body specifications require doses of medication tailored specifically to them. In conventional continuous production lines in biomanufacturing processes, humans need to work in three shifts for 24 hours, frequently resulting in worker lethargy and thus low productivity. On the other hand, AI and robots are capable of working on the production line 24/7, enabling an assembly line to be more responsive to the demands of customers in a timely manner with a readiness to change. Industry 5.0 can cater to these demands through 3D printing. In other words, 3D printers revolutionize and enable full implementation of agile manufacturing (Kuliś 2017). 3D printers are able to produce drugs from digital designs via layer by layer assembly. This increases flexibility over complex, time-consuming conventional methods such as tableting. On-demand 3D printing also circumnavigates the problem of expired drugs. Research into 3D printing has been ongoing for over 30 years, but the first FDA approval for a 3D-printed tablet, SPRITAM®, occurred in 2015. The drug SPRITAM®, produced through 3D printing, has a highly porous structure to increase its solubility upon consumption and this unique feature cannot be achieved using the conventional tabletting method of compression. A simplified schematic diagram of the inkjet printer configuration for pharmaceutical 3D printing can be observed in Figure 3.1.3 (Norman et al. 2017, 39–50). The drug formulation is sprayed onto a powder bed in droplets at a specific rate and in precise movements. The drug will be printed layer by layer, up to 30 or 40 times, depending on the size of the tablet. This production approach not only allows for the manufacture of drug formulations with high complexity but can also create incredibly precise drug structures.

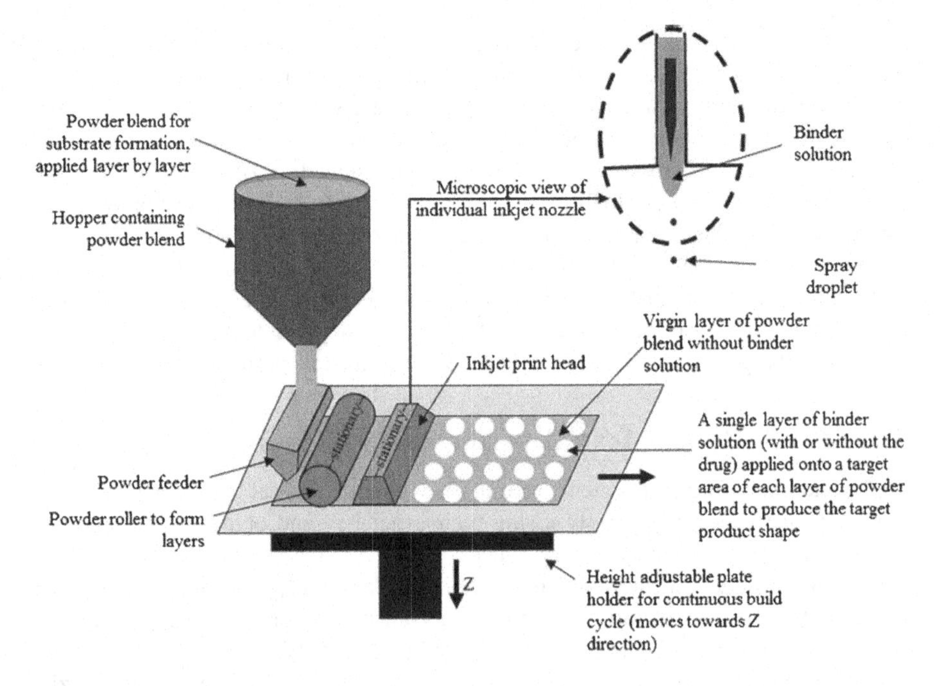

FIGURE 3.1.3 Inkjet configuration for pharmaceutical 3D printing. Used with permission from Elsevier.
Credit: Norman et al. 2017, 39–50.

Furthermore, 3D printing can create lattices, allowing the drug to disperse in the mouth within seconds after being in contact with liquid. This can benefit children, the elderly and other patients who have problems with swallowing pills. It also allows very large doses to be included in a single small tablet (Notman 2018). 3D printing can also produce multiple, small batches of highly personalized medication that is financially viable because swapping between the digital designs requires fewer resources than the modifications of particular equipment for each batch. The personalization or mass customization that is emphasized in agile manufacturing not only allows for more accurate dosing based on patient weight, gender, genetics and metabolism but can also be used for the production of "polypills". Polypills are bilayer tablets comprising of multiple drugs that contain all the medications needed for different ailments or diseases in a single tablet (Khaled et al. 2014, 105–111). This may minimize the amount of tablets a patient with various medical conditions needs to take. 3D printing can overcome the problems of drug compatibility, accidental dose skipping, drug release rate and timescales by allowing multiple drugs to be compartmentalized within a single tablet at which the drugs are released at the designed time with no interactions between different drugs. In other words, 3D printing allows the distribution of medication in a single tablet by changing its concentration and release time (Notman 2018). The speed and ease associated with 3D-printed medication will allow home printed medication to be realized in the future. This will allow patients with low mobility to access drugs from the comfort of their home. As discussed previously, the data, in terms of medication prescribed, can be collected, monitored and sent remotely from wearable technology to the 3D printer for periodic production at the necessary dosing times. On-demand 3D printing can also be applied in operating theaters, where specific tissue scaffolds can be printed directly onto the patients to reduce the chances of rejection by the body (Han et al. 2014, 1–5). To sum up, Industry 5.0 utilizes 3D bioprinting technology to produce 3D-printed fully customizable drug tablets, advancing the realization of personalized medication through agile manufacturing to create medications tailored to meet a patients' specific needs.

3.1.5 DIGITAL THERAPEUTICS

The medical industry in Industry 5.0 is also expected to experience the advent of new therapies known as digital therapeutics, vastly different from the conventional and traditional treatments. Digital therapeutics is a treatment method that uses evidence-based software to deliver treatments to prevent or manage a disease or as a complement to existing treatment. The digital therapeutics market is expected to be worth approximately $9 billion by 2015 and expand by 21% annually (LaRock 2019). There are some digital therapeutics companies, such as Big Health, Roche, Omron, Novartis, Diabeto, Novo Nordisk, Pear Therapeutics and Sanofi, that are already providing this software for practical use. Digital therapeutics can reduce inefficiencies, reduce costs, improve quality and personalize or customize medication for patients, thus transforming the healthcare sector. Digital therapeutics is significantly different from digital care in aspects such as target demographic, regulatory approval needed and others as shown in Table 3.1.2 (Duffy and Lee 2018, 104–6).

To give an example, type 2 diabetes mellitus can be significantly reduced by behavioral interventions such as changes in diet and exercise (Knowler et al. 2002,

TABLE 3.1.2
The Differences between Digital Therapeutics and Digital Care

Aspect	Digital Therapeutics	Digital Care
Fundamental Concept	Personalized treatment to produce a specific biomedical effect	System of both diagnostic and therapeutic modules to produce measured outcomes
Target Demographic	Very specific patients with certain clinical disorders	General population with no specific medical eligibility
Main Purpose	To target and treat a specific outcome through software intervention	Can be loosely set to targets depending on patient's general needs and circumstances
Regulatory Approval	FDA approval required	Regulated by state and federal laws

393–403). However, this method encounters several complications in the frequency of follow ups needed and the problem of scheduling for activities requiring supervision (Delahanty and Nathan 2008, 66). To overcome these issues, the concept of delivering digital intervention for this condition was developed by Omada Health, San Francisco. Through this program, medical devices were incorporated into a network to monitor the nutritional intake, physical activity and weight fluctuations of a patient in order to provide personalized health advice. After three years of running this program, it was reported that the blood sugar levels of diabetic patients reduced significantly and regressed from the diabetes-susceptible range to a normal range (Sepah et al. 2017, 1–9). Furthermore, in 2019, Novo Nordisk collaborated with Flextronics for the production of connected insulin pens to solve the problems of patients skipping injections or not using the correct specific dose. The insulin pens relay data to connected electronic devices which are integrated with diabetes management platforms. It is easier for diabetic patients to manage and administer insulin drugs through this platform. Thus, people with diabetes mellitus and their associated healthcare providers will be able to track glucose monitoring and insulin dosing of the patient automatically, enabling those with diabetes mellitus to have daily management of their condition.

Digital therapy can also be adapted for the treatment of mental health conditions such as schizophrenia, insomnia and depression, for instance, through the digital implementation of cognitive behavioral therapy (CBT) to treat depression and anxiety disorders. In 2017, Pear Therapeutics in Boston partnered with Sandoz to develop an app called reSET to deliver CBT for substance-abuse disorders and drug addiction. ReSET therapy was the first prescription digital therapeutic or mobile medical app authorized for use by the FDA and is intended to be used with outpatient therapy to treat opioid use disorder (OUD). This system works fundamentally through a smartphone application that monitors cravings, triggers and medication to complement the prescribed medical treatments for OUD. Psychiatrists have access to the data for better monitoring of patient progress. This system runs constantly and is an intensive and repetitive therapy to strengthen the neural circuits in the brain to subside cravings. While these applications are known to provide better adherence to the treatment as well as access to mental health resources and user autonomy, there are challenges faced in maintaining patient confidentiality and increasing user competence (Prentice and Dobson 2014, 282–90). Therefore, these applications must have password protection and other security features to prevent electronic records being stolen by a third party.

The COVID-19 crisis debilitated the whole world, placing particular strains on healthcare systems. The weaknesses and inefficiencies in healthcare systems have become obvious and a new solution is needed to reduce points of inefficiency. In Iceland, Nordic startup SideKickHealth together with Reykjavik-gaming group CCP have provided a digital therapeutics platform for COVID-19 patients. This system works in tandem with national emergency services to manage large numbers of people in isolation or in quarantine. The quarantined individuals are required to self-report on their symptoms which will be monitored every 12 hours and recorded via a smartphone app multiple times a day. The individuals in isolation will receive targeted information and support such as prompts, videos and messages from the clinical teams. An algorithm also has been created to classify the patients by disease severity and alert healthcare workers if their condition deteriorates (Lovell 2020).

Furthermore, the improvements in Virtual Reality (VR) technology and the reduced costs associated with it are raising expectations that its use in medicine will become more common. VR technology has been shown to be more effective in the treatment of mental health and evaluation of paranoia and hostility levels, for instance, in the use of VR to treat schizophrenia by the Freeman Company. VR is used to measure anxiety by presenting neutral social situations to patients and observing their reactions to stimuli. By experiencing real-world scenarios created by VR, people can learn to tackle fear, aggression and anxiety. The gameChange clinical trial in July 2019 was the largest trial of a VR schizophrenia therapy. The VR therapy was developed by computer programmers and designers that working side-by-side with people who have experienced psychosis. The participants chose one scenario from a total of six with different difficulty levels, such as the settings of a cafe, pub, bus, street scene, GP waiting room or newsagent. The 30-minute therapy sessions were administered a total of six times. A virtual coach guided the person to overcome his/her fears, playing the role of a real life therapist, which was animated using motion capture and voices of an actor, to offer the recommendations on how their anxiety could be overcome.

As VR headsets are gradually becoming more affordable and mass-produced, the possibility of having access to this technology in one's own home will soon become a reality. However, these digital and VR therapies need to get approval from the respective government and regulatory authorities before they can be sold on the market. In the USA, the FDA classifies these digital therapies as medical devices. This means companies need to follow the regulatory pathways developed for the marketing of medical devices to consumers (Makin 2019). As a result, more stringent clinical trials are required which is a notoriously slow process, resulting in a long wait before these therapies are widely available to the world. In short, digital therapy can reduce the cost of therapy and provide personalized dosage recommendations based on an individuals' condition and relevant environmental factors.

3.1.6 CHALLENGES

3.1.6.1 Ethical Issues

The advent of healthcare apps and monitoring systems installed in electronic devices such as smartphones and the use of AI for remote prescriptions are becoming increasingly popular because treatment options, such as the AI clinician have, in some cases, been found to be more reliable than human clinicians (Komorowski et al. 2018, 1716–20). Nevertheless, the accuracy of predictions and data evaluation by AI is not always completely accurate and AI bias has been found in criminal prediction software where it shows bias against minority races because AI system learning is fundamentally a product of human programers. Therefore, the data needs to be analyzed in a neutral and morally sensitive manner (Angwin et al. 2016).

Big Data is defined as incredibly large datasets that cannot be processed, analyzed, searched or interpreted using conventional methods of data processing. Consequently, they need to be analyzed computationally to identify patterns, trends and other associations. AI is able to sift through this big data from multiple electronic devices on a single patient and compare the obtained data in terms of genetic sequences, gender, age and medical conditions among others in order to prescribe the most appropriate treatment to the patient. However, concerns arise when the machine itself makes mistakes and who is to be responsible for this mistake as the errors may due to device design or susceptibility to software bugs and viruses. Therefore, software quality assurances have been devised to monitor all software activities in order to reduce software failures in medical devices although this does not eliminate the failures completely especially considering the additional levels of complexity produced through frequent technological revolutions (Harrison et al. 2017, 1140–51).

Furthermore, predictive algorithm-driven AI cannot convey the reasoning that led it to its eventual decision and the decision-making process is unclear to the users, the developers and the manufacturers (Bleicher 2017). Considering this, manufacturers have to consider risk management strategies carefully with respect to the design of AI machines either allowing complete machine control or offering room for more human input in the decision making process after the data has been collected, processed and analyzed. A recent review found that current legal models were insufficient to address the harm, injuries or damage caused by the medical use of AI, so the legalities associated with these novel concepts have to be addressed in order to prevent malpractice (Sullivan and Schweikart 2019, 160–66).

The examination of vast quantities of medical data, also known as data mining, has raised issues in the areas of data ownership, privacy and security. In terms of data ownership, the issue of who is entitled to deal with the data collected or sell the data to a third party is a matter for concern despite the act of selling personal information to third party being considered unethical (Cios and Moore 2002, 1–24). Therefore, seeking informed consent from the patients before the collection of data or personal information for medical use or for research purposes is imperative. A recent review found that a majority of medical app developers often share the data without informing or obtaining consent from patients (Grundy et al. 2019, 1–11). Hence, it is essential to maintain physician-patient confidentiality when designing further technological integration.

Moreover, ethical dilemmas also arise in the application of human. The medical necessity of bionic body parts might be hindered by the rush to human augmentation out of want and not need. Bionic limbs are being designed to be stronger and more durable than human legs which may be exploited in manufacturing industries to do repetitive heavy lifting, which can dehumanize workers. Furthermore, most of the research into bionic limbs are funded by military organizations and this will raise the possibility of soldiers being armored with these bionic body parts, creating dangerous robot soldiers reminiscent of the "Iron Man" mechanics for warfare. The role of human bionics in sport has been debated greatly over the past few years, bringing into question the fairness of competition between augmented athletes and those without such enhancement. In the future, as more multiple artificial organs and bionic body parts are being created and are able to function together in a human body, the question arises of whether a human with bionic body parts or artificial organs can still be considered human. Additionally, with the possible creation of an artificial brain and artificial heart, a person is fitted with a semi-organic super-computer that is able to function beyond the ability of a normal human brain or heart and may contribute to extraordinary longevity. It is unclear if such individuals can continue to be defined as simply "human" and if the act is too close to playing God.

Lastly, a recent study published by the Worcester Polytechnic Institute showed that robotic upper limb prosthetics cost approximately $20,000–$120,000 (Morrison and Topping 2012, 1–63) whereas the cost of multi-grip bionic hands was between £25,000 to £60,000 per hand (Fanning and Austin-Morgan 2018). Therefore, only those with adequate financial resources are able to afford these bionic limbs which may create inequity issues in terms of opportunity. In summary, the relevant authorities should take these ethical issues into consideration to prevent the misuse of patient data and the creation of a "superhuman" using advanced human bionics.

3.1.6.2 Challenges in Data Processing

There are some challenges in the processing and storage of large datasets. Among the current available medical health records, only some are in machine-readable formats. Thus, a platform that is able to normalize and standardize the heavy influx of random, unstructured data in order to make it actionable for analysis by a machine is needed. Furthermore, different platforms are created and used for various stages of healthcare and pharmaceutical manufacturing, causing difficulties in rapid data transfer and exchange of information due to the differences in interfaces. In other words, medical devices, EHRs and other IT systems lack interoperability and consistency. Subsequently, this reduces productivity because without a seamless process chain that does not require excessive human intervention, full automation cannot occur (Cantwell and McDermott 2016, 70–76). On a larger scale, international cooperation is required for consistent data collection and comparability in order to observe medical patterns across continents.

Additionally, data collected from various sources in different formats needs to undergo a process known as data cleaning to ensure all the data collected is consistently formatted, compatible with the system and not corrupted. Due to the availability of automatic data cleaning tools, further developmental work is needed to increase the sophistication and precision of these tools to support all the data. This unique problem faced by medical big data collection and analysis is not found in classical statistical analysis. Due to limitations on storage capacity and memory, only a few batches of data can be processed at one time. Therefore, more healthcare firms choose to store their data in the cloud as it is a low-cost solution equipped with cloud disaster recovery.

Furthermore, when dealing with the processing of large quantities of data, the issue of data security must be addressed as it is a matter of client confidentiality. A 2016 study on cybersecurity in healthcare organizations showed that these institutes had experienced cyberattacks at least once a month which resulted in the exposure or release of sensitive patient information. More investment is needed to develop more stringent cybersecurity systems because distributed denial-of-service (DDoS) attacks have already caused healthcare organizations losses of almost $1.32 million in a single year (Ponemon Institute 2016, 1–32). Unsecure medical devices and mobile devices are major areas of concern because data is being accumulated and collected constantly from these electronic devices. Cybercriminals are expending more resources in the exploitation of healthcare data as medical data is non-perishable and can easily be held for ransom. Thus, the FDA has issued guidelines to address the security vulnerability problems on these devices with stricter security measures being required. There is a recommended guideline of safety protocols for medical data storage named the HIPAA Security Rule that covers data security aspects including access controls, auditing, transfer security and authentications (AMA 2020).

Moreover, programs such as the AI Clinician enhance the overall healthcare system by aiding clinicians and providing them with reasonable predictive and diagnostic tools. However, in the context of IBM Watson Health's program for oncology, the AI algorithm has prescribed incorrect treatments to the cancer patients (Topol 2019, 44–56). This happened because the oncologists obtained only a small input of "real data" with the majority of data originating from synthetic and non-real cases for final decision making and analysis. This proves that humans should be engaged in the decision-making process with the help of software as there is still great potential to bring harm to a patient by AI due to flawed algorithms or the "black-box problem" where machine learning renders the algorithms decision-making process unreadable (Harrison et al. 2017, 1140–51).

Thus, while it can be argued that optimizing the collection of big data is the key to a successful transition to Industry 5.0 systems, the challenges arising from the actual data processing stage need to be overcome. Data collected needs to be consistent across all platforms to prevent resource expenditure on reformatting and processing speeds need to be enhanced to prevent the need for bulky local storage as well as fast decision making.

3.1.6.3 Designing for Human–Computer Interactions

Despite the positive attributes of Industry 5.0 through the invention of more electronic medical devices, manufacturers need to consider the design of these devices before widespread implementation as, according to the FDA, medical devices errors caused more than 10,000 injuries between 2008 to 2017 in the United States (Stowers and Mouloua 2018, 88–91) due to faulty device design and user error. Devices need to incorporate user interfaces that are easy to understand and respond to, as many patients have varying levels of medical knowledge. As medical devices are becoming more personalized and mostly used for outpatient care, the operation of these devices should be simplistic, user-friendly and understandable enough to be operated by patients from different backgrounds and not only by medical professionals. Inoperability has become a challenge to users as they have varying levels of understanding of their condition, mobility and cognitive abilities which may affect their capability to use these devices correctly. Therefore, in 2012, the FDA released documentation recommending medical device designers to consider the literacy and emotional levels of potential users during design to ensure operation is user-friendly.

Similarly, the environment in which these medical devices will be used must also be put into consideration. Previously, medical devices were designed for the sterile and more controlled settings of hospital environments but with the coming of Industry 5.0, these portable devices will also be used for care outside of hospitals. Therefore, medical devices should be designed to withstand many environmental factors such as noise, lighting and space limitations. This is the reason why medical device manufacturers need to consider the availability of power sources and frequency of charging needed in case the devices use a battery as a power source. Even in the pharmaceutical manufacturing industry, the devices anticipatory behavior will need to be improved upon on the transition to Industry 5.0. The current state of computer vision and deep learning is not advanced enough to use emotional intelligence to sense the unnatural, spontaneous events in a workplace and make judgments. Hence, sensory technology and analysis methods must be developed to mimic how a human operator would react to certain stimuli. Deep learning algorithms in a deep neural network (DNN) have shown more promise than conventional learning methods for robotic vision.

Lastly, another design challenge lies in bionics technology, particularly in reference to the bionic eye. The retina of the eye contains photoreceptors cells that are responsible for visual recognition. The bionic vision system works by transmitting high-frequency radio signals from a camera to a microchip implanted in the retina or back of the brain. The bionic implant will stimulate the retina and excite all the cells. This may cause over-stimulation which results in blurred vision, fuzzy contours, indistinct shapes or loss of visual input for a fast-moving object. Misinterpretation could also occur due to the inability of patients to read or interpret numbers, fine text, facial expressions and street signs, putting users in harm.

Considering these challenges, it is clear that conventional medical design standards can no longer be applied in Industry 5.0, and medical devices should be designed with focus on simplicity without being dependant on the user having prior medical knowledge. The challenges concerning user acclimatization to this new technology will also have to be addressed and overcome.

3.1.6.4 Job Security

As the main premise behind Industry 5.0 is human-machine integration, a primary concern among healthcare workers is the availability of job opportunities due to increased digitalization and use of robotics in the medical field. In the pharmaceutical manufacturing industry, repetitive and labor-intensive tasks are gradually being replaced by robots or AI, for example robotic arms. AI will also potentially replace many white-collar tasks, particularly at the manufacture level, to increase operational efficiency, reduce production costs and make faster, more informed decisions. On the other hand, human workers are needed for innovation, customization, cognitive computing and maintenance of the machines as well as the AI systems. To prevent occupational hazards and injury cases, a restructure of the workforce with AI and robotic technology would be beneficial as it provides value-added tasks to the production line and increases productivity. Considering these points, it is understandable why employees are worried that automation will be a threat to job security as more tasks are replaced by AI in the future.

Instead of causing unemployment in the long run however, automation only replaces the need for humans to perform repetitive and monotonous tasks and thus cannot substitute all jobs completely. This will also create opportunities for high-skill or high-value jobs in the industry, including the manufacturing stages. This system of functioning, when applied to a biomanufacturing process, has been found to be more productive, efficient and durable (Au-Yong-Oliveira et al. 2019, 348–57), creating more demand for employees in certain fields such as chemical engineers, physicists, artificial intelligence developers, market-research analysts, data scientists, machine learning engineers and research scientists. In short, automation creates job opportunities for roles that require human intelligence and innovation and replaces unskilled job tasks. It is important to keep in mind that while robots and machines can co-exist with humans, AI or automation cannot replace humans completely.

3.1.7 FUTURE PROSPECTS

In general, this chapter covered research and innovations in the pharmaceutical field that are already in developmental stages or in small-scale use, but there are still other promising areas which are in the early research or designing stages and will become fundamental to Industry 5.0. As previously discussed, 3D printing is extremely convenient for the production of on-demand pharmaceuticals and even human tissue. 3D bioprinting has been suggested as a means to overcome the existing issues with the high demand for organ transplants as there are more than 100,000 people in USA on the waiting list for organ transplants. Precise and highly specific 3D bioprinting is being developed to dispense specific types of cells into bio-scaffolding in specific locations in order to construct organs. This process uses microelectromechanical systems (MEMS) to construct certain structures but problems still lie in creating biological tissue with multiple layers on a large scale (Yoo 2015, 507–11). In the process of printing, cell viability may decrease and the system should be able to maintain its spatial accuracy. Specific bioreactors are also needed after the printing stage to support the organ while its cells experience additional growth before implantation. Besides this, 3D printing is still not capable of creating the fine structures of organs on a large scale or with full functionality. In 2019, a 3D bioprinting technique called projection stereolithography was used to print vessels less than a third of a millimeter wide needed to construct lungs (Grigoryan et al. 2019, 458–64). While this development is promising, there are several fine structures such as blood vessels and bile ducts that operate in independent networks that need to be synthesized before complete organ printing is realized. As of yet, 3D-printed organs are not likely to be developed for widespread use in the current decade; however, the concepts behind this can still be applied to medical research such as in the creation of artificial skin or tissue models for experimentation.

The advances in human bionics exemplifies the human-machine interactions that are unique to Industry 5.0, yet a more ambitious project is on the horizon: robotic exoskeletons. From a medical standpoint, exoskeletons are robotic devices that can restore full mobility to patients with disabilities or the elderly. Exoskeletons require rigorous control with position or force sensors, actuator control and high-speed signal processing in order to produce motion by the actuators (Bogue 2015, 5–10). While sensor and processing technologies are currently adequate, the power source and hydraulic actuators add too much weight onto the exoskeleton. To overcome these problems, remote charging through wireless energy transfer has been considered yet this is still an emerging technology. Nanomaterials, carbon fibers and metal or polymer composites are being investigated as a lightweight but strong material to build the main structure. It is predicted that the technology should ideally evolve into a stage where the exoskeleton is able to be used and controlled using thoughts rather than small movements signalling how they are expected to move. A global research effort of creating a brain computer interface (BCI) is currently ongoing to help the severely disabled to regain their mobility. Furthermore, these exoskeletons can also help to reduce workplace injuries among manual workers who perform tasks involving significant physical exertion. The advancement of bionic technology can be seen in the progress of identification via facial recognition technology in bionic eyes as well as in the detection of potentially harmful radiation in the atmosphere through microchips inserted under the skin.

As personalization is one of the main tenets of the Industry 5.0 revolution, cancer vaccines deserve a mention as an effective prospective technology. Cancer immunotherapy is a novel technique as it manipulates the immune system to produce immune cells to kill tumor cells instead of targeting the tumor directly. As tumor cells are constantly evolving and differ greatly from patient to patient, personalization of medicine is instrumental in developing this therapy. Studies on prostate cancer therapy where algorithms were tested using patient data before treatment, was used to formulate the personalized prostate cancer vaccines showed that this method of personalized treatment is feasible (Kogan et al. 2012, 2218–27).

Many developments are still occurring to enable constant monitoring through wearable technology (Chen, 2018), most recently in the development of a glucose monitoring contact lens fitted with a graphene sensor. As blood glucose testing is still an uncomfortable procedure necessitating the drawing of a blood sample by a prick, this contact lens would be a non-invasive method to monitor glucose levels as they can be measured through tears. While previous versions have been unwearable due to the use of less flexible materials that can cause eye discomfort, a model developed by the Ulsan National Institute of Science and Technology deconstructs the graphene sensor, with each piece enrobed in soft polymer yet still connected through a flexible mesh (Park et al. 2018, 1–11). This flexibility not only provides comfort but also enables the lens to be bent and removed like conventional lenses. The device consists of a sensor, rectifier, LED display and stretchable antenna, ensuring no external power source is needed. Furthermore, this device could also be implemented for use by glaucoma patients as the presence of dielectric layers enables the monitoring of intraocular pressure.

Prediction technology in Industry 5.0 allows for smart sensing networks that are able to use the human brain as a source of signals through functional near-infrared spectroscopy (fNIRS). These are wireless headsets that can capture brain waves and can be used to predict intent and for contextual awareness (Nahavandi 2019, 1–13). Data obtained by the fNIRS is sent to a deep learning algorithm to process and determine the intent of the user. In this way, an operator can request a secondary robotic arm to complete procedures ranging from handing over specific instruments to performing simple operations on bodies through brain function control. While this technology is still far from being realized, it is a prime example of healthcare in Industry 5.0 as the human operator is not removed from the procedure but the process efficiency of said procedure is improved. Furthermore, remote diagnostic procedures will be aided through this technology as a human operator will not be required to be in the same room as the patient. In summary, AI and automation are progressing rapidly, enabling the medical and pharmaceutical industry to go farther and provide more efficient treatments for the betterment of patients' lives.

3.1.8 CONCLUSION

In conclusion, Industry 5.0 will emphasize the concepts of automation and personalization via Internet of Things, big data and AI. The Fifth Industrial Revolution is on the horizon with the expectation of integration between humans and machines for autonomous manufacturing. This revolution comes with increased opportunities for the custom tailoring of products for different consumers' needs. Subsequently, this phenomenon will starkly affect the medicine and pharmaceutical industry as individual personalization concepts based on each patient's needs is introduced. As discussed in this chapter, the key to data collection lies in the network of sensors installed in electronic devices. With the aid of AI and IoT, data is able to be stored directly in the cloud to prevent bulky local storage hardware and for monitoring purposes without the waste of human resources. Moreover, there have been great advances in pharmaceutical biomanufacturing processes through the introduction of 3D printing for the production of pills or tablets, advancements on the factory floor as well as agile manufacturing. Nevertheless, there are still some unprecedented challenges facing the world today due to human-machine integration, such as the ethical issues arising from human bionics, challenges in processing large datasets and cybersecurity issues. Future prospects will focus more intently on furthering customization, bioprinting of organs and the creation of fine and miniscule biological structures with high precision. The healthcare industry is sure to be aided by the coming of such technology as the biosensing contact lenses for glucose monitoring and the development of more ambitious wireless headsets for machine control. The possible integration of human and machine (AI and robots) in minute aspects of daily life displays how Industry 5.0 can be applied to improve health and well-being on a fundamental level. It will also open up new avenues of innovation for humans as menial tasks are taken up by machines and AI. This human-machine interaction will minimize occupational hazards and speed up manufacturing processes too. In the long run, this will create more job opportunities as more human resources are needed for the upkeep of intelligence systems including programming, training and maintenance. Although it is a concept in the distant technological horizon for now and we are still in the process of realizing the true vision of Industry 4.0, it is clear that Industry 5.0 or the Fifth Industrial Revolution will revolve around the collaboration between man and machine and bring major positive changes to the medical and pharmaceutical industry.

REFERENCES

Ali, Abid, Mirza Jahanzaib, and Haris Aziz. 2014. "Manufacturing flexibility and agility: A distinctive comparison." *Nucleus* 51 (3): 379–384.

AMA. 2020. *HIPAA Security Rule & Risk Analysis*. American Medical Association. https://www.ama-assn.org/practice-management/hipaa/hipaa-security-rule-risk-analysis.

Angwin, J., J. Larson, S. Mattu, and L. Kirchner. 2016. *Machine Bias—ProPublica*. https://www.propublica.org/article/machine-bias-risk-assessments-in-criminal-sentencing.

Au-Yong-Oliveira, Manuel, Diogo Canastro, Joana Oliveira, João Tomás, Sofia Amorim, and Fernando Moreira. 2019. "The role of AI and automation on the future of jobs and the opportunity to change society." *Advances in Intelligent Systems and Computing*. Springer Verlag. 348–357.

Avery, Matthew, and Dan Liu. 2011. "Bringing smart pills to market: FDA regulation of ingestible drug/device combination products." *Food and Drug Law Journal* 66, 329–352.

Bleicher, A. 2017. *Demystifying the Black Box That Is AI* Scientific American. https://www.scientificamerican.com/article/demystifying-the-black-box-that-is-ai/.

Bloch, Edward, Yvonne Luo, and Lyndon da Cruz. 2019. "Advances in retinal prosthesis systems." Therapeutic Advances in Ophthalmology 11: 251584141881750.

Bogue, Robert. 2015. "Robotic exoskeletons: A review of recent progress." *Industrial Robot* 42 (1): 5–10.

Brooks, Kristin. 2020. *The Future of Pharmaceutical Manufacturing*. Contract Pharma. https://www.contractpharma.com/contents/view_online-exclusives/2020-02-12/the-future-of-pharmaceutical-manufacturing/.

Brucher, Luc, Carlo Duprel, Alexandra Georges, and Yasmin Kilders. 2018. "Digitalization of clinical trials; How new technologies enhance the future of health care." Inside magazine Issue 19, Part 02-From a core transformation/technology perspective, DeloitteWebsite: https://www2.deloitte.com/lu/en/pages/life-sciences-and-healthcare/articles/digitalization-clinical-trials.html.

Cantwell, Ed, and Kerry McDermott. 2016. "Making technology talk: How interoperability can improve care, drive efficiency, and reduce waste." *Healthcare Financial Management: Journal of the Healthcare Financial Management Association* 70 (5): 70–76.

Chen, Wei Ting, Alexander Y. Zhu, Vyshakh Sanjeev, Mohammadreza Khorasaninejad, Zhujun Shi, Eric Lee, and Federico Capasso. 2018. "A broadband achromatic metalens for focusing and imaging in the visible." *Nature Nanotechnology* 13 (3): 220–226.

Cios, Krzysztof J., and G. William Moore. 2002. "Uniqueness of medical data mining." *Artificial Intelligence in Medicine* 26 (1–2): 1–24.

Coravos, Andy. 2018. *Software-Enabled Clinical Trials*. https://blog.andreacoravos.com/software-enabled-clinical-trials-8da53f4cd271.

Delahanty, Linda M., and David M. Nathan. 2008. "Implications of the diabetes prevention program and Look AHEAD clinical trials for lifestyle interventions." *Journal of the American Dietetic Association* 108 (4 Suppl.): S66.

Deloitte Luxembourg. 2019. "Luxembourg Towards a Smart Nation." MarCom at Deloitte LuxembourgWebsite: https://www2.deloitte.com/lu/en/pages/public-sector/articles/luxembourg-towards-smart-nation.html.

Daniel, Ari. 2012. *Engineering Extra Senses: Technology and the Human Body | The World from PRX.* https://www.pri.org/stories/2012-11-14/engineering-extra-senses-technology-and-human-body.

Du, Xiaoyu, Shengyang Fu, and Yufang Zhu. 2018. "3D printing of ceramic-based scaffolds for bone tissue engineering: An overview." *Journal of Materials Chemistry B*. Vol. 6. no. 27. Royal Society of Chemistry, 11 7. 4397–4412.

Duffy, Sean, and Thomas H. Lee. 2018. "In-person health care as option B." *New England Journal of Medicine*. Vol. 378. no. 2. Massachussetts Medical Society, 11 1. 104–106.

Edetek. 2018. *EDETEK to Showcase Digital Clinical Trial Solutions at DIA 2018*. https://www.edetek.com/edetek-to-showcase-digital-clinical-trial-solutions-at-dia-2018/.

Fanning, Paul, and Tom Austin-Morgan. 2018. *Getting to Grips with Bionic Costs*. https://www.eurekamagazine.co.uk/design-engineering-features/technology/getting-to-grips-with-bionic-costs/173342/.

GNS Healthcare. 2020. *Causal Machine Learning: Healthcare Artificial Intelligence (AI) – REFS Platform by GNS Healthcare*. https://www.gnshealthcare.com/refs-platform/.

Grigoryan, Bagrat, Samantha J. Paulsen, Daniel C. Corbett, Daniel W. Sazer, Chelsea L. Fortin, Alexander J. Zaita, Paul T. Greenfield, et al. 2019. "Multivascular networks and functional intravascular topologies within biocompatible hydrogels." *Science* 364 (6439): 458–464.

Grundy, Quinn, Kellia Chiu, Fabian Held, Andrea Continella, Lisa Bero, and Ralph Holz. 2019. "Data sharing practices of medicines related apps and the mobile ecosystem: Traffic, content, and network analysis." *BMJ Online* 364.

Han, Yu Long, Jie Hu, Guy M. Genin, Tian Jian Lu, and Feng Xu. 2014. "BioPen: Direct writing of functional materials at the point of care." *Scientific Reports* 4 (1): 1–5.

Harrison, Richard P., Steven Ruck, Nicholas Medcalf, and Qasim A. Rafiq. 2017. "Decentralized manufacturing of cell and gene therapies: Overcoming challenges and identifying opportunities." *Cytotherapy*. Vol. 19. no. 10. Elsevier B.V., 1 10. 1140–1151.

Heiskanen, M. 2019. *Can You See the Future of Bionic Body? Nordic Business Report*. https://www.nbforum.com/nbreport/can-you-see-the-future-of-bionic-body/.

Henschen, D. 2014. *Merck Optimizes Manufacturing with Big Data Analytics*. InformationWeek. https://www.informationweek.com/strategic-cio/executive-insights-and-innovation/merck-optimizes-manufacturing-with-big-data-analytics/d/d-id/1127901.

Hui, Xiaonan, and Edwin C. Kan. 2018. "Monitoring vital signs over multiplexed radio by near-field coherent sensing." *Nature Electronics* 1 (1): 74–78.

Humayun, Mark S., Eugene de Juan, and Gislin Dagnelie. 2016. "The bionic eye: A quarter century of retinal prosthesis research and development." *Ophthalmology* 123 (10): S89–S97.

Khaled, Shaban A., Jonathan C. Burley, Morgan R. Alexander, and Clive J. Roberts. 2014. "Desktop 3D printing of controlled release pharmaceutical bilayer tablets." *International Journal of Pharmaceutics* (Elsevier) 461 (1–2): 105–111.

Knowler, William C., Elizabeth Barrett-Connor, Sarah E. Fowler, Richard F. Hamman, John M. Lachin, Elizabeth A. Walker, and David M. Nathan. 2002. "Reduction in the incidence of type 2 diabetes with lifestyle intervention or Metformin." *New England Journal of Medicine* (Massachusetts Medical Society) 346 (6): 393–403.

Kogan, Yuri, Karin Halevi-Tobias, Moran Elishmereni, Stanimir Vuk-Pavlovi C., and Zvia Agur. 2012. "Reconsidering the paradigm of cancer immunotherapy by computationally aided real-time personalization." *Cancer Research*, 72, 2218–2227.

Komorowski, Matthieu, Leo A. Celi, Omar Badawi, Anthony C. Gordon, and A. Aldo Faisal. 2018. "The artificial intelligence clinician learns optimal treatment strategies for sepsis in intensive care." *Nature Medicine* (Nature Publishing Group) 24 (11): 1716–1720.

Kuliś, Michał. 2017. *How 3D Printers Revolutionized Agile Manufacturing*. https://zortrax.com/blog/3d-printers-agile-manufacturing/.

Kumar, Arun, Sumit Kaushal, Shubhini A. Saraf, and Jay Shankar Singh. 2017. "Cyanobacterial biotechnology: An opportunity for sustainable industrial production." *Climate Change and Environmental Sustainability* (Diva Enterprises Private Limited) 5 (1): 97.

LaRock, Z. 2019. *Digital Therapeutics Explained: DTx Trends & Companies in 2020.* Business Insider. https://www.businessinsider.com/digital-therapeutics-report?IR=T.

Li, Qiao, Li-Na Zhang, Xiao-Ming Tao, and Xin Ding. 2017. "Review of flexible temperature sensing networks for wearable physiological monitoring." *Advanced Healthcare Materials* (Wiley-VCH Verlag) 6 (12): 1601371.

Lovell, Tammy. 2020. *SideKickHealth to Provide Digital Platform for COVID-19 Patients in Iceland* | MobiHealthNews. https://www.mobihealthnews.com/news/europe/sidekickhealth-provide-digital-platform-covid-19-patients-iceland.

Lunit Inc. 2020. *AI Product*| Lunit Inc. https://www.lunit.io/en/product/insight_cxr3/.

Makin, Simon. 2019. "The emerging world of digital therapeutics." *Nature*. Vol. 573. no. 7775. Nature Publishing Group, 26 9. S106–S109.

Mirochnik, Rebecca M., and John S. Pezaris. 2019. "Contemporary approaches to visual prostheses." *Military Medical Research*. Vol. 6. no. 1. BioMed Central Ltd., 5 6. 1–9.

Mishra, Anand K., Thomas J. Wallin, Wenyang Pan, Patricia Xu, Kaiyang Wang, Emmanuel P. Giannelis, Barbara Mazzolai, and Robert F. Shepherd. 2020. "Autonomic perspiration in 3D-printed hydrogel actuators." *Science Robotics* (American Association for the Advancement of Science) 5 (38), eaaz3918.

Morrison, Benjamin, and Daniel Topping. 2012. "Robotic Prosthetic Availability Analysis." Interactive Qualifying Projects (All Years).

Murthy, Vivek H., Harlan M. Krumholz, and Cary P. Gross. 2004. "Participation in cancer clinical trials: Race-, sex-, and age-based disparities." *Journal of the American Medical Association* 291 (22): 2720–2726.

Nachtwey, James. 2019. *The Worst Opioid Addiction Crisis in U.S. History* | Time. https://time.com/james-nachtwey-opioid-addiction-america/.

Nahavandi, Saeid. 2019. "Industry 5.0—A human-centric solution." *Sustainability* (MDPI AG) 11 (16): 4371.

Nørfeldt, L., J. Bøtker, Magnus Edinger, Natalja Genina, and J. Rantanen. 2019. "Cryptopharmaceuticals: Increasing the safety of medication by a blockchain of pharmaceutical products." *Journal of Pharmaceutical Sciences*. Vol. 108. no. 9. Elsevier B.V., 1 9. 2838–2841.

Norman, James, Rapti D. Madurawe, Christine M.V. Moore, Mansoor A. Khan, and Akm Khairuzzaman. 2017. "A new chapter in pharmaceutical manufacturing: 3D-printed drug products." *Advanced Drug Delivery Reviews*. Vol. 108. Elsevier B.V., 1 1. 39–50.

Notman, Nina. 2018. *3D Printing in Pharma | Feature* | Chemistry World. https://www.chemistryworld.com/features/3d-printing-in-pharma/3008804.article.

Oh, Sam S., Joshua Galanter, Neeta Thakur, Maria Pino-Yanes, Nicolas E. Barcelo, Marquitta J. White, Danielle M. de Bruin, et al. 2015. "Diversity in clinical and biomedical research: A promise yet to be fulfilled." *PLOS Medicine* 12 (12): e1001918.

Park, Jihun, Joohee Kim, So Yun Kim, Woon Hyung Cheong, Jiuk Jang, Young Geun Park, Kyungmin Na, et al. 2018. "Soft, smart contact lenses with integrations of wireless circuits, glucose sensors, and displays." *Science Advances* (American Association for the Advancement of Science) 4 (1): eaap9841.

Plant Automation Technology. 2020. *The Future of Artificial Intelligence in Manufacturing Industries*. https://www.plantautomation-technology.com/articles/the-future-of-artificial-intelligence-in-manufacturing-industries.

Ponemon Institute. 2016. "The State of Cybersecurity in Healthcare Organizations in 2016."

Prentice, Jennifer L., and Keith S. Dobson. 2014. "A review of the risks and benefits associated with mobile phone applications for psychological interventions." *Canadian Psychology*. Vol. 55. no. 4. 282–290.

Sarkar, Bikash Kanti. 2017. "Big data for secure healthcare system: A conceptual design." *Complex & Intelligent Systems* 3 (2): 133–151.

Schmidt, J. 2016. *How Big Data Is Transforming Pharmaceutical Manufacturing*. https://www.nbforum.com/nbreport/can-you-see-the-future-of-bionic-body/.

Sepah, S. Cameron, Luohua Jiang, Robert J. Ellis, Kelly McDermott, and Anne L. Peters. 2017. "Engagement and outcomes in a digital Diabetes Prevention Program: 3-Year update." *BMJ Open Diabetes Research & Care* 5 (1): e000422.

Stowers, Kimberly, and Mustapha Mouloua. 2018. "Human computer interaction trends in healthcare: An update." *Proceedings of the International Symposium on Human Factors and Ergonomics in Health Care* (SAGE Publications) 7 (1): 88–91.

Sullivan, Hannah R., and Scott J. Schweikart. 2019. "Are current tort liability doctrines adequate for addressing injury caused by AI?" *AMA Journal of Ethics* 21 (2): 160–166.

Tan, Daniel W., Matthew A. Schiefer, Michael W. Keith, James Robert Anderson, Joyce Tyler, and Dustin J. Tyler. 2014. "A neural interface provides long-term stable natural touch perception." *Science Translational Medicine* (American Association for the Advancement of Science) 6 (257), 257ra138.

Taylor, Christopher. 2019. *Continued Process Verification, 3rd Stage of FDA Process Validation Guidelines | Pharmaceutical Engineering*. https://ispe.org/pharmaceutical-engineering/ispeak/continued-process-verification-3rd-stage-fda-process-validation.

Topol, Eric J. 2019. "High-performance medicine: The convergence of human and artificial intelligence." *Nature Medicine*. Vol. 25. no. 1. Nature Publishing Group, 1 1. 44–56.

Wang, Liangliang, Junjie Ding, Li Pan, Dongsheng Cao, Hui Jiang, and Xiaoqin Ding. 2019. "Artificial intelligence facilitates drug design in the big data era." *Chemometrics and Intelligent Laboratory Systems*. Vol. 194. 103850.

Yoo, Seung-Schik. 2015. "3D-printed biological organs: Medical potential and patenting opportunity." *Expert Opinion on Therapeutic Patents* (Informa Healthcare) 25 (5): 507–511.

You, Minli, Min Lin, Shurui Wang, Xuemin Wang, Ge Zhang, Yuan Hong, Yuqing Dong, Guorui Jin, and Feng Xu. 2016. "Three-dimensional quick response code based on inkjet printing of upconversion fluorescent nanoparticles for drug anti-counterfeiting." *Nanoscale* (Royal Society of Chemistry) 8 (19): 10096–10104.

Zhang, Mian, and Yuhong Ji. 2018. "Blockchain for healthcare records: A data perspective." *PeerJ* 6, e26942v1.

3.2 Food and Beverage Bio-manufacturing – Industry 5.0

Deepshika Deepak, Wen Yi Chia, Kit Wayne Chew, and Pau Loke Show

CONTENTS

3.2.1 INTRODUCTION

The food and beverage (F&B) industry has been tagged as one of the largest growing markets of the 21st century. The main aim of the industry is to be able to provide nourishment to all consumers, while consistently improving the quality of the food and ensuring that food provided is safe and of a high nutritional value. Consumption of nutritious food is extremely crucial for the well-being and health of humans, but nowadays many factors come into play when consumers choose the type of food they want to eat. Instead of focusing on having a balanced diet, less nutritious, high cholesterol, processed fatty food is consumed by a certain group of people due to changes in taste and the industry. This, however, is the least of humanity's problems when it comes to the F&B industry.

This changing era where technology dominates the leisure time has led to less physical activity coupled with greater intake of starch and sugar. The World Health

Organization (WHO) reported that 1.9 billion adults are obese, while 462 million are underweight (Branca 2019). It is also evident that nutrition, or lack thereof, is the main cause of death and disease in the world. Consequently, there is a rise in obesity and other health conditions caused by oxidative stress – neuro-degeneration due to an imbalanced defence mechanism of antioxidants, leading to a range of neural disorders linked with old age such as Alzheimer's disease, Parkinson's disease as well as cardiovascular disease (Uttara et al. 2009, 65–74).

According to a compilation of studies by Saadi et al. (2014), a strong link has been determined between biopeptides and scavenging oxidative stress, as the relevant biochemical and biophysical properties of biopeptides are able to modulate immune disorders once they exist within the body. The manufacturing of biopeptides should thus be prioritized, as well as addition of these compounds to consumer food; however, this poses a difficulty due to the absence of a major linkage between immunology, pharmacy, biotechnology and biochemical engineering. Through the implementation of elements of Industry 4.0, such as the IoT (Internet of Things), this issue could be solved as biological data can freely be interpreted throughout these different industries.

With such pressing health issues, there is also a rise in the health consciousness found in consumers. Firstly, more individuals are conscious about the environmental impacts of the meat and dairy industry. The growth of the global food crisis is brought upon by the change in the climate which is indirectly caused by industrial agriculture, with a supply that overshoots beyond human needs, while still managing to have a hungry population. The greatest link between the food industry and climate change lies in beef. The rearing of cattle takes up 60% of agricultural land, making it the most ecologically destructive food. Shifting the focus from beef into plant-based proteins could free up millions of square miles of agricultural land and reduce global greenhouse gas emissions by 8–10% (Harrabin 2019). With the current industrial revolution, the focus may be shifted to optimizing the growth of other crops to replace beef or to grow meat industrially.

There is also an increased awareness and proper diagnosis for lactose intolerance in bovine milk. The food industry is responding to this by switching from bovine milk to plant-based milk and lactose-free milk alternatives, such as almond, soy, oat, coconut and rice. Plant-based milks are either derived through their natural derivatives or can be assembled by homogenizing oil, water and emulsifier together to form these oil-in-water milk emulsions (McClements, Newman and McClements 2019, 2047–67).

Furthermore, consumers are eager to learn about how food is processed. The chemicals, preservatives and additives that are added to keep food fresh are questioned. There is a fear of not being able to recognize the names of the chemicals used when reading the labels on the back of food products, raising concern about toxicity. Therefore, it is important for the food companies to take initiative to inform the public about the additives in food and the reasons behind the addition. This information is typically available but accessing and publicizing of the information must be prioritized in order to educate the customers about the food they consume, while feeding their curious minds.

Another serious issue that is present in the global food industry is food waste. The underlying issue behind food waste is that food is being produced but does

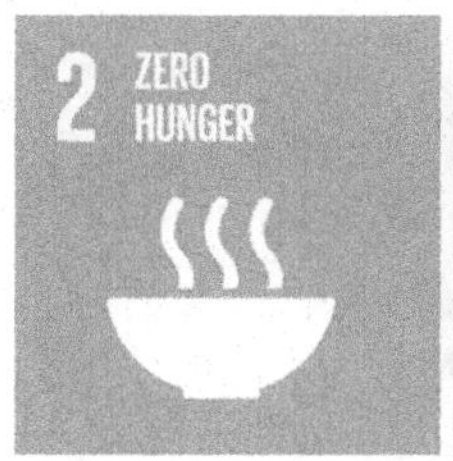

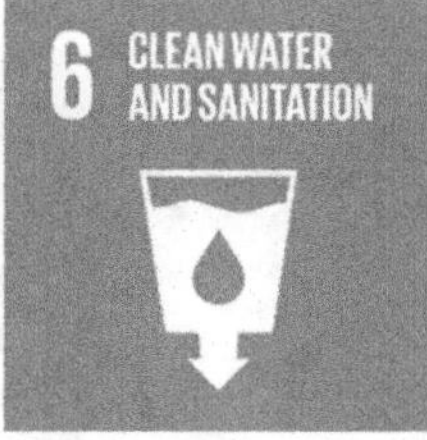

FIGURE 3.2.1 Sustainable Development Goals for 2030 by the United Nations (United Nations, 2016).

not reach the hungry population and ends up being wasted. This issue can be tackled by the use of a well interconnected system at the industry scale which analyzes how much food is being consumed and disposed of as well as controls the production rate based on the amount of food which is being spoilt and eventually wasted. Industry 5.0 boasts elements such as big data, machine learning and artificial intelligence, which can be put to good use to eliminate a large-scale food crisis to solve the world's issues regarding food. The United Nation has released Sustainable Development Goals that it wishes to achieve to tackle many issues, including Goal #2 which is Zero Hunger as well as Goal #6 which is to provide clean water to all, as demonstrated in Figure 3.2.1 (About the Sustainable Development Goals 2016). Both the goals could be achieved more easily with certain aspects from Industry 5.0.

Nations are adopting policies, such as the National Research Strategy Bioeconomy 2030 initiative in Germany, which has aims for the integration of goals striving towards a natural cycle oriented biobased economy that is in accordance with advancements in technology and ecology, global food supplies, bio-based energy and climate change. These policies do not only focus on one issue, but how prioritizing a bio-based economy, or bioeconomy can be advantageous in solving many critical global issues, including food waste issue. Bio-based markets have been significant in the United States, representing more than 2.2 percent of the gross domestic product (GDP) in 2012, or more than $353 billion in economic activity in 2012. The European Commission estimated that the European bioeconomy (excluding health applications) is worth more than €2 trillion annually and employs more than 21.5 million people (National Research Council of the National Academies, 2015).

The bioeconomy spans a wide range of sectors and advancements in the bioeconomy in primary sectors such as agriculture, forestry, horticulture, fisheries and aquaculture. This will lead to developments in their respective secondary sectors such as nutrition and beverage, as well as wood, paper, textile and biochemical industries. For example, for the fishing industry, some governments are providing satellite navigation systems that are able to detect regions where fish are present, reducing the time spent navigating to a region where they may be.

Advancements in Industry 4.0 are not yet widespread in these primary sectors because the use of technology in these types of primary sector is limited by the cost, the complexities of data management, transfer of data between sectors and the provision of training for the workers in these sectors. Therefore, it is imperative that advancements need to occur in primary sectors of these bio-industries in order to establish a well linked and interconnected system for the transition into Industry 5.0. For instance, the labourers of these primary sectors tend to possess a certain

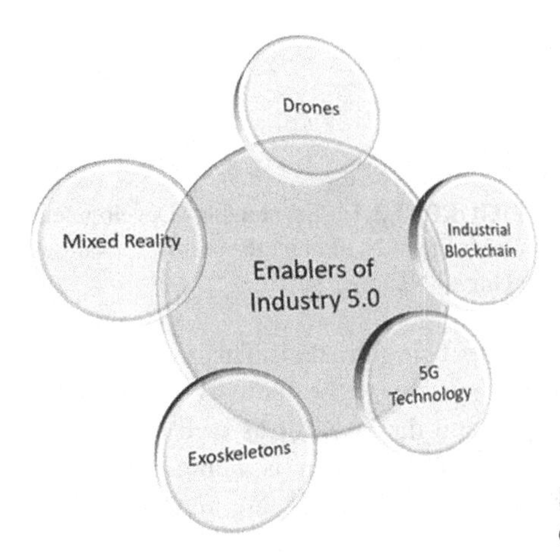

FIGURE 3.2.2 Greatest technological changes brought about by Industry 5.0.

skillset which would need to change in order to accommodate for the changes in the type of skillset required by these industries (Girard and Payrat 2017).

In order to understand Industry 5.0 and how it will be able to revolutionize the food processing industry, it is first important to understand Industry 4.0 and how it differs from Industry 5.0 – which is a highly interconnected system of industries that effectively integrates data while still focusing on the important aspects which Industry 4.0 has neglected, such as environmental protection, sustainability and the collaborative efforts between humans and robots, termed "cobots." The synergy created by humans and robots will be powerful and advanced as man and machine work side by side (Nahavandi 2019, 4371). Some other aspects of Industry 5.0 include additive manufacturing which can be seen in the food industry as 3D-printed food and meat. Besides, the introduction of 5G is said to bring significant changes by creating a wireless and flexible backbone that can make end-to-end monitoring of the entire production line in food processing very simple and fast (Beasley 2020). The other key features linked to Industry 5.0 are highlighted in Figure 3.2.2.

In this chapter, we will review the current trends and developments present in the F&B industry, as well as the future developments in the upcoming Fifth Industrial Revolution. It includes trends which are not widespread in the industry, such as the use of cyber-physical systems, as well as more established bio-technological trends such as genetically modified food which are leading into the new era of food processing technology. The chapter also covers challenges that may be present with these rising technologies, coupled with solutions to overcome them to go forth and ensure a smooth transition to the upcoming industrial revolution.

3.2.2 CURRENT TRENDS AND DEVELOPMENTS

3.2.2.1 Digitalization of the Food Processing and Manufacturing Industry

There is a shift in the types of challenges faced by the food processing industry. The challenges faced stem from the alterations in demand and changes in requirements from consumers and suppliers. For example, food has become very individualistic and widely produced consumer foods do not attract the same masses as they once did. The busy lifestyle and increased awareness towards good quality food have caused consumers to seek an increasingly customized product. Due to this, the industry has shifted its focus from a supply-based approach to a demand-based approach in order to provide to the consumers what they really prefer to eat, as there has been an observed change in tastes and eating habits (Hasnan et al., 2018). These changes are made possible through the advancements in Industry 4.0, as showcased in Table 3.2.1. The healthy competition between large food corporations has pushed them in seeking to use latest advanced technologies in order to achieve high levels of productivity while delivering consumer's needs and capitalizing on it.

The autonomous behaviour between machines, storage systems and utilities will be important to store these unique demands and cater to the needs of consumers (Demartini et al. 2018, 1371–78), since Industry 5.0 emphasizes the "age of personalization." The industrial revolution also brings about efficiency to the existing manufacturing systems resulting in the increase in productivity, leading to the growth of revenues benefitting the industry as a whole. Furthermore, the automation aspect of it allows for less physical human involvement and "hands-on skills" on the factory floor, replacing this type of involvement with creative skills, problem-solving techniques and critical thinking.

The use of Cyber-Physical Production Systems (CPPS) is one of the highlights that is currently dominating the food industry. Since food is product centric, "smart products" are endowed with intelligence in order to perform self-configuration, with the ability to steer production by itself based on data. This can be done through the use of embedded systems which are able to communicate and relay information gathered from the masses – i.e., Big Data, through the forms of surveys, polls or simply sales and marketing trends to the machines which are pre-programmed to run the production line based on this data.

Advancements in sensing technology also lead to this abundance of processing data and through the use of continuous development of CPPS, this information can be used to leverage the interconnectedness between machines (Lee, Bagheri, and Kao 2015, 18–23). This would mean that the machines are able to understand and communicate with one another, analyzing data generated from the production line and being able to solve these issues with minimal human contribution. For example, on the factory floor, machines monitor processes and detect deviations from the process based on data collected and stored from previous similar operations and correct for any discrepancies without the involvement of a human operator. Such Artificial Intelligence (AI) technology can either be applied to batch processes or continuous production.

3.2.2.2 Augmented Reality

Through the execution of Augmented Reality (AR), human intervention can truly be minimized apart from cases of extreme situations such as emergency shutdowns and safety alarms. It can help workers in training to deal with emergency situations, such as a fire or chemical leaks, and provide steps and protocol to follow in these

TABLE 3.2.1
The Major Changes in Tech That the Food Industry Is Currently Seeing from the Fourth Industrial Revolution

Technology	Description	Sources
Intelligent manufacturing	Applying cyber-physical systems, Industrial Internet of Things (IIoT) and cloud computing and create a consistent digital linkage of all production units – resulting in a "Smart Factory."	Lee, Bagheri and Kao (2015, 18–23)
Quality control	Food inspection using sensors, camera and other visioning systems for accurate determination of food quality.	Karoui (2015, 567–72)
Food traceability system	The ability to follow the history of a food product and link it back to its source using recorded identifications – such as Quick Response (QR) codes and Radio Frequency Identification (RFID) tags.	Costa et al. (2013, 353–66)
Manufacturing design	Fabricating a virtual model of the process in order to perform testing, analysis and optimization before implementing changes in the physical system, plant or production line.	Gerbert et al. (n.d.)
Automation	Repetitive tasks that require human effort can be replaced by robots as they are able to perform these tasks not only effectively but also meeting the requirements for a specific standard of safety and hygiene that manual human intervention may not bring about.	Hasnan et al. (2018)
Gastronomy	Chef Robots and serving robots are taking over and being able to replicate actions of a human chef and server through a 3D camera.	Zoran (2019, 1467–73)
Marketing	Augmented Reality (AR) technology can be used to market the products to consumers, allowing for close examination of the product and boosting sales due to personalization and customization.	Chatzopoulos et al. (n.d.)
Training	Training provided using Augmented Reality (AR) is more effective in teaching participants as it provides a hands-on approach for the operators as well as others employed in the food and beverage manufacturing industry.	Akçayır and Akçayır (2017, 1–11)
Customization and personalization	Being able to implement individualistic customer needs with additive manufacturing such as 3D printing.	Sun et al. (2015, 1605–15)

unfortunate situations. Training sessions through virtual reality have been more useful than conventional learning through classrooms and 2D learning techniques as it provides a better hands-on practical and immersive experience. In fact, participants of the training sessions are able to complete tasks eight times faster through AR learning than the typical methods (Akçayır and Akçayır 2017, 1–11). It also significantly reduces the cost of the training, as a single video and screen can be accessed and utilized by many trainees.

Apart from training, it is also able to market food products to consumers and allow them to see the products through technology found in smartphones (Carmigniani and Borko 2011). This enables the customer to closely examine the product, as well as details such as nutritional information, before purchasing it. They are also able to personalize the product and engage with it through games which will help in decision making. This type of technology may further be developed to recognize the individual preferences of each customer without requirement to conduct a post-purchase survey (Chatzopoulos et al. n.d.).

Another key element is known as the Industrial Internet of Things (IIoT) which is able to provide a well-linked system where machines are able to communicate with each other as well as humans. The ease of monitoring production line increases through these well-linked systems as well as the possibility of being able to track and control the sequence of events. This allows the production facility to be environmentally conscious too, by being able to implement circular economy solutions in the food chain. For example, IIoT is able link the food from the farm, through its production process right to the fridge of the individual consumer. This will be effective in the present day where consumers are becoming more aware about the additives that are present in food for preserving and making it last. The ease of food traceability is possible with such a well-linked system.

Traceability ensures ease of monitoring processing aspects such as harvesting in agriculture as well as food safety control procedures. The real value of traceability comes into light when information about the supply chain can easily be shared and the time taken to make changes in a food safety incident is shortened as the root cause of the problem is able to be located quickly and accurately. The rising technology used is known as Radio Frequency Identification (RFID) technology, and it is slowly becoming widespread as it is fairly easy to use and inexpensive. RFID tags are adhered on to the food product and the complete chain is able to be tracked. This information is not only available to retailers, but also to the public and consumers whereby they would be able to view the entire history of the product by entering the RFID tag code onto a smartphone application (Costa et al. 2013, 353–66). A cheaper alternative to this RFID tag system is the use of Quick Response (QR) codes, which are also able to be scanned through applications installed on smartphones.

3.2.2.3 Customization and Personalization

Consumers that are health conscious, and curious to identify the products used in their food, may benefit from a novel food scanning device that has been on the market. TellSpec food scanner, launched in 2013, utilizes spectral technology such as near infrared spectroscopy (NIRS) to identify the food, while being able to identify the amount of fat, protein, sugar and total energy content of the food. This is done through the classification of a sample of food using the spectra obtained by a user and comparing it to the spectra produced when calibrating the device. This information is available through a cloud-based system, and the device is linked to an application on mobile phones that have access to this cloud. Information is then displayed on the application developed by the same company, easily identifying the nutritional value of the food in question (Prasad et al. 2019).

These devices, by TellSpec, are retailing at $1500 (Prasad et al. 2019). They are not cheap, as the technology NIRS is still at a relatively early stage of development. Since this technology is associated with computational complexity, there is demand for more developments in the link between theoretical and applied spectroscopy. Advancements in this field are anticipated, especially through the involvement of data from large biological systems and directly applying theories of NIRS into common laboratory analytical routines (Beć and Huck 2019, 1–2). When more laboratories and scientific institutions are able to exploit this technology in handheld form, it will become cheaper on the market. It becomes especially useful in the identification of allergens and intolerances in food, and many consumers will benefit from carrying a device like this in their pockets, rather than risking a trip to the hospital, especially in the cases of extreme sensitivity to certain foods.

There are also 3D printers for food which are available in the market today, which is a form of additive manufacturing. One such example is the "Foodini" produced by the company Natural Machines (Sun et al. 2015, 1605–15). This state of the art 3D printer retails for $4000 on Natural Machines website, and it is capable of producing customized food products, such as patterned chocolates and pastries of different geometries. The latest generation of food printers are fitted with nozzles, lasers, syringes and sprays in order to customize orders and recipes to meet the taste, nutritional value, texture and colour desired by the consumer.

3.2.2.4 Quality Control

There are difficulties in ensuring food is of a certain quality prior to selling it to the market, particularly with food prone to spoilage. Quality control of food is a mandatory regulatory activity enforced through national and corporate food laws in order to protect customers from bad-quality food as well as from being cheated in terms of the weight and quality of food they are paying for. The conditions for handling, storage and processing must all be apt and comply with the requirements in order for the food to be deemed safe to consume.

Determining the quality of the food produced is critical and is done through time-consuming analytical methods, such as microscopic, rheological, sensory and physicochemical, with the latter being the most widely used technique. In all of these methods, both destructive and non-destructive techniques are employed, although destructive techniques, such as high-performance liquid chromatography (HPLC) and gas chromatography are not preferred as they tend to be tedious, time consuming and require highly skilled operators (Karoui 2015, 567–72). Preferably, an online analysis would be more convenient and cost effective, where techniques such as Infrared

Spectroscopy and Fluorescence Spectroscopy come into effect. These are relatively low cost and can be applied on the factory floor. In fact, it has been put to effect in the dairy industry for process monitoring and product assessment.

A camera can also be used to inspect the food, through determination of the shape and colour as well as the presence of foreign bodies in the food. This form of monitoring can also activate the necessary changes if deviations in product quality are detected, and this is done quickly to ensure that produced food is not being wasted. Human inspection may not always be accurate, and using these visual sensors, the quality of the food is standardized and can be recorded in the case of any complaint with respect to food quality, health and safety.

Food packaging is required to keep food fresh, protect it from bacteria and becoming spoilt, as well as providing information about the product. Food wastage from spoilage can be avoided through the use of intelligent packaging, based on a compilation of studies (Müller and Schmid 2019, 3–7). While food companies test their products prior to delivery to the supermarket, intelligent packaging is set to close the gap that leads to avoidable food wastage due to spoilage.

As temperature is one of the governing factors of shelf life and product quality, making time temperature indicators (TTIs) is important in smart packaging. These indicators will show the deviations in the temperature profile of the product and it is imperative in determining whether it is spoilt. Based on this temperature, it can be determined whether the food has undergone any biological changes with indication on the packaging, using a polymerization reaction depending on the temperature range. These indicators are simple and inexpensive gadgets which are attached to the packaging. Freshness indicators are also available, through measurements using an electrochemical sensor. The indicator typically utilizes colorimetry based on pH to display the freshness of the food product.

Gas sensors are also employed to determine the quality of the food, but this is based on the indoor atmosphere within the packaging. Biological activity, such as gas generation from microorganisms can be used to indicate whether the food has gotten spoiled. Typically, gases such as oxygen and carbon dioxide are monitored, as well as water vapour, ethanol and hydrogen sulphide. Based on the amount of gas detected, the indicator displays freshness level on a UV-activated colorimetric indicator, as some dyes are prone to leaching due to moisture content inside the packaged food.

3.2.2.5 Genetic Engineering and Systems Metabolic Engineering

Through genetic engineering, the DNA of organisms, e.g., plants, animals or microorganisms, is able to be altered in a way that does not occur through natural means such as reproduction or natural recombination. This is done for a variety of reasons, to increase the yield of crop because of advanced genetics that leads to an increased resistance to pests and weeds, leading to decreased costs of production since the amount of herbicides and pesticides used and land space are reduced where an estimate of 300 million additional acres of land are necessary in order to meet the same crop harvest, of 370 million tonnes through the years 1996 to 2012 (Brookes and Barfoot 2014, 65–75).

All of these factors have led to savings and economic benefits where the income for the farming industry for genetically modified (GM) food has tripled between the years 2006 and 2012, making it a $116 billion industry. There is also necessity to provide nutritious food and some genetic modification aims to do so by specifically targeting to increase the nutrients, especially in the case where the food contains substances that possess healthy and therapeutic properties (Zhang, Wohlhueter, and Zhang 2016, 116–23).

An example of GM food is the GM-modified potato variety known as Amflora. Amflora has modified levels of carbohydrates through the alteration of the amino acid composition of proteins. Only one of the two types of starch found in potatoes are useful in non-food applications, namely, amylose and amylopectin. Through the elimination of a granule bound starch synthase (GBSS), which has the primary function of producing amylose, producing potatoes which were low in amylose but had a high content of amylopectin. This method of modification is known as "gene silencing," due to the suppression of the GSSB (Kramkowska, Grzelak, and Czyzewska 2013, 413–9).

Another successful and widely used example of GM is the success of "Flavr Savr" tomatoes that possess a long shelf-life. By genetic alteration through the addition of an antisense known to decrease production of the polygalacturonase enzyme, the shelf-life increases by slowing down the ripening process (Kramkowska, Grzelak, and Czyzewska 2013, 413–9). Nearly two decades after the successes of the "Flavr Savr" tomatoes, genetic engineering has come a long way. Genetic modification today includes genetically modified salmon (refer to Figure 3.2.3), which is the first time a GM food has been sold in the open food market (Waltz 2017, 148). With over 25 years of research and development, Altantic salmon species S*almo salar* has been modified so that it grows quicker than non-GM salmon. This poses a great advantage for the salmon fishery industry, that is able to half the time taken for the fish to reach its adult size (Smith and Asche 2010, 330).

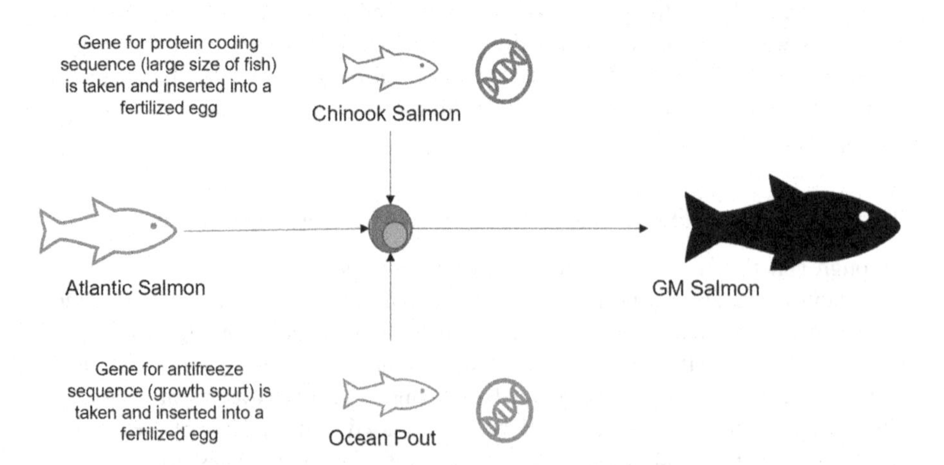

FIGURE 3.2.3 The procedure through which GM salmon was created – using specific gene sequences from Ocean pout and Chinook salmon.

There is a significant amount of funding going into more ambitious projects, such as the Bill and Melinda Gates Foundation that has currently provided $15 million to fund genetically modified organism (GMO) research. Gates himself believes that "genetically modified organisms are perfectly healthy and an important tool in the fight to end world hunger and malnutrition". The foundation funded a project that is researching into creating and modifying cereal crops which are able to provide their own nitrogen as a fertilizer. This would revolutionize the industry and the entire biological pathway that crops utilize to grow (Nesbit 2017).

Furthermore, new types of technology applied in genetic engineering are the true game changers of biotechnology. An example is clustered, regularly interspaced, short palindromic repeat (CRISPR) technology. In essence, CRISPR is a genome editing tool that allows greater precision in modification of the genome. These technologies use physical, chemical and biological mutagenesis and have significant contributions in the study of biological mechanisms for the improvement of the plant species. With tools such as Big Data, these large masses of data are speeding up the development of new drugs and crop species.

Paired with CRISPR, Cas 9 is CRISPR associated protein 9, which plays an essential role in the immunological defence of certain bacteria, leading to many breakthroughs in genetic engineering. A shining example of the application of CRISPR-Cas9 technology combined with big data and machine learning is by CropsOS, an American genetic engineering company. They have created a genome editing system with the help of machine learning-based analytics and this is able to effectively improve properties in the plant such as flavour, nutrient density and sustainability.

Systems metabolic engineering is an up-and-coming evolutionary engineering which is facilitating the development of high performance strains that can be used to cultivate cells and be exploited by food, pharmaceutical and biotechnology industries. The integration of tools and strategies of systems biology, which models biological systems through computational and mathematical methods, along with metabolic engineering, is a discipline of bio-engineering that genetically modulates living cells and organisms to produce desired products and allows for the development of industrially competitive high performance strains.

Through the help of bio-Big Data, more varieties of micro-organisms are being used as "host" strains in order to develop these commercially viable strains. Datasets of bio-Big Data are obtained typically from conventional omics data and the experimental results of serial repetitive or high-throughput experiments, as well as simulation data that is obtained from downstream fermentation, recovery and purification processes (Choi et al. 2019, 817–37).

In order to battle the rising emissions caused by the rearing of livestock, for the meat and dairy industry, alternative meat options are slowly becoming the norm in the industry. Novameat is a startup which has been the first of its kind to utilize a 3D printer to fabricate very realistic meat which is completely vegan. Technology behind this lies in the ability of the plant-based proteins to replicate a 3D matrix which is present in meat, giving the final product an extremely realistic feel. This technology can be extremely useful to tackle food security, climate change, as well as animal-carried food-related diseases. Another company, MosaMeat, founded in the Netherlands, is currently developing cultured ground meat which is rumoured to

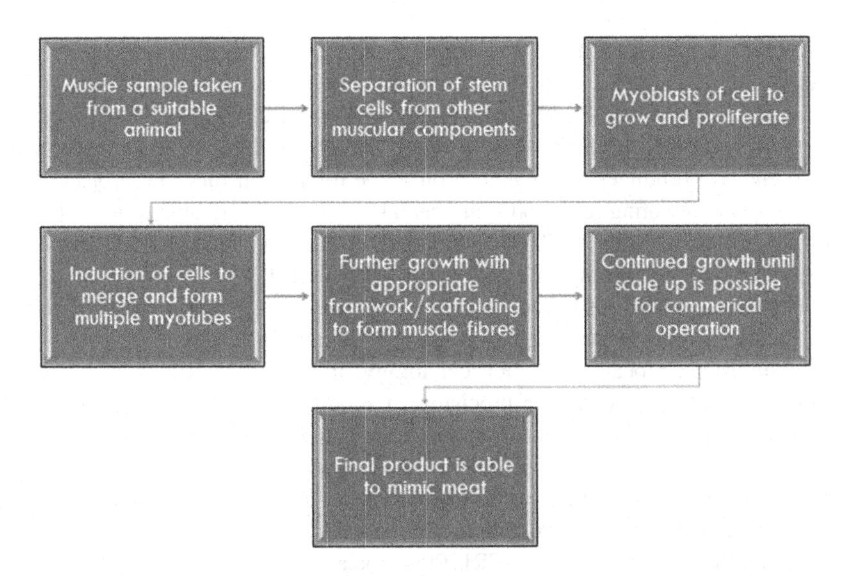

FIGURE 3.2.4 Steps to synthesize commercial scale cultured meat.

hit the market in the upcoming years. Growing concerns of animal rights issues and the rise of veganism can be tackled through this, because lab-grown meat avoids the common issues that are present in conventional meat production (Lynch and Pierrehumbert 2019, 3).

With the help of advancements in tissue engineering and "cellular agriculture," cells and cell lines are obtained from livestock, such as myosatellite cells and are cultivated to grow and proliferate under the right growth conditions such as temperature, oxygen demand and culture medium composition. After the cells have merged to form nuclear myotubes, they are then introduced to some form of framework, typically collagen-based in order to facilitate the formation of muscles, and then extend the production in order to deliver a commercially viable large-scale production resulting in the final product that mimics meat, as shown in Figure 3.2.4 (Kadim et al. 2015, 222–33).

3.2.3 CHALLENGES AND FUTURE DEVELOPMENTS

There are many challenges to viably implement Industry 5.0. Many years of testing are required to fully eliminate the errors and even then it may not be commercially doable. Highly integrated systems are vulnerable to systemic risks such as total network collapse. This form of extreme connectivity also creates new social and political structures. If left unchecked, they might lead to authoritarian governance.

3.2.3.1 Network Failures

A mass network failure could be particularly devastating when dealing with bio-products, as failure in the system could lead to mass food wastage of a large scale due to sensitive nature of bio-products. Warning systems and layers of protection through alarms are the only way to alert operators and personnel to be informed about the shutdown, or any other emergencies which could lead to food wastage. In manufacturing, these problems can be overcome by planning, preparing and equipping the workers and staff with the right knowledge and solutions to welcome the inevitable, in the case of total network failures.

It is fundamental to understand that outages are beyond the control of the engineers and operators, however, most Internet and network failures can be prevented through good design and employee education. For example, the placement of network equipment must be far away from a dangerous environment. In the current food and beverage plants, the production line is not affected by the Internet, but in a more interconnected system, the network will play a major role in making decisions based on data being sent to a centralized location.

A method of tackling this is through having an alternative Internet service provider (ISP) and perhaps even through the implementation of 5G. The biggest focus of the implementation of 5G has been on improving the wireless experience of consumers. However, this technology is bringing much more to the table as the food industry gains access to a fast and flexible method of connecting the production line, providing a wireless support system for the entire supply chain.

3.2.3.2 Job Security

The loss of jobs is one of the largest concerns of any industrial revolution, as observed in all previous industrial revolutions. However, the loss of jobs is considered to be temporary as there is a change in the skillset and a different set of skills will be required as the technology transitions from Industry 4.0 to 5.0. It is a common misconception that robots, automation and intelligent machines are going to take over human's job and cause a downfall in the economy but that is incorrect, as it is only going to cause a shift in the types of jobs people do.

This may be an issue for jobs involving physical labour, data collection and processing, as well as manufacturing and retail, but at the same time it will open up many opportunities in information technology. An example to consider is what occurred in 1980 during the previous industrial revolution: the introduction of computers caused the obsoletion of 3.5 million jobs but created 19.2 million new opportunities in various sectors.

"If history is any guide, we could expect eight to nine percent of 2030 labour demand will be in new types of occupations that have not existed before," says the McKinsey Institution in their article "Jobs Lost, Jobs Gained: Workforce Transitions in a time of Automation" (2017). Additionally, the World Economic Forum (WEF) have made predictions that positions will certainly open up in fields with emerging technologies such as AI, Blockchain, Robotics and Big Data, and also in other customer service–oriented industries and marketing, as well as training for technical jobs in the new industrial revolution.

For the agricultural industry, the average age of farmers can be quite old. This means that they may not be able to adapt so easily to new technology and may be more comfortable in doing things through traditional approaches. Hence, incentives and special training should be given by the government to the farmers so that more young people with bright minds and the ability to learn would join the industry and be very beneficial.

3.2.3.3 Customer Preferences and Lifestyle Changes

When it comes to a customized pill that consumers can take, it does pose significant concerns. One of these may be that consumers stop eating fresh fruit and vegetables and may solely depend on pills to govern nutritional health. They may get carried away and stray away from more traditional methods of having a balanced diet. They would not be able to reap the benefits provided by the advancements in crop technology and the farming industry which would be able to produce a better quality and yield of fresh fruit and vegetables.

Plant-based meat may not be nutritious and may pose drawbacks as this technology still needs testing and trials to ensure that this meat is safe to consume. Consumers may not easily accept the idea of eating meat that was cultured in a lab, as some are still having ethical concerns of eating genetically modified food. Nutritionists take it a step further by saying that these lab-grown meats may lead to more health issues as the nutritional content of meat is not clear, especially in terms of micronutrition and iron (Stehfest et al. 2009, 83–102).

As for the environmental concerns that are to be eliminated through switching to cultured meat, less land would definitely be used although it is not yet confirmed that this would reduce the amount of greenhouse gas emissions to a significantly less level. Experts argue that switching completely to veganism or vegetarianism would show greater positive impacts to the environment with regards to climate change. In order for the commercializing plant-based lab cultivated meat, more research must be conducted on the nutrients present in this meat as well as comparing the carbon footprint with normal meat in order to determine whether it is sustainable in reducing greenhouse gas emissions.

3.2.3.4 Technological Advancements and Drawbacks

Cobots are what will be prioritized in the upcoming revolution. These machines are meant to cooperate with humans and offer assistance when required. They have human-like qualities and decision-making artificial intelligence mechanisms built into their system. Cobots can mimic human action where it is able to gauge the actions of an operator on the factory floor, and decide by itself whether it should assist the human in that particular task (Nahavandi 2019, 4371).

Furthermore, automation on the factory floor especially in food processing is preferred. Mundane and repetitive tasks can be quickly performed by robots, primarily, loading, unloading, assembly, packaging, sorting, piling and arranging. Some of the aforementioned tasks require precision which is easy for the robot to achieve, as well as strength which the average human may have difficulty performing. This could even lead to injuries for the operators which could be avoided completely. Additionally, there is the issue of food hygiene. It is not always certain that the standard for food hygiene is being met, and therefore with an automated system it eliminates that problem as a whole.

In customer service, too, robots and automation are taking over. Waitstaff are being replaced with serving robots and checkout counters with self-checkout scanning kiosks with voice activation and instructions. Even in kitchens, Chef Robots are replacing the way that cooking is done traditionally. This is another environment where cobots could be implemented successfully where chefs are assisted by these cobots where precision is essential, such as in a fine dining restaurant. These cobots should be able to track the movement of the human chefs and replicate it, while also monitoring cooking conditions to ensure the perfect quality and taste that the recipe calls for. In January of 2020, Samsung introduced a Bot Chef that is capable of performing a range of menial kitchen tasks that no home chef is keen on doing. It functions through voice commands and underlying Artificial Intelligence (AI) and machine learning technology hidden under an ultra-sleek exterior.

Yet another challenge of the transition from IR 4.0 to 5.0 is the availability of non-invasive sensors which are able to remotely measure. The use and implementation of handheld scanners may not be as easy as one may assume. First of all, they can be expensive as the technology utilized by these devices is known as Near Infra Red Spectroscopy (NIRS) and is only feasible at a theoretical stage (Dale et al. 2013, 142–59). Secondly, food and allergies are also closely linked to the medical industry, so in the case where unknown allergies are present, advancements in the medical industry such as allergen testing data need to be input into the handheld scanner automatically to personalize the device for each individual consumer allowing them to accurately identify and avoid foods which they may be allergic to. This indicates that different industries, F&B industry and medical industry in this case, must work closely together to see advancements in Industry 5.0.

The interconnectedness within an industry between sectors is what will rule the next industrial revolution. Taking the fishing industry as an example, as demonstrated in Figure 3.2.5, the boat can be fitted with navigation equipment and mapping systems which can relay to fishermen regarding the location of fish, the species of fish and the amount to be retrieved. This information is then relayed to the processing centre where the fish can be tracked and counted. Through the use of sensors and imaging, the quality of the fish can be analyzed. One of the safety concerns may be the presence of microplastic which is ingested by the fish, and a scanning device can ensure that there are no foreign or toxic objects in the fish assuring that it has the seal of approval.

All of these data, the date, time and location from where the fish is retrieved could be made available to consumers in supermarkets, as well as additional nutritional information so that consumers are able to make an informed decision about their choice in food. If the fresh fish is not sold to consumers at a supermarket, it is sent to a processing facility where it may be canned or preserved for future use. Food traceability drawback is that every supply chain is different so there will be challenges in adaptation of the designs and implementing them with respect to each industry and its needs.

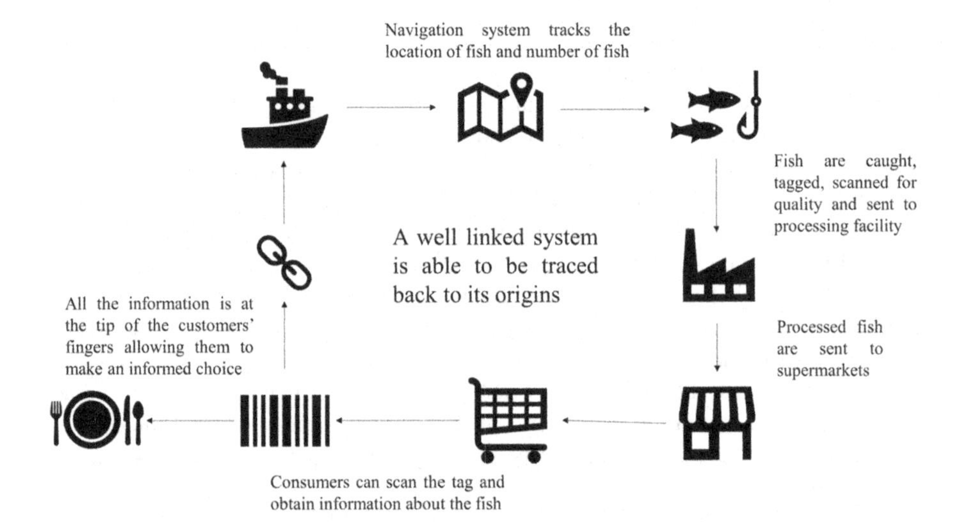

FIGURE 3.2.5 Food traceability diagram for the fishery industry and fish supply chain.

A highly integrated system with a similar concept can be used to tackle food waste. At a smaller scale, crowd-farming may be done, where food and fresh produce can be shared among small communities. This is already being done in organization such as Oilo, where neighbours and local farmer's markets are able to share their excess produce so that waste is not produced. At a larger scale, through the use of databases, factories may be able to predict how much food is going to be wasted and may arrange to deliver this food to the hungry population, or avoid the wastage from occurring to begin with, by preserving the biological product or not accepting it into the production facility (De Clercq et al., 2018).

The downside is that most industries in the primary sector in developing countries may find it difficult to utilize this hard technology. Many rural areas do not have access to electricity, let alone an Internet connection so most of this technology may not be able to be applied there. The more developed countries, can however, develop systems and practice them at an industry level, and implement the same systems in these developing countries and introduce the technology to them slowly. These are the gaps between Industry 4.0 and 5.0 where some plants still rely on machinery and technology from previous industrial revolutions and have not yet updated the technology.

3.2.4 CONCLUSION

Advancements in the latest technology are truly revolutionizing the market across industries, and it is especially prevalent in the agricultural industry and the food manufacturing industry. This chapter reviewed the research and developments in the Food and Beverage industry including new technologies that have been developed and as well as other promising areas which are currently in the infant stage of research and will be fundamental to Industry 5.0. Industry 5.0 has the ability to bridge the gap between these industries and utilize new technology not simply because it is available, but for the purpose of addressing and tackling the issues that are present including food wastage and spoilage.

The digitalization of the food processing industry will provide more flexibility by enabling customers to pick and choose to make informed decisions about food with the mass amounts of information available to them, allowing for personalization and customization of food products. This food will be of a high quality through smart packaging and quality control techniques. With an interconnected and well linked system, the issue of food shortages will be eased by delivering the food to where it is needed based on a demand and supply system. The use and optimization of big data will allow for more biological discoveries in the cellular agriculture sector, while being able to harvest automation will become more ubiquitous in this new era of Industry 5.0 with the smooth collaboration of humans and robots, ensuring production while making lives of human operators easier and less risky.

Stepping into Industry 5.0, however, the mindset of change must be adopted across the enterprise, from the corporate board room meetings of food and beverage giants, to the floor of the factory where the processing takes place. The issue of funding also cannot be ignored, as all these technologies are expensive and developing nations are yet to implement innovations from the previous industrial revolutions. It is predicted that emerging technologies such as 5G will help to bridge this gap as it could eliminate the use of bulky equipment, which is typically required in other conventional networking methods. The job market is also predicted to shift, where new skills need to be acquired in order to accommodate for the changes in skillset necessary with the relevant technology, however this may be difficult for senior members of the workforce to adapt to.

The Fifth Industrial Revolution, i.e., Industry 5.0, will arise in the years to come and will consist of an amalgamation of intelligent devices, systems and automation as well as human creativity and intelligence. The food and beverage processing industry will see efficiency and top-quality food, while being able to cater to individual needs of consumers in the provision of highly nourishing food to its consumers. With the correct implementation of the technology, long-standing issues such as climate change and world hunger can be eliminated, if not eradicated completely, bringing numerous significant benefits to human beings.

REFERENCES

Akçayır, Murat, and Gökçe Akçayır. 2017. "Advantages and challenges associated with augmented reality for education: A systematic review of the literature." *Educational Research Review* 20: 1–11.

Beasley, Kevin. 2020. "How 5G will transform the food industry." *Food Manufacturing*. https://www.foodmanufacturing.com/capital-investment/article/21115679/how-5g-will-transform-the-food-industry#:~:text=Food%20processing%20facilities%20can%20retrofit,recalls%20made%20headlines%20in%202019

Beć, Krzysztof B., and Christian W. Huck. 2019. "Breakthrough potential in near-infrared spectroscopy: Spectra simulation. A review of recent developments." *Frontiers in Chemistry*. 7.

Branca, Francesco. 2019. *Malnutrition is a World Health Crisis*. World Health Organization. https://www.who.int/news/item/26-09-2019-malnutrition-is-a-world-health-crisis

Brookes, Graham, and Peter Barfoot. 2014. “Economic impact of GM crops: The global income and production effects 1996-2012.” *GM Crops & Food* 5 (1): 65–75.

Carmigniani, Julie, and Furht Borko. 2011. Augmented Reality: An Overview. 10.1007/978-1-4614-0064-6_1.

Chatzopoulos, Dimitris, Carlos Bermejo, Zhanpeng Huang, and Pan Hui. n.d. “Mobile augmented reality survey: From where we are to where we go.” *IEEE Accesss* 5: 6917–6950.

Choi, Kyeong Rok, Woo Dae Jang, Dongsoo Yang, Jae Sung Cho, Dahyeon Park, and Sang Yup Lee. 2019. “Systems metabolic engineering strategies: Integrating systems and synthetic biology with metabolic engineering.” *Trends in Biotechnology.* 37: 817–837.

Costa, Corrado, Francesca Antonucci, Federico Pallottino, Jacopo Aguzzi, David Sarriá, and Paolo Menesatti. 2013. “A review on agri-food supply chain traceability by means of RFID technology.” *Food and Bioprocess Technology.* 6 (2): 353–366.

Dale, Laura M., André Thewis, Christelle Boudry, Ioan Rotar, Pierre Dardenne, Vincent Baeten, and Juan A. Fernández Pierna. 2013. “Hyperspectral imaging applications in agriculture and agro-food product quality and safety control: A review.” *Applied Spectroscopy Reviews* 48 (2): 142–159.

De Clercq, Djavan, Wen Zongguo, and Fan Fei. 2017. “Economic performance evaluation of bio-waste treatment technology at the facility level.” *Resources, Conservation and Recycling* 116: 178–184.

Demartini, Melissa, Claudia Pinna, Flavio Tonelli, Sergio Terzi, Cinzia Sansone, and Chiara Testa. 2018. “Food industry digitalization: From challenges and trends to opportunities and solutions.” *IFAC-PapersOnLine* 51 (11): 1371–1378.

Gerbert, Philipp, Markus Lorenz, Michael Rüßmann, Manuela Waldner, Jan Justus, Pascal Engel, and Michael Harnisch. n.d. *Industry 4.0: The Future of Productivity and Growth in Manufacturing Industries.* https://www.bcg.com/en-sea/publications/2015/engineered_products_project_business_industry_4_future_productivity_growth_manufacturing_industries.aspx.

Girard, Pierre, and Thomas Du Payrat. 2017. “An inventory of new technologies in fisheries.” OECD Greening the Ocean Economy, Paris.

Harrabin, Roger. 2019. “Plant-based diet can fight climate change – UN.” BBC News-Science. https://www.bbc.com/news/science-environment-49238749

Hasnan, Noor, Noor Zafira, and Yuzainee Md Yusoff. 2018. “Short review: Application areas of Industry 4.0 technologies in food processing sector.” In *2018 IEEE 16th Student Conference on Research and Development, SCOReD 2018.* Institute of Electrical and Electronics Engineers Inc. 8711184.

Kadim, Isam T., Osman Mahgoub, Senan Baqir, Bernard Faye, and Roger Purchas. 2015. “Cultured meat from muscle stem cells: A review of challenges and prospects.” *Journal of Integrative Agriculture* 14 (2): 222–233.

Karoui, R. 2015. “Quality control in food processing.” In *Encyclopedia of Food and Health,* edited by R. Karoui, 567–572. Elsevier Inc.

Kramkowska, Marta, Teresa Grzelak, and Krystyna Czyzewska. 2013. “Benefits and risks associated with genetically modified food products.” *Annals of Agricultural and Environmental Medicine* 20 (3): 413–419.

Lee, Jay, Behrad Bagheri, and Hung An Kao. 2015. “A cyber-physical systems architecture for Industry 4.0-based manufacturing systems.” *Manufacturing Letters* 3: 18–23.

Lynch, John, and Raymond Pierrehumbert. 2019. “Climate impacts of cultured meat and beef cattle.” *Frontiers in Sustainable Food Systems* 3. https://doi.org/10.3389/fsufs.2019.00005.

McClements, David Julian, Emily Newman, and Isobelle Farrell McClements. 2019. “Plant-based milks: A review of the science underpinning their design, fabrication, and performance.” *Comprehensive Reviews in Food Science and Food Safety* 18 (6): 2047–2067.

Müller, Patricia, and Markus Schmid. 2019. "Intelligent packaging in the food sector: A brief overview." *Foods* 8(1).

Nahavandi, Saeid. 2019. "Industry 5.0—A human-centric solution." *Sustainability* 11 (16): 4371.

Nesbit, Rebecca. 2017. *The Future of GMO Food.* https://blogs.scientificamerican.com/observations/the-future-of-gmo-food/.

Prasad, K.V.S.V., Yonas Asmare, A. Melesse, Frederic Kosmowski, V.P. Padmakumar, and Michael Blümmel. 2019. "Mobile and hand-held near infrared spectrometers in feed evaluation—Solutions to challenges?" International Livestock Research Institute.

Saadi, S. Saari, N. Anwar, F. Abdul Hamid, and H. Ghazali. 2015. "Recent advances in food biopeptides: Production, biological functionalities and therapeutic applications." *Biotechnology Advances* 33 (1): 80–116. https://doi.org/10.1016/j.biotechadv.2014.12.003

Smith, Martin D, and Frank Asche. 2010. "Genetically modified salmon and full impact assessment." *Science* 330 (6007): 1052–1053.

Stehfest, Elke, Lex Bouwman, Detlef P. van Vuuren, Michel G. J. den Elzen, Bas Eickhout, and Pavel Kabat. 2009. "Climate benefits of changing diet." *Climatic Change* 95 (1–2): 83–102.

Sun, Jie, Weibiao Zhou, Dejian Huang, Jerry Y.H. Fuh, and Geok Soon Hong. 2015. "An overview of 3D printing technologies for food fabrication." *Food and Bioprocess Technology* 8 (8): 1605–1615.

Uttara, Bayani, Ajay Singh, Paolo Zamboni, and R. Mahajan. 2009. "Oxidative stress and neurodegenerative diseases: A review of upstream and downstream antioxidant therapeutic options." *Current Neuropharmacology* 7 (1): 65–74.

United Nations. 2016. The Sustainable Development Agenda. https://www.un.org/sustainabledevelopment/development-agenda/.

Waltz, Emily. 2017. "First genetically engineered salmon sold in Canada." *Nature* 548 (7666): 148.

Zhang, Chen, Robert Wohlhueter, and Han Zhang. 2016. "Genetically modified foods: A critical review of their promise and problems." *Food Science and Human Wellness* 5 (3): 116–123.

Zoran, Amit. 2019. "Cooking with computers: The vision of digital gastronomy [Point of View]." *Proceedings of the IEEE* 107 (8): 1467–1473.

3.3 Fuel and Biofuels

Incorporation of Industry 5.0 to Biofuel Industry

Mei Yin Ong, Saifuddin Nomanbhay, Kuan Shiong Khoo, and Pau Loke Show

CONTENTS

3.3.1 INTRODUCTION

Since the era of Second Industrial Revolution, our mother Earth has experienced a massive increase in environmental pollution and non-renewable fossil fuel depletion issues. Hence, tremendous efforts are required to reduce the adverse environmental impact, particularly in renewable energy development and waste management. The current trend of all industries requires an effective production to minimize any environmental damage. Government policies have also been implemented in the recent years in many countries to support the renewable energy development, for example, certain share of energy demand should be fulfilled by renewable energy. Hence, rapid and substantial development in renewable energy generation, especially in terms of technological innovation and cost reduction, has been driven under the close cooperation of government and the business community. Recent events, such as the nuclear accident in Fukushima, Japan, where massive oil spills and severe climate changes, have highlighted the need of further development and enhancement of renewable energy generation and utilization. However, institutional, technological and societal change remain as the real challenge in up scaling its implementation. Although numerous AI algorithms have been developed from the view of sustainability, unfortunately, there is still lack of a strong focus on environmental protection in Industry 4.0 (Nahavandi 2019). Hence, Industry 5.0 will envisage the solution needed to protect the environment and save the Earth, especially in bioenergy industry such as biofuel production.

According to BP Statistical Review of World Energy 2019, the global primary energy consumption grew at a rate of 2.9% in 2018, which is the highest growth rate since 2010 (BP 2019). In the words, the global energy consumption is expanding rapidly, driven by all fuels, especially natural gas and renewable energy in 2018. As a result, carbon emissions in 2018 also increased by 2%, the fastest growth for seven years (BP 2019). The global increased of energy demand is mainly due to the industrialization and urbanization. Among the available energy resources, fossil fuel plays an important role, which meets almost 85% of the total energy demand in 2018 (BP 2019). Nevertheless, it is well-known that energy generation system from fossil fuel creates several problems, including high greenhouse gas (GHG) emission, fossil fuel depletion, environmental pollution and others.

Greenhouse gases, such as carbon dioxide (CO_2), methane (CH_4), nitrous oxide (N_2O) and fluorinated gases (F-gases), trap heat within the Earth's atmosphere, and eventually lead to global warming and climate change. Human activities, particularly burning of fossil fuel for electricity generation, industrial usage and transportation, are accountable for almost all the GHGs emission, in which around 80% is made up of CO_2 (EPA 2019). Figure 3.3.1 shows the annual CO_2 emission from different fuel types since 1800. In fact, almost 65% of current global electricity generation and over 90% of transportation is still dependent on non-renewable resources, fossil fuel (IEA 2019a). Based on the present consumption rate, it is estimated that fossil fuel will be depleted by 2029 (Malaysiakini 2019). Henceforth, a major shift in utilizing alternative renewable and sustainable energy sources is needed.

The formation of fossil fuel, such as coal, natural gas and oil, took hundreds of million years, and hence, it is considered as non-renewable energy sources and will run out based on the current consumption rate. On the other hand, renewable energy are produced from the renewable sources that are naturally replenished on a human timescale. There are several renewable energies that are available at present, such as solar energy, tidal energy, wind energy, hydro-energy, geothermal energy, biofuel and so on. These renewable energy technologies convert natural phenomena/resources on the Earth into useful forms of energy. For example, hydro-energy is generated by utilizing the falling water, while solar energy is produced through the solar radiation. The ability of renewable energy to meet the global energy demand partially, up to 11% (i.e., 1,510 million tonnes oil equivalent) in 2018 has been fully demonstrated (BP 2019). However, significant improvement can be done by enhancing the efficiencies of renewable energy conversion and collection, reducing the

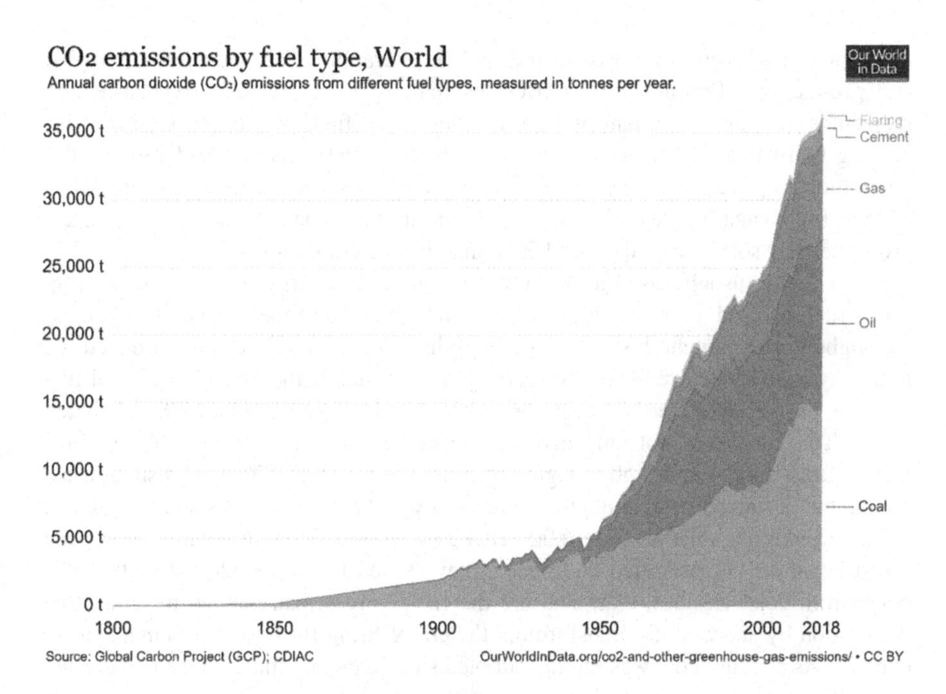

FIGURE 3.3.1 Annual CO_2 emission produced from different fuel types since 1800.
Source: Adapted from Hannah and Max (2017).

installation, operating and maintenance costs, and improving the system reliability and applicability. Hence, several studies have been done with the aim to upscale, improve yield and lower the overall production cost, and so able to commercialize and replace higher fraction of conventional non-renewable energy in meeting the global energy demand (Castello, Pedersen, and Rosendahl 2018; Chen et al. 2016; Perea-Moreno, Samerón-Manzano, and Perea-Moreno 2019; Rodrigues et al. 2017). It is believed that the benefits of renewable fuel will be intensified once the renewable energy production technology become mature and cost-effective. In achieving this target, Industry 5.0 plays an important role as human brainpower with the assist of AI algorithms is very important in developing better technological solution.

3.3.2 FUEL

In fact, fuel is one of the most useful Earth resources. Fuel refers to any materials that can react and release energy, such as heat energy, for mankind activities. Hence, fuel is also known as energy source. Other than chemical reaction (e.g., combustion), nuclear reaction (fission and fusion) is also one of the current available technologies to convert fuel into energy. The main difference between the chemical reaction and nuclear reaction is that the chemical reaction releases energy by breaking the chemical bonds that holds the fuel molecules together and involves only rearrangement of electron. However, the later one release energy by altering the structure of atomic nucleus of the fuel (i.e., uranium-235 and plutonium-239) and producing different element. Besides that, hydrocarbon and oxygen-related molecules are very important and are considered as fuels for living organism, including human. These substances are consumed by the cells and undergo cellular respiration to produce energy for living organism. In short, there are various kinds of fuels but basically, they can be categorized into three main groups based on their properties: (i) solid fuel, (ii) liquid fuel and (iii) gaseous fuel.

Solid fuel is usually used to produce heat and light energy through combustion. Solid fuel is used in many applications, including solid-fuel rocket technology. Throughout the human history, solid fuel has been discovered and utilized by humanity to produce fire for many years. Wood or stick is the first-known solid fuel that was burned by *Homo* at nearly three million years ago (Schobert 2013; Gowlett 2016). This discovery not only give human being warmth, cooking, but also protection from animal and higher degree of power over nature. This has distinguished the unique of human from animals. Charcoal, a wood derivative, was then introduced for metal melting since at least 6,000 BCE. At around the 18th century, European forest began to be exhausted and hence, they started to derive alternative fuel, the coke, from coal. Besides, that, coal are the fuel sources that enabled the Industrial Revolution by successfully transforming the era of firing furnace into running steam engines. As a result, coal was rapidly adopted since then and finally have become the major energy source for power generation in most of the countries nowadays.

Liquid fuel, however, is commonly used to create mechanical energy. As its name implies, liquid fuel is in liquid form, but its flammable part is the fume rather than the fluid itself. Currently, the liquid fuel, that is broadly used, is mainly the derivative of crude oil, which is non-renewable and plays an essential part especially in transportation sector. Crude oil is formed through the intense heating and pressurization of organic materials (i.e., remains of plants and animals) over a long period of time beneath the Earth's surface. The crude oil is then extracted and introduced into a distillation tower in order to refine and break down the crude oil into various petroleum-based products, such as diesel, kerosene and gasoline. Basically, there are three main stages of refining process, which are separation, conversion and treating. The main concept of the separation is based on different molecular weight and boiling point. During the process, the crude oil is heated at temperature 350–400°C, causing it to vaporize. Light portion rises to the top while the heavy fraction remains on the bottom. Then, the molecule condenses at different temperatures in the distillation column and forms different petroleum products. For the second stage, the heavy hydrocarbon molecules that remain after the separation are further converted into lighter and more value-added products through catalytic cracking or hydrocracking. Lastly, the products collected from the previous processes are treated to remove the molecules that are corrosive and have negative impact to the environment, particularly sulphur. Figure 3.3.2 shows the percentage yield of different petroleum products in United States.

Gaseous fuel is the fuel in gaseous state under normal condition, which primarily consists of hydrocarbon, hydrogen and/or carbon monoxide. Unlike solid fuel, gaseous fuel can be easily transported and supplied directly to the point of consumption via piping. Besides, they also can be liquefied and stored in a tank. However, there is

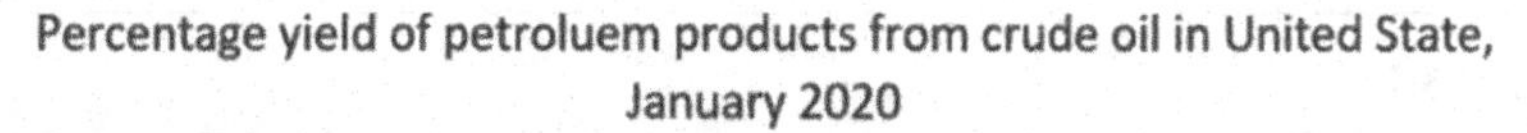

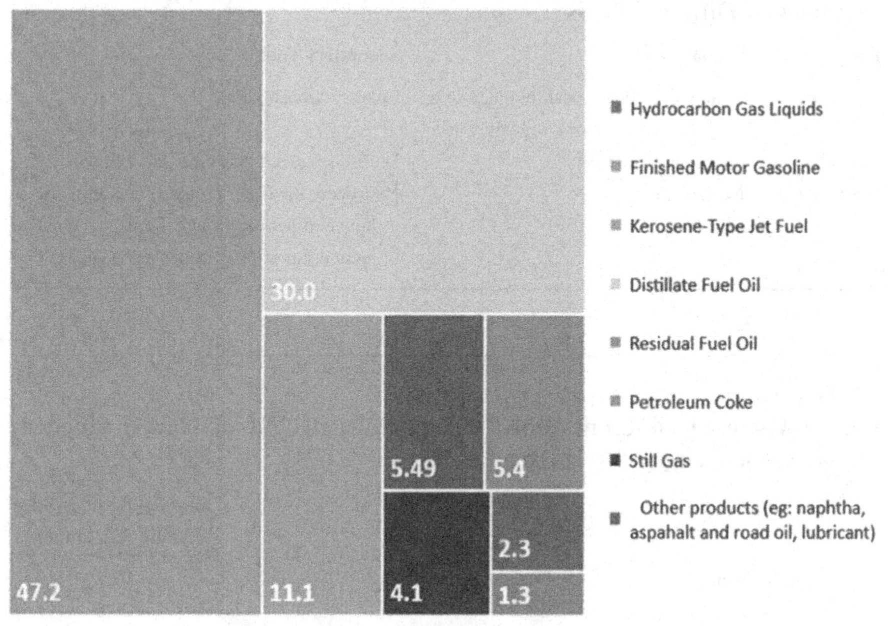

FIGURE 3.3.2 Percentage yield of different petroleum product in the United States.
Source: U.S. EIA 2020.

a limitation as some of the gaseous fuels are odourless and undetectable. Hence, most of the gaseous fuel are odorized with a distinct smell, which is very essential in detecting gas leakage to avoid the danger of gas explosion.

Furthermore, other than categorizing the fuels based on their properties, fuels can also be grouped into two, depend on the way they occur: (i) primary fuel and (ii) secondary fuel. Primary fuel describes the fuel that occurred in nature while secondary fuel refers to the derivatives of the primary fuel. Table 3.3.1 indicates the examples of different fuels, while Table 3.3.2 shows the calorific value of different fuels. Calorific value describes the energy stored in a fuel, which is commonly determined by measuring the total energy released as heat through complete combustion. The conventional fossil fuel, including petroleum, coal and natural gas, consists of higher calorific value and mature processing technology in comparison to renewable fuel source. Hence, fossil fuel contributes to the largest portion of energy supply nowadays in most of the countries. Nevertheless, fossil fuel is non-renewable energy source, and the extensive usage of fossil fuel has risen the fossil fuel depletion issue. Moreover, burning of fossil fuel also lead to environmental pollution, such as global warming, climate change and others, as mentioned previously. Therefore, the current trend has moved towards the development of renewable fuel, which is also known as biofuel and will be discussed in the Section 3.3.3.

TABLE 3.3.1
Examples of Different Fuels

Fuel Types	Primary Fuel	Secondary Fuel
Solid fuel	Coal, wood, dung, peat, biomass (e.g., wheat, corn, straw), organic waste	Coke, charcoal, pellet
Liquid fuel	Petroleum/crude oil	Diesel, kerosene, gasoline, tar, ethanol
Gaseous fuel	Natural gas	Hydrogen, methane, propane, coal gas, liquefied petroleum gas (LPG), compressed natural gas (CNG), water gas, syngas

TABLE 3.3.2
Calorif Value of Different Fuels [Information: (Digest of United Kingdom Energy Statistics (DUKES) 2018)]

	Fuels	Average Net Calorific Value (GJ/tonne)
Non-renewable sources	Coal	27.2
	Coke	29.8
	Crude oil	43.4
	Liquified petroleum gas	45.9
	Ethane	46.6
	Aviation turbine fuel	43.9
	Motor spirit	44.7
	Diesel oil	42.6
	Natural gas	35.7
Renewable sources	Wood (Domestic)	14.7
	Wood (Industrial)	19.0
	Straw	13.5
	General industrial waste	15.2
	Municipal solid waste	7.0
	Tyres	30.4
	Wood pellets	16.9
	Biodiesel	37.2
	Bioethanol	26.8

3.3.3 BIOFUELS

Biofuels refer to any renewable and biological energy-enriched material that can be used as fuel. The direct utilization of solid biofuel, such as wood or straw, to release energy is the well-known concept. Recently, the definition of biofuel has been narrowed down to the transport fuel derived from biomass. However, the current available biomass conversion methods are not as mature as the conventional fossil fuel processing technologies. The complexity of the biomass conversion process is greatly dependent on the chemical composition of the feedstock (Williams, Emerson, and Tumuluru 2017). The more complex the biomass used, the more complicated the biomass conversion process needed, and as the result, the higher the cost of biofuel production.

Biomass is the organic material that comes from plants and animals. Photosynthetic organism, such as vascular land plant, algae and photosynthetic bacteria, converts the solar energy into carbohydrates, which form the building blocks of biomass. There are various biomass sources, including corn, rapeseed, potato, grain, wood, straw, animal manure, algae, municipal solid waste, agriculture waste and industrial effluents. Hence, in order to have a better understanding on the type of biofuels produced, it is vital to categorize the diversity of biomass source. Generally, biofuels can be classified into three groups based on the biomass used and generation technologies, which are (i) first-generation biofuel, (ii) second-generation biofuel and (iii) third-generation biofuel. First-generation biofuel mainly includes bioethanol from sugar- and starch-based biomass (i.e., fermentation), biodiesel from edible crop oil and/or animal fat (i.e., transesterification), and biomethane from wet biomass (i.e., anaerobic digestion). Most of the biomass feedstocks used for first-generation biofuel production includes food crops, such as potato, corn, sugarcane, sunflower oil and coconut oil, and hence, it creates conflict with food interest. Therefore, second-generation biofuel has been introduced as it is produced from non-edible biomass, such as Jatropha, agriculture waste (e.g., rice husk, palm seed, coconut shell and sugarcane bagasse), forest residue (e.g., stem, bark and cone) and wood processing residue (e.g., sawdust, woodchips, pellets and tree barks). Most of the second-generation biomass are energy crops that consists of cellulose, hemicellulose and lignin composition. Hence, they are also known as lignocellulosic-based biomass. To produce second-generation biofuel, thermochemical method, including pyrolysis, gasification and liquefaction, is one of the most suggested biofuel conversion techniques. This is because thermochemical method converts the whole lignocellulosic-based biomass into biofuel, unlike fermentation (Latif et al. 2019). Fermentation is a metabolic process of converting sugars, such as glucose, fructose and sucrose, into cellular energy and at the same time, producing alcohol (biofuel) as a by-product through the action of yeast, bacteria or other microorganism. It is noted that first-generation biomass is mostly sugar- and starch-based feedstock, and hence, fermentation has been applied commercially on a large scale in producing first-generation biofuel (bioethanol). On the other hand, second-generation biomass consists mostly lignocellulosic-based feedstock, which requires a series of pre-treatment to recover the fermentable sugar before being directed into biorefineries for biofuel production through fermentation. As the result, the production of second-generation biofuel through fermentation requires additional pre-processing action, and so, increases the overall operating cost (Toor et al. 2020). Besides, fermentation also utilizes the fermentable part of the lignocellulosic biomass only, while other remains wasted.

The third-generation biofuels, however, generally include the biofuel production that still under development. The third-generation biomass usually has high growth rate with less nutrient requirement, such as food waste, animal manure, municipal solid waste, industrial effluent and sewage sludge (Picazo-Espinosa, Gonzalez-Lopez, and Manzaner 2011). It also refers to the biomass that could be related to carbon dioxide (CO_2) utilization and mitigation, such as aquatic biomass. Other than CO_2 utilization, aquatic biomass, including macroalgae and microalgae, has a high potential to be used as feedstock for biofuel production, especially biodiesel, due to its perennial and inherent growth, no arable land consumption, high lipid content and high growth rate (Nanda et al. 2018). Aquatic biomass can be used to produce several types of biofuels, such as bioethanol, biodiesel, syngas and biohydrogen. Animal manure and food waste, however, are potential candidates to produce biofuel through anaerobic digestion due to their high organic matter content (Zhang 2018).

In addition, biofuels can also be categorized into two groups based on the commercialization status of biofuel technologies, which are (i) conventional biofuels and (ii) advanced biofuels. The conventional biofuels refer to the biofuel that are widely available at present, which mostly first-generation biofuels, such as bioethanol and biodiesel. Advanced biofuels, however, mainly refer to second- and third-generation biofuels that are currently under demonstration and research stages with the potential to be fully commercialized in the future. There are also some advanced biofuels that already available in the market but still at early commercial phase, such as hydrotreated vegetable oil (HVO) and hydrotreated esters and fatty acids (HEFA). HVO and HEFA, also known as green diesel, are diesel substitute fuels that are produced by treating the vegetable oils and animal fats with hydrogen. Table 3.3.3 presents the examples of conventional and advanced biofuels, and their respective blending characteristics for biofuel application in the transportation sector.

There are various biofuel conversion technologies, but basically, they can be divided into three main groups, which are (i) chemical method, (ii) biochemical method and (iii) thermochemical method. Figure 3.3.3 summarizes different biofuel conversion techniques with their respective biofuel obtained. Chemical method refers to the use of chemical agents to convert biomass into liquid fuel, which is mostly biodiesel, such as acid-/base-catalyzed transesterification and hydrotreating process. The biochemical conversion method, however, involves the utilization of microorganisms or enzyme to transform the biomass or waste into useful biofuels, whereas thermochemical method involves the breakdown of biomass components using heat energy. Conversion by means of biochemical method includes anaerobic digestion, fermentation and enzymatic transesterification. On the other hand, thermochemical method comprises gasification, liquefaction and pyrolysis. It is noted that transesterification can be either considered as chemical or biochemical conversion method depend on catalyst or enzymes used.

TABLE 3.3.3
Different Conventional and Advanced Biofuels with Their Respective Blending Ratio [Information: (IEA 2011)]

Biofuel			Blending Characteristics
Conventional biofuels	Commercial stage	Sugar-based bioethanol	Conventional gasoline vehicle: usually E10-E15, but up to E25 in BrazilFlexible-fuel or ethanol vehicle: E85-E100
		Starch-based bioethanol	Similar with sugar-based bioethanol
		Conventional biodiesel, FAME (by transesterification)	Conventional diesel engine: Up to B20
		Biogas (anaerobic digestion)	After upgrading: fully compatible with existing vehicles and fuelling infrastructure
Advanced biofuels	Early commercial stage	Hydrotreated vegetable oil (HVO)	Well suited with current vehicle and distribution infrastructure
	Demonstration stage	Cellulosic bioethanol	Similar with sugar-based bioethanol
		Bio-synthetic gas	Similar with biogas
		Other biomass-to-liquid biodiesel	Similar with HVO
	Research stage	Algal-oil-based biodiesel/ jet fuel	After hydrotreating: fully compatible with existing vehicle and distribution infrastructure
		Sugar-based diesel/jet fuel	Similar with HVO

3.3.3.1 Biodiesel

The exploration of alternatives to conventional diesel began with the direct utilization of vegetable oil into the diesel engines without any modification (Knothe, Dunn, and Bagby 1997). Although vegetable oil is more environmentally friendly, such as sulphur-free and high ash point, some properties of vegetable oil have limited its usage in the diesel engine directly (Mumtaz et al. 2017). For instance, the high viscosity, poly-unsaturation properties, low volatility and poor fuel atomization of vegetable oil has led to the incomplete combustion and unwanted carbon formation in the combustion chamber. Besides, the unwanted deposit will stick on the piston ring, causing injector coking and delay the ignition process (Mumtaz et al. 2017; Agarwal 2007). Hence,

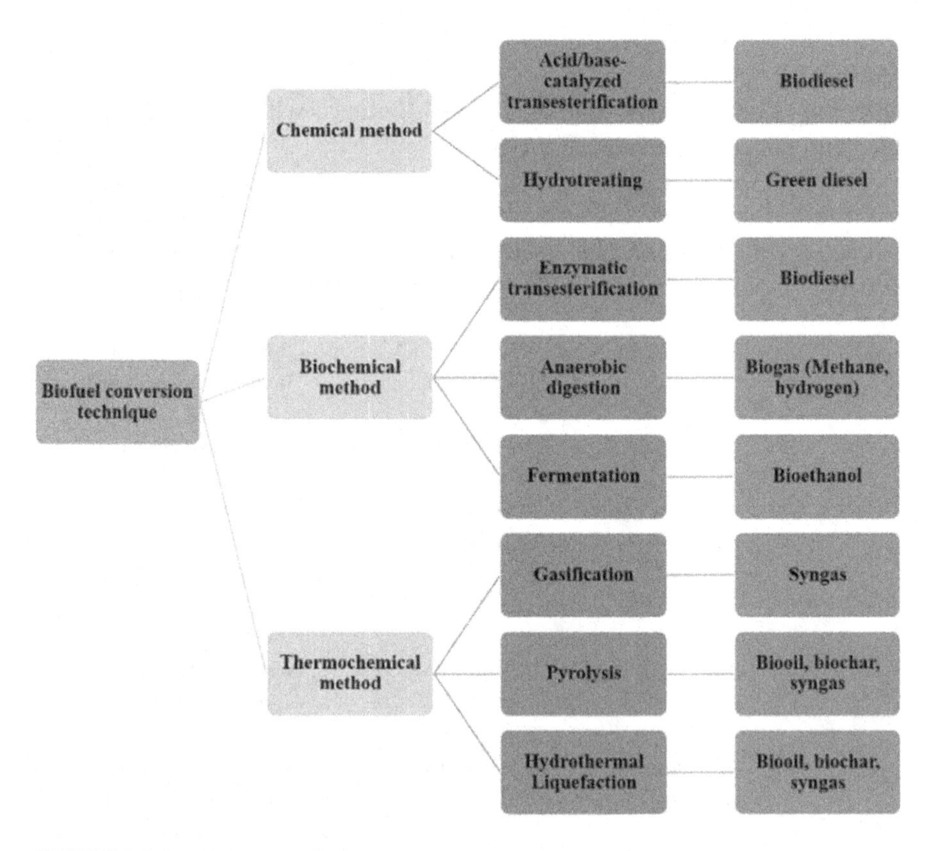

FIGURE 3.3.3 Various biofuel conversion techniques.

studies have been done and discovered that transesterification is one of the methods that can used to lower down the barriers that related to the direct use of vegetable oil as petroleum diesel replacement in diesel engines (Math and Chandrashekhara 2016). Transesterification is a process in which a carboxylic acid ester is converted into another carboxylic acid ester. The transesterification process usually involves the breakdown of triglyceride (i.e., oils or fats) into fatty acid alkyl esters (FAAE), also known as biodiesel, by using alcohol (mostly methanol or ethanol) in the presence or absence of catalysts. Although biodiesel performs like a petroleum diesel, however, they have different chemical structures resulting in different physical and chemical properties with each other. Table 3.3.4 summarizes and compares the properties of petroleum diesel, biodiesel and green diesel (will be explained in section 3.3.3.2) (Aatola et al. 2009; Kaya, Kutlar, and Taskiran 2018; Labeckas, Slavinskas, and Kanapkienė 2019; Sanjid et al. 2013; Szabados and Bereczky 2015; Pandey et al. 2019). As shown, petroleum diesel and biodiesel have different chemical compound and structure, hence, this has resulted in numerous notable variations between both of them. For example, biodiesel has higher flash point and cetane number, which in turn causes the storage and transportation of biodiesel to be safer and has a better ignition quality than petroleum

TABLE 3.3.4
Comparison of Properties between Petroleum Diesel, Biodiesel and Green Diesel

	Petroleum Diesel	Biodiesel	Green Diesel
Carbon (%)	86.8	79.6	84.9
Hydrogen (%)	13.2	10.5	15.1
Oxygen (%)	0	8.6	0
Nitrogen (%)	0	1.3	0
Carbon to hydrogen ratio, C/H	6.6	7.6	5.6
n-Aliphatics (%)	67.4	15.2	100 (paraffinic)
Olephenics (%)	3.4	84.7	0
Aromatics (%)	20.1	0	0.2
Naphtens (%)	9.1	0	0
Sulphur content (mg/kg)	3.6–15	1.54	<5
Density at 15 °C (kg/m^3)	796–841	820–897	770–790
Kinematic viscosity at 40 °C (mm^2/s)	1.9–4.1	2.9–11	2–4
Flash point (°C)	50–148	100–180	>59
Cloud point (°C)	Down to −40	Down to −13	Down to −34
Calorific value (MJ/kg)	42–46	32–43	43.7–44.5
Iodine value (J$_2$g/100g)	6	110	–
Cetane number	45–55	46–66	>70
Air Fuel Ratio, AFR	15.54	12.47	15.12

diesel. In contrast, biodiesel more likely to be thicken and solidified at low temperature in comparison to petroleum diesel as biodiesel consists of higher cloud point. This has limited the deployment of biodiesel especially for the countries with cold winters. As stated before, transesterification can reduce the viscosity of vegetable oil, but the viscosity of the reaction product (biodiesel) is still higher than the conventional petroleum diesel. As a result, the higher viscosity of biodiesel causes unfavourable impact on the fuel spray atomization. To balance the negative effect of biodiesel utilization, biodiesel is commonly blended with petroleum diesel at a certain ratio, up to B20 (20% biodiesel with 80% petroleum diesel) before being commercialized (Morone and Cottoni 2016). Overall, biodiesel is a promising petroleum diesel alternative as it can be directly used in diesel engine (e.g., car engines, home heating, mining equipment and railway locomotive) without any modification, particularly in warm climate areas. In addition, the biodiesel is renewable, biodegradable and environmentally friendly due to its lower greenhouse gases emission and lower sulphur content.

3.3.3.2 Green Diesel

The global biodiesel production has increased form 3.66 billion litres in 2005 to 41.3 billion litres in 2018 (World Bioenergy Association 2019; IEA 2019b). This significant growth of biodiesel production is mainly due to the policy priorities (i.e., economic subsidies) as its production cost is relatively high. Besides that, the production of biodiesel through transesterification creates problems due to the excessive co-production of crude glycerol. In general, the ratio of crude glycerol produced from biodiesel production is around 1:10. In other words, roughly ten pounds of crude glycerol are generated for every 100 pounds of biodiesel produced. Hence, various method has been attempted to utilize and dispose these crude glycerol (Binhayeeding, Klomklao, and Sangkharak 2017; Hammond et al. 2011). As stated earlier, biodiesel has several shortcomings compared to petroleum diesel, such as high oxygen content, high viscosity, high cloud points and others. Therefore, biodiesel has been blended with petroleum diesel to balance its disadvantages. Nevertheless, the utilization of biodiesel blend still results in higher nitrogen oxide (NO_x) emission, lower energy output and lower engine thermal efficiency in comparison to petroleum diesel (Hosseinzadeh-Bandbafha et al. 2018; Noor, Noor, and Mamat 2018; Saluja, Kumar, and Sham 2016).

Recently, a new generation of biofuel has been introduced, which is green diesel. Green diesel is also known as hydrogenated vegetable oil (HVO), or hydrogenated esters and fatty acid (HEFA), and is usually produced from vegetable oil and other biomass source such as animal and fish fats. Green diesel is composed of straight chain and branched saturated hydrocarbons (typically C15 to C18). This composition has made it similar with the petroleum diesel, and so, can be direct utilized in the compression ignition engine/diesel engine in pure form or as a blend (Eleana Kordouli et al. 2018). Green diesel is a paraffinic fuel, which is a clean transport fuel with near zero sulphur and aromatics. The properties of green diesel and its comparison with petroleum diesel and biodiesel can be found in Table 3.3.4. As shown in the table, green diesel consists of higher cetane number and lower density, which in turn can enhance the performance of diesel engine. Similar with biodiesel, green diesel also allows cleaner combustion and produces less carbon dioxide (CO_2) emission. Besides that, one of the major advantages of green diesel as compared to biodiesel is green diesel does not contain oxygen, and so, it is more stable, not corrosive and has same heating value with petroleum diesel. Moreover, the drawbacks of biodiesel, such as higher NO_x emission and poor ignition ability in diesel engine, have been solved by using green diesel. Furthermore, propane, a valuable gaseous fuel, instead of low-value crude glycerol, is produced as by-product during green diesel production through hydro-processing of triglycerides. Hence, due to these advantages, the production of green diesel has become more economically attractive in comparison to biodiesel production (Eleana Kordouli et al. 2017; E. Kordouli et al. 2017).

Hydrotreating process is one of the methods used to produce green diesel, in which the triglycerides of the biomass lipids react with hydrogen and being converted into saturated hydrocarbons liquid fuel in the presence catalysts (Douvartzides et al. 2019). Commonly, the hydrotreating of triglycerides into green diesel is conducted at temperature ranged between 280–450 °C, under pressure 1–5 MPa, and using heterogeneous mild-acid catalysts, such as sulphided Ni-Mo/Al_2O_3 and Co-Mo/Al_2O_3. One of the major advantages of using hydrotreating method for green diesel production is it can be well-integrated in the existing refinery

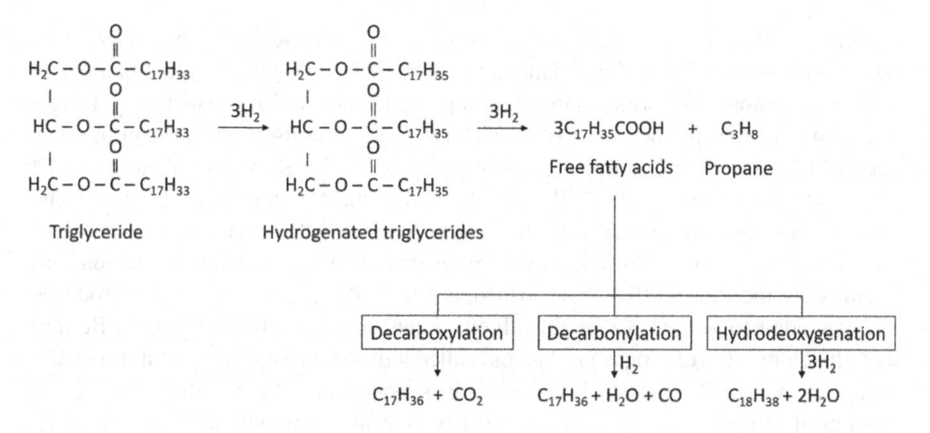

FIGURE 3.3.4 Reaction pathway of hydrotreating process for green diesel production.
Source: Adapted from Heriyanto et al. (2018).

infrastructure that operated for hydro-processing of petroleum distillates. The green diesel production consists of two main steps: (i) hydrogenation, in which the double bond of the fatty chains of a triglyceride is saturated by hydrogen (H_2); (ii) selective deoxygenation (SDO), where the oxygen molecules in the triglyceride are removed, and eventually forms saturated hydrocarbon fuel (green diesel). Generally, SDO can be further categorized into hydrodeoxygenation (HDO), decarbonylation (deCO) and decarboxylation (deCO_2). Figure 3.3.4 shows a possible reaction pathway of hydrotreating a sample triglyceride.

3.3.3.3 Biogas

Anaerobic digestion is a biological method of utilizing bacteria or other microorganisms to break down the organic portion of the biomass feedstock in the absence of oxygen. The main product of anaerobic digestion is biogas, which usually consists of 50–75% methane (CH_4), 25–50% carbon dioxide (CO_2), 1–10% nitrogen (N_2) and trace gases such as hydrogen sulphide (H_2S), hydrogen (H_2) and oxygen (O_2) (Anukam et al. 2019; Parawira et al. 2004). Methane is the major combustible component of the biogas, and the composition of gases produced are affected by several factors, such as the pH and water content of the biomass feedstock, the digestibility of the organic matter, digestion time and digestion temperature (Paul, Farcas, and Florentina (Radoi) 2014; Ruan et al. 2019). In the 1930s, biogas was used, mainly in domestic and agriculture areas, as a sludge stabilizer. Eventually, the advantages of biogas have been recognized and biogas production was successfully up-scale into industrial scale, especially in Europe and North America (IRENA 2018). Commonly, the biogas produced can be used to produce heat or electric power for domestic heating, cooking, lighting and others. Moreover, biogas also can be upgraded or purified into natural gas (biomethane) and used as transport fuel in conventional natural gas vehicles (NGVs). The deployment of NGV is gradually increasing globally due to its outstanding advantages, including lower fuel costs and lower greenhouse gas

(GHG) emissions in comparison to the diesel- and gasoline-driven vehicles (60–80% reduction) (IRENA 2018). For example, biomethane has been used as fuel in a tanker ship by a major Swedish shipping company, Furetank, in 2018 (Bioenergy Insight Magazine 2018a). In the same year, a Norway-based cruise operator, Hurtigruten, decided to invest EUR 742 million into biomethane-fuelled ships, and planned to start to operate them starting in 2021 (Bioenergy Insight Magazine 2018b). Germany, Sweden, Switzerland, the UK and the United States are the largest producer in biomethane production. In Europe alone, more than 500 biomethane installation was operated by the end of 2018. From which, about 50 Petajoule of biogas are produced and upgraded to natural gas quality (biomethane) annually (IRENA 2018). Besides that, the co-product of biogas production, called a digestate, is also a useful product. It is the residual of the feedstock that initially supplied into the digestor after the extraction of biogas (main product). It consists of water, nutrients and organic carbon that fit soils, and hence, it can be used as organic fertilizer to treat the land/sludge. This, in turn, reduces the GHG level in the atmosphere by avoiding additional methane (CH_4) emission from landfilling or manure storage.

The production of methane containing biogas through anaerobic digestion is a mature, reliable and worldwide accepted technology for treatment of organic-rich biomass feedstock, especially wet biomass. Numerous biomass feedstock can be fed into the digestor for biogas production, such as wastewater treatment sludge, animal manure, vegetable by-product, food waste, industrial waste, municipal organic waste and energy crops. Anaerobic digestion is a process that is fully reliant on the mutual and syntrophic interaction of a cluster of microorganisms. Hence, it is crucial to explore and understand its chemical reaction mechanism for optimization purpose.

3.3.3.4 Bioethanol

Bioethanol is chemically known as ethylic alcohol (C_2H_5OH) or ethanol. It has the same organic compound used in alcoholic drinks. Bioethanol is a colourless, less toxic and biodegradable liquid fuel that produces less air pollutant. There are few ways of bioethanol utilization, including direct use in pure form, blend with gasoline to produce gasohol, or blend with diesel to reduce emission from diesel combustion. Table 3.3.5 compares the physicochemical properties between gasoline and ethanol/bioethanol (Ruan et al. 2019; Yüksel and Yüksel 2004). Bioethanol offers several advantages over gasoline, such as higher-octane number, higher flammability limits and higher flame speed. Hence, bioethanol is a good candidate to replace tetraethyl lead in improving the octane level of gasoline, and reducing the tendency of detonation (Demain and Báez-Vásquez 2013). By using fuel with higher octane number, a higher engine compression ratio can be used. Consequently, the thermal efficiency and power of the engine can be improved while reducing fuel consumption (Cruz et al. 2013). Moreover, bioethanol can be used as additives to oxygenate the fuel mixture, leading to a more complete combustion, and hence help to reduce GHG emission (Chin and Hng 2013; García 2016). On the other hand, the lower heating value (LHV) of ethanol is lower than gasoline. Specifically, a gallon of gasoline provides one-third more energy than a

TABLE 3.3.5
Comparison of Physiochemical Properties between Gasoline and Bioethanol

Properties	Gasoline	Ethanol/Bioethanol
Formula	C_4 to C_{12}	C_2H_5OH
Molecular weight	100–105	46.07
Density at 15 °C (kg/L)	0.69–0.79	0.79
Specific gravity at 15 °C (relative to density)	91	106–110
Freezing point (°C)	–40	–114
Boiling point (°C)	27–225	78
Vapour pressure at 38°C (kPa)	48–103	15.9
Specific heat (kJ/kg K)	2.0	2.4
Viscosity at 20 °C (mPas)	0.37–0.44	1.19
Lower heating value (MJ/L)	30–33	21.1
Flash point (°C)	–43	13
Auto-ignition temperature (°C)	257	423
Lower flammability limit (vol%)	1.4	4.3
Higher flammability limit (vol%)	7.6	19.0
Stoichiometric air-fuel ratio	14.7	9.0
Research octane number	88–100	108.6
Motor octane number	80–90	89.7
Cetane number	n/a	0–54
Solubility	Trace	High

gallon of ethanol. In other words, more ethanol is needed to generate the same output as gasoline. Besides that, ethanol might corrode and damage the fuel system and engine that pure gasoline does not. This is because ethanol has a high solubility with water and so, it absorbs water and causes water contamination, eventually corroding the metal parts in the fuel systems and affecting the engine performance. Even worse, the engine might be damaged as fuel separation occurs, especially when the car does not operate for a long time.

The utilization of bioethanol has a long history. Bioethanol was utilized initially by Brazil since 1925. Besides, it was started to be used in internal combustion engines by Germany and France in 1984 (Demirbas and Karslioglu 2007). However, the utilization of bioethanol was ignored after World War II due to its high production cost in comparison to petroleum fuel until the 1970s (Demirbas 2009). This is because an oil crisis occurred in the 1970s, and hence, the bioethanol started to gain interest in many countries. Brazil and the United States (US) started mass production of bioethanol in the 1970s, from sugarcane and corn particularly, and has become the largest contributor (85%) of global bioethanol production (Azhar et al. 2017). Currently, bioethanol can be considered as the most widely used transport biofuel, which accounted for 63% (in terms of energy) of total global biofuel production (REN21 2019).

Bioethanol is mostly produced from the fermentation of sugar or starch from various biomass feedstocks using yeast or bacteria under the absence of oxygen. Sugar- and starch-based feedstocks, such as corn and sugar, are the best option for bioethanol production; however, it creates conflict with food interest. Hence, lignocellulosic-based feedstock is suggested as it is widely available, such as crop residues, food processing waste and municipal organic waste. Nevertheless, bioethanol production from lignocellulosic feedstock requires an additional of pre-treatments to recover fermentable sugar from cellulosic components, which is the major economical deficiency of this technology. Hence, research attention has been given to the development of cost-effective method for sugar extraction from lignocellulosic-based feedstock. There are several pre-treatment methods such as mechanical milling (physical), acid or alkaline hydrolysis (chemical), steaming or ammonia fibre explosion (physiochemical) and biological pre-treatment by using fungus (Kudakasseril Kurian et al. 2013; Azhar et al. 2017).

3.3.3.5 Bio-oil, Bio-char and Syngas

The thermochemical process includes pyrolysis, gasification and hydrothermal liquefaction, and applies a similar basic concept, which is converting the biomass into energy/fuel by heating. However, these mentioned thermochemical methods have different amounts of air supply and energy/fuel output. Gasification requires partial amounts of air; pyrolysis and hydrothermal liquefaction, however, occur in the absence of air.

Gasification is one of the thermochemical methods to process biomass, where syngas is produced in the presence of a gasifying agent under sub-stoichiometric conditions. Syngas, also known as synthesis gas, has wider applications, such as used as fuel in internal combustion engines, gas turbines or fuel cells for heat and electricity generation, or as feedstock for chemical synthesis and biofuel production. Generally, syngas is a gas mixture that is mainly made up of carbon monoxide (CO), hydrogen (H_2), carbon dioxide (CO_2) and methane (CH_4). The quality and yield of the syngas are highly affected by the types and characteristics of feedstock (e.g., cellulose, hemicellulose, lignin compositions, moisture content, particle size), operating condition (e.g., type of gasifying agent, operating temperature and pressure, heating rate) and gasification technology (e.g., fixed bed, fluidized bed, entrained flow) (Farzad, Mandegari, and Görgens 2016; Molino et al. 2018; Sansaniwal et al. 2017).

Hydrothermal liquefaction (HTL) is a hydrothermal processing that operates at a moderate temperature of 150–374 °C with appropriate pressures within the range of 5–20 MPa. It involves the thermochemical conversion of various biomass types in the presence of hot compressed water, producing bio-oil at subcritical condition of water. On the other hand, pyrolysis involves the conversion of biomass at a high temperature of 300–700 °C under atmospheric pressure. Both methods convert biomass into three products, which are solid bio-char, liquid bio-oil and syngas. Solid bio-char is the by-product of the processes and it can be used as soil fertilizer, water filtration substrate, catalysts and carbon sequestration element. Bio-oil, as the primary product, however, is a dark brown liquid with a distinct odour. It usually consists of hundreds of organic compounds that belong to alkanes, aromatic hydrocarbons and phenol derivatives. Bio-oil can be used directly as fuel in boilers for heat and electricity generation (Isahak et al. 2012). However, to use as a commercially viable transportation fuel, upgrading is needed due to its unfavourable properties, such as high oxygen content and water content, high density and high acidity (Mirkouei et al. 2017).

3.3.4 INDUSTRY 5.0 IN BIOFUEL PRODUCTION

To fulfil the increasing energy demand, and at the same time building a sustainable living environment, transport biofuel plays an important role. As mentioned previously, the definition of biofuel has been narrowed down to the transport fuel that derived from biomass. Besides, biofuel is considered a carbon-neutral fuel because the carbon released is balanced by the carbon consumed by biomass during photosynthesis. Hence, it shows a high potential for sustainability and economic growth for industrialized countries as biomass is renewable and is widely available in the local. However, in 2016, almost 96% of global transport energy demands were met by conventional petroleum, with only 3% met by biofuels (REN21 2019). To align with the IEA's Sustainable Development Scenario (SDS), the global transport biofuel consumption should be increased by triple (298 Mtoe), up to 9% of global transport energy demand in 2030 (IEA 2019c). SDS is an integrated approach for energy and sustainable development, which highlights the reduction of carbon dioxide (CO_2) emission while tackling the air pollution, achieving a climate goal, reaching universal energy access and accessing implication for water (Katowice 2018). Nevertheless, with the current expansion rate of transport biofuel production (6% in 2019) and a predicted expansion rate of 3% per annual over the next five years, there is still short of 10% annual growth of biofuel production until 2030 in order to be on track with the SDS. Hence, there is a must to upscale the biofuel production and increase the deployment of biofuels, especially in aviation and marine transport, by fully supporting the sustainable policy and further enhancing the biofuel processing technology to reduce the production cost.

However, upscaling of first-generation biofuels may not be feasible as it conflicts with the food interests and interrupts the usage of land for other important purposes. Hence, the implementation and upscaling of advanced biofuels from second- and third-generation biofuels should be given more attention. Theoretically, the deployment of advanced biofuels in large scale would be possible, especially using biomass feedstock that does not require arable land or those that consume arable lands without affecting the food supply, for instance, algal biomass, food waste, municipal solid waste and forestry and agriculture residue. In the other words, advanced biofuel technology involves the transformation of waste matter into different types of biofuels, as the mentioned biomass are mostly non-edible and useless for human activities. Nevertheless, there are some technical difficulties that limit the commercialization of advanced biofuels, including low biomass-to-fuel conversion efficiency, high energy consumption, limited supply of enzyme for biofuel conversion and dependence on commercially unproven technology (Timilsina and Cheng 2010). Although advanced biofuels have a huge future potential, however, upscaling of advanced biofuel production remains doubtful unless further research and development have successfully overcome or lowered the mentioned barriers. In fact, all advanced biofuel technologies have their own technical barriers that restrict their potential for commercialization. For example, the production of lignocellulosic-based bioethanol requires high-cost pre-treatment to recover the fermentable sugar, expensive enzymes for hydrolysis and has relative low conversion efficiency of five-carbon sugars to bioethanol. Hence, further exploration on these areas or development of new technology should be performed to improve the overall cost and conversion efficiencies and increase its possibility of commercialization.

Technological breakthroughs and the Industry Revolution are leading to advances in manufacturing sectors at unprecedented rates. The First Industrial Revolution (Industry 1.0) started with the utilization of steam power for industrial purposes. With the combination of steam power and mechanization, the human productivity was increased significantly. Next was the discovery of electricity and assembly line production, which were the dawn of the Second Industrial Revolution (Industry 2.0). The concept of Industry 2.0 is mass production, with the aims to manufacture products in a faster and cheaper way. In the last several decades, information technology and electronics started to integrate into industrial production, and hence, began the Third Industrial Revolution (Industry 3.0). In Industry 3.0, automation was achieved by using computers, while in the Fourth Industrial Revolution (Industry 4.0), artificial intelligence technologies were introduced to automate the process further. Basically, the focus of Industry 4.0 is about the automation of physical system with the help of machine-learning algorithms, so that the human labour can be directed into a more value-added field, instead of time-consuming works. However, the fast-growing digital technologies and AI (artificial intelligence)-based solutions have led to the scenario that robots are more important than humans. Challenges from labour unions and politicians are the biggest restriction in fully implementing Industry 4.0 (Nahavandi 2019). Hence, it can be foreseen that the advantages of Industry 4.0 will be neutralized as the pressure of increasing labour employment rises. Furthermore, the advancement in artificial intelligence technologies and human-machine interfaces have further increased the competitiveness between human labour and robot. Therefore, Industry 5.0 has been proposed to bring back human labour to the industrial field, in which robots are introduced as a collaborator of human labour, instead of a competitor. In Industry 5.0, attention will be continuously given on the enhancement of human-machine interfaces, but with the aim to further utilize human brainpower and creativity in enhancing the process efficiency, unlike Industry 4.0 in which human cost is unconsciously overlooked. Hence, robots will always aware of human desire and safety, and at the same time, human labour will work along with robots trustfully and reliability. As a result, higher-value jobs can be created in Industry 5.0 than Industry 4.0 because human labour will be in charge of design responsibility or tasks that involve creative thinking. On the other hand, monotonous and repetitive tasks will be left to the machine and being supervised by the human. In overall, production quality can be improved by taking and combining the best part of both humans and machines in all industry, including the renewable energy area (Nahavandi 2019).

As stated before, Industry 5.0 focus on improving the process efficiency and quality through the collaboration between human and robots. In Industry 5.0, a robot is far more than an autonomous machine. The robots in Industry 5.0 are commonly known as cobots, which provide robotic production with human touch. Cobots, unlike the robots presently used on the production floor, are collaborative robots programmed to interact with humans in shared workplaces. Cobots should already know what to do or are a quick learner in order to assist the human worker in achieving targets. With this revolution, biofuels will be able to cost-compete with the conventional fossil-based fuel. Hence, the benefits of biofuels, such as overcome fossil fuel depletion issues and reduce greenhouse gas emissions, can be maximized. However, the transformation of current biofuel production into next-generation technology is challenging. Currently, several strategies, including the implementation of cyber-physical system, artificial intelligence technique (AI) and machine learning techniques (ML), have been proposed and deployed to advance the biofuel production (Hansen, Mirkouei, and Xian 2019). The cyber-physical system (CPS) combines the physical components (e.g., thermocouples, pressure gauge, moisture metres, sampling probes, and gas flow metre) with a digital interface. It includes a sensing module with a programmable logic controller (PLC) to monitor the process in real time and control the unit. The CPS is able to collect data, analyze it, make a decision based on the history data and finally, develop a prediction model (Lee, Bagheri, and Kao 2015; Wu et al. 2017). Hence, the quality of biofuel can be maintained while optimizing the biofuel production process. Basically, there are two digital interfaces that are integrated into CPS, which are artificial intelligence (AI)/Artificial Neural Networks (ANN). There are various forms of ANN, such as Convolutional Neural Networks (CNN), Deep Neural Networks (DNN) and Fuzzy Logic Modeling (FLM). In the last last decades, ANN has been used in the development of bioprocess that full of variations, including in biofuel production (Betiku and Taiwo 2015; Vassileva et al. 2012; Whiteman and Gueguim Kana 2014). The biggest advantages of the ANN model are that it consists of remarkable learning, analysis and adaptation capability by arithmetically modelling the network structure of human nervous system. In addition, ANNs is entirely data-driven with no prior process-related information needed. CNN and DNN, however, are different forms of ANN with improved datasets and training algorithms. Besides, DNN is found to be more efficient than ANN, especially for large datasets. On the other hand, FLM is useful for applications where an exact mathematical model is impossible. Hence, FLM is usually used in biofuel production to automate and optimize the biofuel production without a clear knowledge of the process parameters (Hansen and Mirkouei 2018). Nevertheless, a deeper understanding of the biofuel production technology is a must to optimize the biofuel conversion technology, scaling up the biofuel production and enhancing the sustainability benefits in the biofuel industry. Hence, AI-based solutions (Industry 4.0) should be collaborated with human intelligence in Industry 5.0 as a tool for humans to explore the reaction mechanism, especially for advanced biofuel production, and utilize human creativity in creating a more responsive biofuel production system. Besides, Industry 5.0 also provides the ability to push the boundaries of physics on the design of the biofuel reactor. For example, Industry 5.0 is able to automate the biofuel production process better. In other words, real-time data is always available from the production floor and hence, can be used by the researcher to enhance the design of the reactor and hence, increase the energy and cost-efficiency of the biofuel production. Overall, the existing AI algorithms will pave the way towards Industry 5.0 Revolution in the biofuel industry.

3.3.4.1 Conversion of Waste into Valuable Biofuel

In Industry 4.0, the existing business and operational methods can be reshaped, and new business can be generated through the digitalization. As for biofuel production, new opportunities to convert waste materials into valuable biofuel can be achieved through digitalization. Waste refers to the useless by-products that would like to be disposed of even though disposal payment is required. Since the era of the Industrial Revolution, the waste generated increases significantly along with the increasing urbanization rate. Waste is a significant global issue, which creates huge environmental impacts. Several epidemics with high death tolls due to the unhealthy waste management habits occurred in human history. Hence, a proper waste management is necessary, particularly in a developing country. However, the nature of waste is subjective, fully dependent on the owners (Amasuomo and Baird 2016). A substance that is considered as waste by one individual may be a resource to another. For example, waste, including municipal solid waste, food waste, agriculture residues and animal manure, consist of huge potential as a feedstock in biofuel production, especially bioethanol and biogas. Since the material source is inconsistent, the biofuel production requires traceability for transparency of raw materials throughout the supply chain. So, the information on the quality and quantity of different batches of waste materials will be available to ensure an efficient and proper processing method. Hence, Industry 4.0 provides the solution to real-time monitor the waste material by using robust autonomous systems. Nevertheless, a robust autonomous system alone is not enough; human brainpower is necessary to further analyze the data collected and make decisions in order to fully utilize the waste material and optimize the biofuel production. So, here comes Industry 5.0, in which a more sophisticated and responsive operational intelligence systems should be used. The artificial intelligence algorithms should be able to advise the human workers, and to collect feedback for the purpose of process enhancement. Indeed, the differentiation and advancement of biofuel technologies cannot be done without the guide of the human mind, especially when dealing with the inconsistent waste materials.

3.3.4.2 Genetic Engineering

The bioengineering industrial revolution started in the latter half of the 20th century when recombinant DNA was used within the health sector, and this was followed by the genetic modification on the agriculture product to promote the food productivity. And now, technological innovation in the genetic engineering of energy crops has been deployed to enhance their agronomical traits for biofuel production. This is because the production of biofuel crops is highly dependent on their agronomic traits and genetic engineering shows high patenting in enhancing the existing genotypes, results in a sustainable and profitable biomass production and eventually, increase and maximize the productivity of large-scale biofuel production. There are several targets for genetic modification of biofuel crops, including optimizing the metabolism of the biofuel crop, overcoming its lignocellulose recalcitrance, enhancing its biomass productivity, increasing its efficiency in terms of harvesting rate and nutrient consumption, increasing its environmental adaptability (e.g., abiotic stress and pest resistances) and increasing its ability to produce value-added products (Akashi and Nanasato 2018).

To investigate the genetical potential of biofuel crops, there is a need to establish an efficient transformation protocol, which involves the design and construct of gene vector, gene delivery, regeneration of transformed cell and selection of stable transgenic plants with desired characteristics (Akashi and Nanasato 2018; Kumar, Ogita, and Yau 2018). However, this establishment of requires huge effort and time. As a result, the transformation technologies are more advanced in traditional edible crops (first-generation biomass), such as maize, soybean and sugarcane (Hoang et al. 2015; Homrich et al. 2012; Que et al. 2014). Lately, a major improvement has been made in transforming second-generation biomass, for instances, Jatropha and switchgrass, and third-generation biomass, such as algae (King et al. 2014; Maghuly and Laimer 2013; Sharma et al. 2018). Other than gene editing on the biofuel crops, different microbes (enzymes and yeasts) are also being modified for biofuel production, especially bioethanol and biogas production, in which microbes plays an important role in their production. Currently, AI has been used in bioengineering for drug test identification, drug screening, image screening and predictive modelling. In Industry 5.0, AI application in biotechnology will be expanded to the gene editing level. AI can be used to analyze mutations and predict the mutation impact based on the hundreds of thousands of mutation examples provided by AI (Allen et al. 2019). Hence, the transformation of biofuel crops with different desired traits can be accelerated as gene editing can be done in a more accurate, cheaper and easier way with the assistance of artificial intelligence.

3.3.4.3 Extremophiles

Conventionally, mesophilic organisms that grow at moderate temperatures within 20 to 45 °C and their enzymes are used for biofuel production. In the recent decades, the application of extremophiles and extremozymes as promising alternatives in producing biofuel have been acknowledged (Amoozegar et al. 2019; Zhu et al. 2020). Extremophiles are the organisms that grow in extreme environmental conditions, where the carbon-based life form is difficult to survive, such as high/low temperature, high/low acidity and alkalinity, high pressure and high salinity. These organisms show unique characteristics that allow them to adapt, colonize and thrive in extreme living conditions. Basically, there are different types of extremophiles according to the physiochemical conditions to which they are adapted (Arora and Panosyan 2019). For example, basophiles are the organisms that can live under high pressure, especially deep under the Earth's surface and water. Acidophilic and alkaliphilic organisms are adapted to acidic (pH 0–5) and basic (pH 8.5–11.5) environments, respectively. On the other hand, thermophiles are the organisms that can survive at temperature above 50 °C. There are also few extremophiles that can adapt to more than two extreme conditions, such as high temperature and high osmotic pressure/pH (Rampelotto 2013). Extremophiles often demonstrate remarkable capability to adapt and deal with the challenges of biomolecule breakdown, due to their harsh living environment, through different strategies, such as a highly efficient DNA repair system, inherent protein stability and cytoplasmic accumulation of salts (Eldie et al. 2014). Extremozymes, however, are the robust enzymes that produced by extremophiles, which show kinetic characteristics that allow integration into processes conducted under extreme conditions (Rathinam and Sani 2018; Taylor et al. 2012). Hence, it can be used to catalyze the biofuel production that involves high temperature and pressure. Furthermore, extremophilic algae also shows potential as the biomass feedstock in biodiesel production as it consists of long-chain hydrocarbon similar to those found in conventional petroleum (Moll et al. 2018). In short, extremophiles, especially the enzyme produced, have a huge potential in overcoming the deficiency of biochemical conversion of biomass to biofuel. It is believed that the next industrial age will begin in the extremes and hence, extremophilic engineering plays an important role in commercializing biofuel in the next industrial age.

3.3.5 CONCLUSION

Environmental problems, such as global warming, climate change and pollution, have dominated the headlines since a few decades ago. One of the main contributors to these problems is the burning of fossil fuel. Nevertheless, the fuel is of great importance in the human life as without fuel, technology will never be developed. As a result, the world will not work as efficiently as it is working nowadays. So, worldwide research and development in the renewable energy area has been conducted to reduce the fossil fuel dependency during the past two decades. Among the available renewable energy technologies, the biomass conversion into biofuels, including biogas, bioethanol, biodiesel, green diesel and bio-oil, have attracted great attention. Biofuels are considered carbon-neutral and do not contribute to global warming, since the carbon dioxide absorbed by plants (biomass) during photosynthesis is equal to the carbon dioxide released when the biofuel is combusted. Moreover, biofuel can be used directly in the conventional transportation system without/with slight modification. There are various biomass-to-biofuel conversion methods, however, they are not as mature as the conventional fossil fuel processing technologies. Therefore, in this paper, several strategies have been highlighted to promote the commercialization of biofuel in the next industrial age (Industry 5.0). The main concept of Industry 4.0 is about the automation of physical systems with the help of artificial intelligence (AI) technologies and consequently, human cost has been overlooked unconsciously. It can be foreseen that the advantages of Industry 4.0 will be neutralized as the pressure of increasing labour employment rises. Therefore, Industry 5.0 has been proposed to bring back human labour to the industrial field, in which robots are introduced as a collaborator of human labour, instead of a competitor. It is significant to notice that Industry 5.0 is an upgrade of

Industry 4.0, not completely new. For instance, the existing AI algorithms that were developed in optimizing and predicting the biofuel production can be used to pave the way towards Industry 5.0 with the option to allow customization and deal with waste feedstock that consists of inconsistent properties. Customization can also be achieved through the collaboration of AI and human brain power in predicting the genetic mutation impact during gene editing of the biofuel crops. In addition, Industry 5.0 should also investigate the "extreme" level, where the extremophilic organisms and their extremozymes have a huge potential in overcoming the deficiency of the biofuel production process, particularly biochemical biomass-to-biofuel conversion.

ACKNOWLEDGEMENTS

This research was funded by AAIBE Chair of Renewable Energy (Project code: 202006KETTHA) and Ministry of Education Malaysia (code: FRGS/1/2018/STG01/UNITEN/01/1). Furthermore, the authors would like to acknowledge UNITEN for the research facilities. M.Y.O would also like to thank UNITEN for the UNITEN Postgraduate Excellence Scholarship 2019.

REFERENCES

Aatola, Hannu, Martti Larmi, Teemu Sarjovaara, and Seppo Mikkonen. 2009. "Hydrotreated vegetable oil (HVO) as a renewable diesel fuel: Trade-off between NOx, particulate emission, and fuel consumption of a heavy duty engine." *SAE International Journal of Engines* 1 (1): 1251–1262. doi:10.4271/2008-01-2500.

Agarwal, Avinash Kumar. 2007. "Biofuels (alcohols and biodiesel) applications as fuels for internal combustion engines." *Progress in Energy and Combustion Science* 33 (3): 233–271. doi:10.1016/j.pecs.2006.08.003.

Akashi, Kinya, and Yoshihiko Nanasato. 2018. "Recent progress in the genetic engineering of biofuel crops." In *Biofuels: Greenhouse Gas Mitigation and Global Warming: Next Generation Biofuels and Role of Biotechnology*, 327–339. Springer India. doi:10.1007/978-81-322-3763-1_18.

Allen, Felicity, Luca Crepaldi, Clara Alsinet, Alexander J. Strong, Vitalii Kleshchevnikov, Pietro De Angeli, Petra Páleníková, et al. 2019. "Predicting the mutations generated by repair of Cas9-induced double-strand breaks." *Nature Biotechnology* 37 (1): 64–82. doi:10.1038/nbt.4317.

Amasuomo, Ebikapade, and Jim Baird. 2016. "The concept of waste and waste management." *Journal of Management and Sustainability* 6 (4): 88. doi:10.5539/jms.v6n4p88.

Amoozegar, Mohammad Ali, Atefeh Safarpour, Kambiz Akbari Noghabi, Tala Bakhtiary, and Antonio Ventosa. 2019. "Halophiles and their vast potential in biofuel production." *Frontiers in Microbiology* 10: 1895. doi:10.3389/fmicb.2019.01895.

Anukam, Anthony, Ali Mohammadi, Muhammad Naqvi, and Karin Granström. 2019. "A review of the chemistry of anaerobic digestion: Methods of accelerating and optimizing process efficiency." *Processes* 7 (8): 504. doi:10.3390/pr7080504.

Arora, Naveen Kumar, and Hovik Panosyan. 2019. "Extremophiles: Applications and roles in environmental sustainability." *Environmental Sustainability* 2 (3): 217–218. doi:10.1007/s42398-019-00082-0.

Azhar, Mohd, Siti Hajar, Rahmath Abdulla, Siti Azmah Jambo, Hartinie Marbawi, Jualang Azlan Gansau, Ainol Azifa Mohd Faik, and Kenneth Francis Rodrigues. 2017. "Yeasts in sustainable bioethanol production: A review." *Biochemistry and Biophysics Reports* 10: 52–61. doi:10.1016/j.bbrep.2017.03.003.

Betiku, Eriola, and Abiola Ezekiel Taiwo. 2015. "Modeling and optimization of bioethanol production from breadfruit starch hydrolyzate vis-à-vis response surface methodology and artificial neural network." *Renewable Energy* 74: 87–94. doi:10.1016/j.renene.2014.07.054.

Binhayeeding, Narisa, Sappasith Klomklao, and Kanokporn Sangkharak. 2017. "Utilization of waste glycerol from biodiesel process as a substrate for mono-, di-, and triacylglycerol production." In *Energy Procedia*, 138:895–900. Elsevier Ltd. doi:10.1016/j.egypro.2017.10.130.

Bioenergy Insight Magazine. 2018a. "Swedish Shipping Company Takesshipping company takes on Liquefied Biogas." liquefied biogas." Bioenergy Insight Magazine. 27 June. Available at: https://www.bioenergy-news.com/news/swedish-shipping-company-takes-on-liquefied-biogas/

Bioenergy Insight Magazine. 2018b. "Cruise firm to invest €742m into biogas fuelled ships." *Bioenergy Insight Magazine*. 19 Nov. Available at: https://www.bioenergy-news.com/news/cruise-firm-to-invest-742m-into-biogas-fuelled-ships/

BP. 2019. "BP Statistical Review of World Energy 2019." 68th edition, pp. 1–57. BP p.l.c., London, UK.

Brito Cruz, Carlos H., Glaucia Mendes Souza, and Luiz A. Barbosa Cortez. 2013. "Biofuels for transport." In *Future Energy: Improved, Sustainable and Clean Options for Our Planet*. Elsevier, Oxford, UK. doi:10.1016/B978-0-08-099424-6.00011-9.

Castello, Daniele, Thomas Helmer Pedersen, and Lasse Aistrup Rosendahl. 2018. "Continuous hydrothermal liquefaction of biomass: A critical review." *Energies* 11 (11): 3165. doi:10.3390/en11113165.

Chen, Meijie, Yurong He, Jiaqi Zhu, and Dongsheng Wen. 2016. "Investigating the collector efficiency of silver nanofluids based direct absorption solar collectors." *Applied Energy* 181: 65–74. doi:10.1016/j.apenergy.2016.08.054.

Chin, K.L., and P.S. Hng. 2013. "A real story of bioethanol from biomass: Malaysia perspective." In *Biomass Now – Sustainable Growth and Use*. InTech. doi:10.5772/51198.

Demain, Arnold L., and Marco A. Báez-Vásquez. 2013. "Biofuels of the present and the future." In *New and Future Developments in Catalysis: Catalytic Biomass Conversion*, 325–370. Elsevier B.V. doi:10.1016/B978-0-444-53878-9.00016-3.

Demirbas, A., and S. Karslioglu. 2007. "Biodiesel production facilities from vegetable oils and animal fats." *Energy Sources, Part A: Recovery, Utilization, and Environmental Effects* 29 (2): 133–141. doi:10.1080/009083190951320.

Demirbas, Ayhan. 2009. "Biofuels securing the planet's future energy needs." *Energy Conversion and Management* 50 (9): 2239–2249. doi:10.1016/j.enconman.2009.05.010.

Digest of United Kingdom Energy Statistics (DUKES). 2018. "Calorific Values of Fuels." Department for Business, Energy & Industrial Strategy, London, UK. https://www.gov.uk/government/statistics/dukes-calorific-values

Douvartzides, Savvas L., Nikolaos D. Charisiou, Kyriakos N. Papageridis, and Maria A. Goula. 2019. "Green diesel: Biomass feedstocks, production technologies, catalytic research, fuel properties and performance in compression ignition internal combustion engines." *Energies* 12 (5): 809. doi:10.3390/en12050809.

Eldie, Berger, Ferras Eloy, Taylor Mark P., and Cowana Don A. 2014. "Extremophiles and their use in biofuel synthesis." In *Industrial Biocatalysis*, edited by Peter Grunwald. Vol. 1. Jenny Stanford Publishing.

EPA. 2019. "Sources of Greenhouse Gas Emissions." Environmental Protection Agency, United States. https://www.epa.gov/ghgemissions/sources-greenhouse-gas-emissions

Farzad, Somayeh, Mohsen Ali Mandegari, and Johann F. Görgens. 2016. "A critical review on biomass gasification, co-gasification, and their environmental assessments." *Biofuel Research Journal* 3 (4): 483–495. doi:10.18331/BRJ2016.3.4.3.

García, I.L. 2016. "Feedstocks and challenges to biofuel development." In *Handbook of Biofuels Production: Processes and Technologies*, 2nd edition, 85–118. Elsevier Inc. doi:10.1016/B978-0-08-100455-5.00005-9.

Gowlett, J.A.J. 2016. "The discovery of fire by humans: A long and convoluted process." *Philosophical Transactions of the Royal Society B: Biological Sciences* 371 (1696). doi:10.1098/rstb.2015.0164.

Hammond, Ceri, Jose A. Lopez-Sanchez, Mohd Hasbi Ab Rahim, Nikolaos Dimitratos, Robert L. Jenkins, Albert F. Carley, Qian He, Christopher J. Kiely, David W. Knight, and Graham J. Hutchings. 2011. "Synthesis of glycerol carbonate from glycerol and urea with gold-based catalysts." *Dalton Transactions* 40 (15): 3927. doi:10.1039/c0dt01389g.

Hannah, Ritchie, and Roser Max. 2017. "CO and Greenhouse Gas Emissions." Our World In Data. https://ourworldindata.org/co2-and-other-greenhouse-gas-emissions.

Hansen, Samuel, and Amin Mirkouei. 2018. "Past Infrastructures and Future Machine Intelligence (MI) for Biofuel Production: A Review and MI-Based Framework." In Proceedings of the ASME 2018 International Design Engineering Technical Conferences and Computers and Information in Engineering Conference. ASME. https://doi.org/10.1115/DETC2018-86150

Hansen, Samuel B., Amin Mirkouei, and Min Xian. 2019. "Cyber-physical control and optimization for biofuel 4.0." In *IISE Annual Conference*.

Heriyanto, Heri, Sd Murti Sumbogo, Septina Is Heriyanti, Inayatu Sholehah, and Ayi Rahmawati. 2018. "Synthesis of Green Diesel from Waste Cooking Oil Through Hydrodeoxygenation Technology with NiMo/γ-Al2O3 Catalysts." In MATEC Web of Conferences Vol. 156. 10.1051/matecconf/201815603032

Hoang, Nam V., Agnelo Furtado, Frederik C. Botha, Blake A. Simmons, and Robert J. Henry. 2015. "Potential for genetic improvement of sugarcane as a source of biomass for biofuels." *Frontiers in Bioengineering and Biotechnology* 3: 182. doi:10.3389/fbioe.2015.00182.

Homrich, Milena Schenkel, Beatriz Wiebke-Strohm, Ricardo Luís Mayer Weber, and Maria Helena Bodanese-Zanettini. 2012. "Soybean genetic transformation: A valuable tool for the functional study of genes and the production of agronomically improved plants." *Genetics and Molecular Biology* 35 (4 SUPPL.): 998–1010. doi:10.1590/S1415-47572012000600015.

Hosseinzadeh-Bandbafha, Homa, Meisam Tabatabaei, Mortaza Aghbashlo, Majid Khanali, and Ayhan Demirbas. 2018. "A comprehensive review on the environmental impacts of diesel/biodiesel additives." *Energy Conversion and Management* 174 (October): 579–614. doi:10.1016/j.enconman.2018.08.050.

IEA. 2011. "Technology roadmap biofuels for transport." *International Energy Agency*. www.iea.org/about/copyright.asp.

IEA. 2019a. "Electricity information 2019." *International Energy Agency*. https://doi.org/10.1787/e0ebb7e9-en

IEA. 2019b. "Oil 2019." *International Energy Agency*. https://www.iea.org/oil2019/.

IEA. 2019c. "Tracking transport 2019." *International Energy Agency*. https://www.iea.org/reports/tracking-transport-2019/transport-biofuels.

IRENA. 2018. "Biogas for road vehicles: Technology brief." International Renewable Energy Agency, Abu Dhabi. https://www.irena.org/-/media/Files/IRENA/Agency/Publication/2017/Mar/IRENA_Biogas_for_Road_Vehicles_2017.pdf

Isahak, Wan Nor Roslam Wan, Mohamed W.M. Hisham, Mohd Ambar Yarmo, and Taufiq Yap Yun Hin. 2012. "A review on bio-oil production from biomass by using pyrolysis method." *Renewable and Sustainable Energy Reviews* 16 (8): 5910–5923. doi:10.1016/j.rser.2012.05.039.

Katowice, Andrew Prag. 2018. "The IEA sustainable development scenario." www.iea.org/COP24.

Kaya, Tolgahan, Osman Akın Kutlar, and Ozgur Oguz Taskiran. 2018. "Evaluation of the effects of biodiesel on emissions and performance by comparing the results of the new European drive cycle and worldwide harmonized light vehicles test cycle." *Energies* 11 (10): 1–14. https://ideas.repec.org/a/gam/jeners/v11y2018i10p2814-d176667.html.

King, Zachary R., Adam L. Bray, Peter R. LaFayette, and Wayne A. Parrott. 2014. "Biolistic transformation of elite genotypes of switchgrass (*Panicum virgatum* L.)." *Plant Cell Reports* 33 (2): 313–322. doi:10.1007/s00299-013-1531-1.

Knothe, Gerhard, Robert O Dunn, and Marvin O Bagby. 1997. "Biodiesel: The use of vegetable oils and their derivatives as alternative diesel fuels." In *ACS Symposium Series* 666: 172–208. doi:10.1021/bk-1997-0666.ch010.

Kordouli, E., C.H. Kordulis, A. Lycourghiotis, R. Cole, P.T. Vasudevan, B. Pawelec, and J.L.G. Fierro. 2017. "HDO activity of carbon-supported Rh, Ni and Mo-Ni catalysts." *Molecular Catalysis* 441: 209–220. doi:10.1016/j.mcat.2017.08.013.

Kordouli, Eleana, Barbara Pawelec, Kyriakos Bourikas, Christos Kordulis, Jose Luis G. Fierro, and Alexis Lycourghiotis. 2018. "Mo promoted Ni-Al_2O_3 co-precipitated catalysts for green diesel production." *Applied Catalysis B: Environmental* 229: 139–154. doi:10.1016/j.apcatb.2018.02.015.

Kordouli, Eleana, Labrini Sygellou, Christos Kordulis, Kyriakos Bourikas, and Alexis Lycourghiotis. 2017. "Probing the synergistic ratio of the NiMo/Γ-Al_2O_3 reduced catalysts for the transformation of natural triglycerides into green diesel." *Applied Catalysis B: Environmental* 209: 12–22. doi:10.1016/j.apcatb.2017.02.045.

Kudakasseril Kurian, Jiby, Gopu Raveendran Nair, Abid Hussain, and G.S. Vijaya Raghavan. 2013. "Feedstocks, logistics and pre-treatment processes for sustainable lignocellulosic biorefineries: A comprehensive review." *Renewable and Sustainable Energy Reviews* 25: 205–219. doi:10.1016/j.rser.2013.04.019.

Kumar, Ashwani, Shinjiro Ogita, and Yuan Yeu Yau. 2018. *Biofuels: Greenhouse Gas Mitigation and Global Warming: Next Generation Biofuels and Role of Biotechnology*. Springer India. doi:10.1007/978-81-322-3763-1.

Labeckas, Gvidonas, Stasys Slavinskas, and Irena Kanapkienė. 2019. "Study of the effects of biofuel-oxygen of various origins on a CRDI diesel engine combustion and emissions." *Energies* 12 (7): 1–49. https://ideas.repec.org/a/gam/jeners/v12y2019i7p1241-d218898.html.

Latif, Abdul, Nor Insyirah Syahira, Mei Yin Ong, and Saifuddin Nomanbhay. 2019. "Hydrothermal liquefaction of Malaysia's algal biomass for high-quality bio-oil production." *Engineering in Life Sciences* 19 (4): 246–269. doi:10.1002/elsc.201800144.

Lee, Jay, Behrad Bagheri, and Hung An Kao. 2015. "A cyber-physical systems architecture for Industry 4.0-based manufacturing systems." *Manufacturing Letters* 3: 18–23. doi:10.1016/j.mfglet.2014.12.001.

Maghuly, Fatemeh, and Margit Laimer. 2013. "Jatropha Curcas, A biofuel crop: Functional genomics for understanding metabolic pathways and genetic improvement." *Biotechnology Journal* 8 (10): 1172–1182. doi:10.1002/biot.201300231.

Malaysiakini. 2019. "Ten Years Before Known Oil, Gas Reserves Run Dry." Malaysiakini. 13 March. Available at: https://www.malaysiakini.com/news/467781

Math, M.C., and Chandrashekhara K.N. 2016. "Optimization of alkali catalyzed transesterification of safflower oil for production of biodiesel." *Journal of Engineering*, 7. Article ID 8928673.

Mirkouei, Amin, Karl R. Haapala, John Sessions, and Ganti S. Murthy. 2017. "A review and future directions in techno-economic modeling and optimization of upstream forest biomass to bio-oil supply chains." *Renewable and Sustainable Energy Reviews* 67: 15–35. doi:10.1016/j.rser.2016.08.053.

Mohd Noor, C.W., M.M. Noor, and R. Mamat. 2018. "Biodiesel as alternative fuel for marine diesel engine applications: A review." *Renewable and Sustainable Energy Reviews* 94: 127–142. doi:10.1016/j.rser.2018.05.031.

Molino, Antonio, Vincenzo Larocca, Simeone Chianese, and Dino Musmarra. 2018. "Biofuels production by biomass gasification: A review." *Energies* 11 (4): 811. doi:10.3390/en11040811.

Moll, Karen M., Todd C. Pedersen, Robert D. Gardner, and Brent M. Peyton. 2018. "Biodiesel (microalgae)." In *Extremophilic Microbial Processing of Lignocellulosic Feedstocks to Biofuels, Value-Added Products, and Usable Power*, 63–78. Springer International Publishing. doi:10.1007/978-3-319-74459-9_4.

Morone, P., and L. Cottoni. 2016. "Biofuels: Technology, economics, and policy issues." In *Handbook of Biofuels Production: Processes and Technologies*, 2nd edition, 61–83. Elsevier Inc. doi:10.1016/B978-0-08-100455-5.00004-7.

Mumtaz, M.W., A. Adnan, H. Mukhtar, U. Rashid, and M. Danish. 2017. "Biodiesel production through chemical and biochemical transesterification: Trends, technicalities, and future perspectives, technicalities, and future perspectives." In *Clean Energy for Sustainable Development: Comparisons and Contrasts of New Approaches*, 465–485. Elsevier Inc. doi:10.1016/B978-0-12-805423-9.00015-6.

Nahavandi, Saeid. 2019. "Industry 5. 0 – A Human-Centric Solution." *Sustainability* 11 (16): 4371. https://doi.org/10.3390/su11164371

Nanda, Sonil, Rachita Rana, Prakash K. Sarangi, Ajay K. Dalai, and Janusz A. Kozinski. 2018. "A broad introduction to first-, second-, and third-generation biofuels." In *Recent Advancements in Biofuels and Bioenergy Utilization*, 1–25. Springer Singapore. doi:10.1007/978-981-13-1307-3_1.

Pandey, Ashok, Christian Larroche, Claude Gilles Dussap, Edgard Gnansounou, Samir Kumar Khanal, and Steven Ricke. 2019. *Biofuels: Alternative Feedstocks and Conversion Processes for the Production of Liquid and Gaseous Biofuels. Biomass, Biofuels, Biochemicals: Biofuels: Alternative Feedstocks and Conversion Processes for the Production of Liquid and Gaseous Biofuels*, 2nd edition. Elsevier. doi:10.1016/C2018-0-00957-3.

Parawira, W., M. Murto, R. Zvauya, and B. Mattiasson. 2004. "Anaerobic batch digestion of solid potato waste alone and in combination with sugar beet leaves." *Renewable Energy* 29 (11): 1811–1823. doi:10.1016/j.renene.2004.02.005.

Paul, Dobre, Nicolae Farcas, and Matei Florentina (Radoi). 2014. "Main factors affecting biogas production – An overview." *Romanian Biotechnological Letters* 19 (3): 9283–9296.

Perea-Moreno, Miguel Angel, Esther Samerón-Manzano, and Alberto Jesus Perea-Moreno. 2019. "Biomass as renewable energy: Worldwide research trends." *Sustainability* 11 (3). doi:10.3390/su11030863.

Picazo-Espinosa, Rafael, Jesus Gonzalez-Lopez, and Maximino Manzaner. 2011. "Bioresources for third-generation biofuels." In *Biofuel's Engineering Process Technology*. InTech. doi:10.5772/17134.

Que, Qiudeng, Sivamani Elumalai, Xianggan Li, Heng Zhong, Samson Nalapalli, Michael Schweiner, Xiaoyin Fei, et al. 2014. "Maize transformation technology development for commercial event generation." *Frontiers in Plant Science* 5: 379. doi:10.3389/fpls.2014.00379.

Rampelotto, Pabulo Henrique. 2013. "Extremophiles and extreme environments." *Life (Basel)* 3 (3): 482–485. doi:10.3390/life3030482.

Rathinam, Navanietha Krishnaraj, and Rajesh K. Sani. 2018. "Bioprospecting of extremophiles for biotechnology applications." In *Extremophilic Microbial Processing of*

Lignocellulosic Feedstocks to Biofuels, Value-Added Products, and Usable Power, 1–23. Springer International Publishing. doi:10.1007/978-3-319-74459-9_1.

REN21. 2019. "Renewables Global Status Report (GSR) 2019." Renewable Energy Policy Network for the 21st Century. https://www.ren21.net/gsr-2019/

Rodrigues, Abel, João Carlos Bordado, and Rui Galhano Dos Santos. 2017. "Upgrading the glycerol from biodiesel production as a source of energy carriers and chemicals – A technological review for three chemical pathways." *Energies* 10 (11). doi:10.3390/en10111817.

Ruan, Roger, Yaning Zhang, Paul Chen, Shiyu Liu, Liangliang Fan, Nan Zhou, Kuan Ding, et al. 2019. "Biofuels: Introduction". *Biofuels: Alternative Feedstocks and Conversion Processes for the Production of Liquid and Gaseous Biofuels*. 3–43. doi: 10.1016/B978-0-12-816856-1.00001-4.

Saluja, Rajesh Kumar, Vineet Kumar, and Radhey Sham. 2016. "Stability of biodiesel – A review." *Renewable and Sustainable Energy Reviews* 62: 866–881. doi:10.1016/j.rser.2016.05.001.

Sanjid, A., H.H. Masjuki, M.A. Kalam, S.M. Ashrafur Rahman, M.J. Abedin, and S.M. Palash. 2013. "Impact of palm, mustard, waste cooking oil and *Calophyllum inophyllum* biofuels on performance and emission of CI engine." *Renewable and Sustainable Energy Reviews* 27: 664–682. doi:10.1016/j.rser.2013.07.059.

Sansaniwal, S.K., K. Pal, M.A. Rosen, and S.K. Tyagi. 2017. "Recent advances in the development of biomass gasification technology: A comprehensive review." *Renewable and Sustainable Energy Reviews* 72: 363–384. doi:10.1016/j.rser.2017.01.038.

Schobert, Harold. 2013. *Chemistry of Fossil Fuels and Biofuels. Chemistry of Fossil Fuels and Biofuels*. Cambridge University Press. doi:10.1017/CBO9780511844188.

Sharma, Prabin Kumar, Manalisha Saharia, Richa Srivstava, Sanjeev Kumar, and Lingaraj Sahoo. 2018. "Tailoring microalgae for efficient biofuel production." *Frontiers in Marine Science* 5: 382. doi:10.3389/fmars.2018.00382.

Szabados, György, and Ákos Bereczky. 2015. "Comparison tests of diesel, biodiesel and TBK-biodiesel." *Periodica Polytechnica Mechanical Engineering* 59 (3): 120–125. doi:10.3311/PPme.7989.

Taylor, M.P., R. Bauer, S. Mackay, M. Tuffin, and D.A. Cowan. 2012. "Extremophiles and their application to biofuel research." In *Extremophiles*, 233–265. Hoboken, NJ, USA: John Wiley & Sons, Inc. doi:10.1002/9781118394144.ch9.

Timilsina, Govinda R., and Jay J. Cheng. 2010. *Advanced Biofuel Technologies: Status and Barriers*. Policy Research Working Papers. The World Bank. doi:10.1596/1813-9450-5411.

Toor, Manju, Smita S. Kumar, Sandeep K. Malyan, Narsi R. Bishnoi, Thangavel Mathimani, Karthik Rajendran, and Arivalagan Pugazhendhi. 2020. "An overview on bioethanol production from lignocellulosic feedstocks." *Chemosphere* 242: 125080. doi:10.1016/j.chemosphere.2019.125080.

U.S. EIA. 2020. "Petroleum Supply Monthly - January." Energy Information Administration, United States. https://www.eia.gov/petroleum/supply/monthly/archive/2020/2020_01/psm_2020_01.php

Vassileva, Svetla, Lyubka Doukovska, and Silvia Mileva. 2012. "AI-based prediction and diagnostic on bioethanol production." In *IS'2012 – 2012 6th IEEE International Conference Intelligent Systems, Proceedings*, 270–274. IEEE. doi:10.1109/IS.2012.6335147.

Whiteman, J.K., and E.B. Gueguim Kana. 2014. "Comparative assessment of the artificial neural network and response surface modelling efficiencies for biohydrogen production on sugar cane molasses." *Bioenergy Research* 7 (1): 295–305. doi:10.1007/s12155-013-9375-7.

Williams, C. Luke, Rachel M. Emerson, and Jaya Shankar Tumuluru. 2017. "Biomass compositional analysis for conversion to renewable fuels and chemicals." In *Biomass Volume Estimation and Valorization for Energy*. InTech. doi:10.5772/65777.

WBA. 2019. "Global Bioenergy Statistics 2019." World Bioenergy Association, Sweden. https://worldbioenergy.org/global-bioenergy-statistics

Wu, Dazhong, Shaopeng Liu, Li Zhang, Janis Terpenny, Robert X. Gao, Thomas Kurfess, and Judith A. Guzzo. 2017. "A fog computing-based framework for process monitoring and prognosis in cyber-manufacturing." *Journal of Manufacturing Systems* 43: 25–34. doi:10.1016/j.jmsy.2017.02.011.

Yüksel, Fikret, and Bedri Yüksel. 2004. "The use of ethanol-gasoline blend as a fuel in an SI engine." *Renewable Energy* 29 (7): 1181–1191. doi:10.1016/j.renene.2003.11.012.

Zhang, Pengchong. 2018. "Biogas recovery from anaerobic digestion of selected industrial wastes." In *Advances in Biofuels and Bioenergy*. InTech. doi:10.5772/intechopen.72292.

Zhu, Daochen, Wasiu Adewale Adebisi, Fiaz Ahmad, Sivasamy Sethupathy, Blessing Danso, and Jianzhong Sun. 2020. "Recent development of extremophilic bacteria and their application in biorefinery." *Frontiers in Bioengineering and Biotechnology* 8: 1–18. doi:10.3389/fbioe.2020.00483.

3.4 Application of Industry 5.0 on Fruit and Vegetables Processing

Xuwei Liu, Jilu Feng, and Yang Tao

CONTENTS

3.4.1 INTRODUCTION

Fruit and vegetables (F&Vs) contain a variety of phytochemicals, which are also found in F&V-derived foods and constitute an important part of the non-nutritional components of the human diet. Their external physical characteristics (including size, color, shape, firmness, texture, etc.) and internal components (including sugar content, acid, soluble solid contents, nutrient contents, secondary metabolites, etc.) are largely influenced by environmental conditions, processing operations, technology level, and storage and transportation. These challenges have put forward new requirements for the supply and function of F&Vs in the future. The future development of F&Vs should become an integrated discipline of systems biology, synthetic biology, the Internet of Things, artificial intelligence, additive manufacturing, medical health, and perception science. On the basis of solving global food supply and quality, food safety, and nutrition issues, the higher demand for better lives can be met in the future. The development of plant-based food is an important direction for the development of food technology in the future.

Industry 5.0 will bring human ideas back to manufacturing. Its theme is human-robot collaboration, which will be a major innovation in society and will greatly influence the way we conduct business (Demir, Alpaslan, and Cicibaş 2018). Industry 4.0 establishes advanced technology at the center of production, while 5.0 actually connects people to work with factory systems (Østergaard 2016). The smart F&V factory of Industry 4.0 connects machines to the Internet, generating and collecting data from the entire supply chain. These data are further analyzed to drive quality improvement, process optimization, cost reduction, and regulatory compliance. The new Industry 5.0 will optimally combine the high speed and accuracy of industrial automation with the cognitive, critical thinking skills of employees (Demir, Döven, and Sezen 2019). Therefore, rather than replacing humans with technology, it enhances the role of robots in manufacturing. Responsibility for repetitive tasks, such as quality screening or data entry, rests on automated collaborative systems. Employees can oversee these systems, make real-time decisions, and take on higher levels of responsibility as they seek to improve quality and production processes.

Cooperative robots are not substitutes for workers, but rather they complement and develop the industry (Birje 2020). Like Industries 1.0, 2.0, and 3.0, this latest wave of industrial automation will result in net job growth, not losses. On the other hand, Industry 5.0 products make people aware of their basic desire to express themselves, even if they have to pay a high price. These products are called humanized goods. Personalized products are the products that consumers need and spend the most. They are products with human care and craftsmanship. Exquisite F&V packaging bags, refined F&V juices, and even special fruit platter from Michelin restaurant or new fruit puree from F&V laboratory. Such products can only be manufactured through human participation. Most importantly, this is what consumers are trying to express, their unique personalities through the products they buy. They favor the personal imprint of human designers and artisans because it is a unique product that they produce through their creativity. This is personalization, the feeling of luxury and the future.

Many tasks in the F&V processing industry are tedious and repetitive. Collaborative robots in Industry 5.0 not only contribute to perform heavy tasks such as transporting materials, cleaning products and equipments, but also interacting with humans to perform task selection, product optimization, and design as needed. On the other hand, collaborative robots can help people package fresh-cut F&V in a completely sterile environment, eliminating the risk of contamination. Machines will make human lives easier, but to do so, they must be taught how to collaborate and provide them with algorithms that replicate human perception, understanding, and tendencies, while retaining decision-making power (Birje 2020). In the next section, current and future issues and challenges related to F&V processing will be discussed. In the third section, we focus on the application of F&V processing in Industry 5.0, namely human-robot co-working. Finally, we briefly discuss future research trends.

3.4.2 ISSUES AND CHALLENGES

This section summarizes the key issues and challenges of current F&V processing manufacturing (Table 3.4.1).

TABLE 3.4.1
Key Issues and Challenges of the Current F&V Processing Manufacturing

	Pre-Production	Post-Production	Processing	Distribution	Consumption
Value chain stage	Agricultural inputs, tillage operations	Sorting or grading, storage	Blanching, dehydration, sterilization, excursion and packaging	Retail, transportation	Preparation, dining table
Key issues or challenges	Diminished quality, decreased yields	Physical damage, infection, by-products (F&V losses)	Quality and nutrition loss, structure change, overprocessing, by-products (F&V losses)	Quality loss, infection, by-products (F&V losses)	By-products (F&V waste)
Cause	Climate changes (e.g., elevated temperature, atmospheric CO_2, and O_3 concentration)	Handling techniques, microbial spoilage, storage technologies	Manufacturing processes, overproduction	Transportation technologies, high quality standards	Extra supply and/or preparation, spoilage

3.4.2.1 Climate Change

Climate change is defined as "a change of climate which is attributed directly or indirectly to human activity that alters the composition of the global atmosphere and which is in addition to natural climate variability observed over comparable periods," according to the United Nations Framework Convention on Climate Change (UNFCCC). Different climatic variables, including elevated temperature, increased atmospheric carbon dioxide (CO_2) levels and ozone (O_3) concentration, largely affect the quantity and quality of food crops around the world, becoming a major challenge in fruit and vegetable production. Therefore, understanding the impact of climate change on fruit and vegetable crops is extremely important for future adaptation in processing parameters and techniques, and also, climate change mitigation approaches.

1. Effect of carbon dioxide. Atmospheric CO_2 concentration has raised from 280 ppm (in pre-industrial levels) to 414 ppm (in February, 2020), and is predicted to reach 568–590 ppm in the 2080s (Hoegh-Guldberg et al. 2018). Elevated atmospheric CO_2 level has been confirmed to be able to alter the growth and physiology of vegetable and fruit plants, such as net photosynthesis, biomass production, nutritional quality, seed yield, etc. (Moretti et al. 2010). However, how the elevated CO_2 affects F&V plants remains controversial.

Rising atmospheric CO_2 could positively influence certain plants by enhancing photosynthesis. On one hand, increased CO_2 positively affects the C_3 plants. C_3 plants fix the carbon dioxide from the air only through the Calvin cycle, which means that CO_2 is limited in these species. Rising carbon dioxide concentration can, therefore, promote the net photosynthesis of these plants, ultimately increasing the accumulation of carbohydrates in leaves. The greater availability of carbohydrate reservoirs can enhance the metabolism and the production of secondary metabolites

(Balasooriya et al., 2019). For instance, a strawberry under elevated CO_2 had a higher strawberry yield, antioxidant content, flavor compounds, and enhanced fruit characteristics (e.g., number, size, and shape). Likewise, an increased CO_2 level also stimulates photosynthesis of potato plants, but as the level increases, the photosynthesis rate will reduce. On the other hand, as compared to C_3 plants, C_4 plants are more effectively concentrating CO_2, so photosynthesis might be CO_2-saturated even at low concentrations. As a consequence, C_4 plants will not benefit a lot by increasing CO_2 concentration.

Higher atmospheric CO_2 concentration could also alter flowering time. Springer and Ward (2007) summarized that with elevated CO_2 levels, most plants have earlier flowering time, while unchanged or delayed flowering time was observed for some plants. The controversial results could be due to the different experimental methodology used, the Open-Top Chambers (OTCs) or the Free-Air Carbon Enrichment (FACE) CO_2-enrichment technology. Nevertheless, Craufurd and Wheeler (2009) reviewed that an increase in CO_2 concentration has no or little change in the flowering time. Furthermore, other climatic variables, e.g., temperature, might interactively affect the growth rate and yield of the plants. Hence, we will discuss the combined effect of different climatic variables hereinafter.

It is also worth noting that agriculture by itself can affect climate change, contributing 30%–40% of anthropogenic greenhouse gas emissions (Mattos et al. 2014). Therefore, future approaches (e.g., reduce deforestation and improve production efficiency) should also be involved to mitigate climate change.

2. Effect of temperature. The expansion of the greenhouse effect has already caused global warming of more than 1°C above the pre-industrial level, which is expected to have a negative impact on F&V production and quality. The temperature change can affect the physiological, biochemical, and metabolic activities of plants. For example, the increased temperature can promote the sterility of stigma and stamen in papaya, causing flower drops and sex exchange in female and hermaphrodite flowers (Haokip, Shankar, and Lalrinngheta 2020).

Higher temperatures can reduce plant photosynthesis owing to the reduced activity of rubisco activase or the limitation of electron transport to regenerate ribulose-1,5-bisphosphate (Sage, Way, and Kubien 2008). Moreover, elevated temperatures lead to an increase in leaf temperature, changing the leaf-to-air vapor pressure difference, and causing stomatal closure, which also reduces the photosynthesis process because less carbon dioxide could be adsorbed (Moretti et al. 2010). As a result, the photosynthesis/respiration ratio decreases, reducing the F&V yields. If the high temperature (40/35 °C day/night) is applied, the net photosynthesis and strawberry yield could reduce by 44% and to 0, respectively (Kadir, Sidhu, and Al-Khatib 2006).

Exposure of the crops to high temperatures can affect the qualities of the F&V, including flavor, dry matter content, micronutrient content, and firmness. For instance, at elevated temperature, the carbohydrate, as well as sugar contents significantly decreased in strawberries, the tartaric acid content reduced by 50% in grapes, affecting the flavor and sensory quality of fruits. Furthermore, increasing the temperature decreased the anthocyanin accumulation in apple skin, citric acid, and ellagic acid contents in strawberries (Lin-Wang et al. 2011). The sun fruits were generally firmer than the shade fruits, as cell wall enzyme activity, which is negatively correlated with fruit firmness, increased at a higher temperature.

A rise in temperature could also increase the incidence of some physiological disorders and plant diseases, e.g., granulation in citrus (Haokip, Shankar, and Lalrinngheta 2020). The increase in pest infestations was also observed in some plants as a consequence of elevated temperature (Parajuli, Thoma, and Matlock 2019).

3. Effects of air pollutants and UV level. Air pollutants like sulfur dioxide (SO_2), carbon monoxide (CO), and ozone(O_3) can damage plant tissue and eventually reduce crop yields. For instance, O_3 can be absorbed into plant tissues via the stomates of leaves, causing direct cellular damage, which might be because of the changes in membrane permeability. This might also lead to visible injury, reduce growth, and eventually decrease yield. Moreover, F&Vs are sensitive to UV radiation, which can reduce photosynthesis and increase vulnerability to viruses (Parajuli, Thoma, and Matlock 2019).

4. Interactive effects of various climatic variables. The previous sections demonstrated the independent impact of a single climatic variable on F&V. Nonetheless, as these climatic variables (e.g., CO_2 concentration, temperature) will change simultaneously, therefore, their interactive effects on F&V may be different. For instance, under elevated CO_2, the production (yield and quality) of the strawberry was improved at low temperatures but decreased at high temperatures. This finding implies that other changes like increased temperature could offset the positive effect of elevated CO_2 concentration. Additionally, under enhanced temperature and water deficit, the pH of the grape berry juice significantly increased as a result of the increase in malic acid and tartaric acid in grapes; however, when elevated CO_2 was applied, the increase of pH was inhibited (Kizildeniz et al. 2015). These observations indicate that enhanced CO_2 levels may compensate for the negative impact of other climatic changes. In a nutshell, it should be emphasized that when designing future techniques and approaches, not only the independent effect, but the interactive effects should also be taken into account.

3.4.2.2 Storage and Transportation

Globalization leads to an increase in international trade of fresh F&Vs, resulting in rapidly raised distances traveled of these goods. However, since most F&V have relatively high moisture content, high perishable nature, and a low tolerance for long-term preservation, special care or treatment is required during the storage and transportation process (Wang et al. 2018).

Deterioration of F&V, including microbial spoilage, physiological aging, and nutrient loss, is still a main challenge through the supply chain. Traditional approaches such as controlled atmosphere and cold chain logistics have been applied to slow down the respiration, moisture loss, and disease decay of fresh F&V. Nonetheless, there are still several drawbacks to these approaches. The major weakness is the temperature fluctuation during the cold chain (especially ground operations during transportation and storage at the retail shelf), which leads to a detrimental effect on F&V quality and safety (Mercier et al. 2017). Temperatures higher than the optimal temperature range will increase the metabolic activity, accelerating decay or tissue dearth; while temperatures lower than the optimal range would result in chilling damage. These could result in large losses; for instance, postharvest losses of mango in the global market can reach 30% (de Mello Vasconcelos et al. 2019). Consequently, ensuring the integrity of the cold chain is of importance. Moreover, as different F&Vs have temperature requirements, it would be more complicated to maintain a suitable temperature if mix loads are present. On the other hand, a controlled atmosphere technique is being used to control the respiratory metabolism of some F&Vs. However, increased carbon dioxide concentration in the package would favor certain microflora like lactic acid bacteria, which would also shorten the shelf-life of these F&Vs. Though several novel techniques have been published to overcome the drawback of the current approaches, most of these techniques are purely based on scientific principles, and hence, the possibility of industrial scale still needs to be studied.

Energy consumption of the cold chain is another issue. Refrigerated storage and transportation are energy-intensive and rely largely on non-renewable energy sources, which could emit a large volume of greenhouse gas (Lo-Iacono-Ferreira et al. 2020). The future trend should also focus on a more sustainable and efficient means of storage and transportation.

3.4.2.3 Processing Technology

For more than a century, various F&V processing technologies have been explored to provide safe, fresh, and nutritious products. The priorities for F&V processing are safety (by inactivating microorganisms) and quality (inactivating enzymes, decolorization). Thermal processing technology is still the most popular technology, but emerging processes (such as cold plasma, pressurized fluid, pulsed electric field, ohmic heating) and technologies (radio frequency electric field, ultrasound and supersonic speed, ultra-high pressure) have attracted widespread attention. Conventional F&V processing techniques usually result in undesirable changes in terms of color, texture, flavor, and/or and nutrient content, which means that their fresh quality is adversely affected. This is conflicting with the consumers' trend toward fresh foods. The novel food processing technology not only can preserve nutritional value and sensory properties, but also significantly reduce the overall processing time, while saving energy and water, while ensuring the safety of F&Vs and bringing rich benefits to the industry. F&Vs are generally processed by a range of process flow, such as washing, blanching, dehydration, cooling or freezing, sorting, and grading. These pre-processed F&V can then be transformed into value-added F&V-based products (e.g., fresh-cut F&V and canned F&V) using traditional and novel techniques, thereby extending the supply chain (Boye and Arcand 2013). Traditionally, nutrition has not been a major driver of optimizing F&V processing or product innovation, which still presents challenges for consumer acceptance. In the following section, we will discuss how these process flow operations affect the quality of F&Vs.

Blanching is an important step to loosen skins and inactivate enzymes to avoid browning and other reactions. Steam and hot water are frequently used approaches. Thus, these thermal treatments usually reduce the nutritional quality of F&Vs.

Reducing blanching time might not be a good option, since the enzymes cannot be properly inactivated, resulting in a shorter shelf-life of F&V (Nayak, Liu, and Tang 2015).

The dehydration process is to decrease a water activity of F&V, thereby reducing the activity of the microorganisms and prolonging shelf-life. Grabowski, Truong, and Daubert (2008) found that beta-carotene and vitamin C contents were significantly reduced after sweet potato spray drying into powder. Hence, the key challenge of dehydration is to retain the heat-sensitive compounds.

The sterilization process is to eliminate pathogens to extend the shelf-life of F&V products, and can either use thermal and non-thermal methods. Conventional thermal sterilization is being widely used by the food industry, but it is known that this technique has a severe effect on the nutritional and organoleptic quality of the food. Novel non-thermal techniques (such as high-pressure processing, pulsed electric field processing, irradiation, and ultrasound processing) have also been developed to minimize the processing effect on F&V quality, but some other issues like high cost and acceptability might occur (Priyadarshini et al. 2019). For instance, the use of high-pressure treatments on F&V can cause complete loss of enzymatic activity when the pressure reached a certain level. However, microbes may survive when lower pressure is applied. Irradiation, the high capital cost technique, might induce localized risks from radiation, and high dose irradiation can also degrade F&V products (Priyadarshini et al. 2019).

Extrusion process plasticizes and cooks the food products at high temperatures under pressure and mechanical shear. This process changes the structure of food matrices as well as the content of nutrients, resulting in molecular transformation and chemical reactions in foods. For instance, Korus, Gumul, and Czechowska (2007) found that extrusion could decrease the phenolic content thereby the antioxidant activity of dry beans of *phaseolus vulgaris* L.

Packaging is vital in minimizing the quality loss of F&V to obtain optimal shelf-life. Conventional packs (such as plastic, paper, and metal) are commonly applied in F&V packaging. Plastic packaging, including polyethylene, polypropylene, and polyamide, is widely used owing to its low price, low weight, and high versatility. However, plastic additives and residual monomers could migrate into F&V, and plastic packaging could also absorb aromas and flavors from F&V, leading to quality loss (Albrecht et al. 2013). Paper-based packaging is normally collapsible and approvable for direct contact with F&V, but it is poorly sealable and easily permeable to water, and other aqueous solutions, air, and volatile flavors and aromas. Metal cans have a robust form of packaging that allows sterilization and proper seal of F&V to achieve a relatively long shelf-life. Nonetheless, the dissolution of tin and iron from the cans to F&V could cause deterioration in flavor. Moreover, polymeric films with a controlled atmosphere (lowered O_2 and raised CO_2 levels) can reduce the respiration of F&V and hence extend their shelf-life. However, if the O_2 amount falls too low, it would lead to off-odors from the fermentation of some tissues. To overcome the limitation or drawbacks of the traditional packaging, some innovative packaging (such as edible coatings and films, biobased materials, nanocomposite materials) has been developed, but its safety, acceptability, cost, and feasibility for production should be extensively studied.

In summary, innovative techniques that can retain the nutritional and sensory properties of F&V need to be developed.

3.4.2.4 By-products

The F&V, comprising the highest wastage rates (may up to 60%) among all types of foods, generate millions of tons of losses and waste per year (Alexandre et al. 2018; Sagar et al. 2018). These losses and waste occur in each section of the supply chain, including agricultural production, post-harvest handling, processing, storage and transportation (F&V losses), and distribution as well as consumption (F&V waste). The losses are mainly the unintended results of the overproduction and the failure to meet the retailers' quality standards, while the waste is mostly related to retailers' and consumers' behavior. Both losses and waste would lead to a loss of valuable biomass (e.g., pomace, skin, seed, and rind), an economic cost, and adverse effects on the environment. Nevertheless, the commercial exploitation of the wasted F&V is still limited, probably due to their a) high moisture content; b) potentially microbiologically contaminated; c) perishable properties resulting in difficulties with storage; d) high enzyme activity that can accelerate spoilage; and e) additional cost of drying, shipping, and storage (Trigo et al. 2020). As a result, only a few methods are currently offered on the market, including livestock feed, biofertilizer, and biogas. However, fruit and vegetable losses and waste are rich in nutrients and extra nutritional compounds, so they have a large potential to be reintroduced back to the food chain. New ways have been proposed to re-purpose wasted vegetables in food products (Trigo et al. 2020), but food safety (e.g., microbiological safety and toxicity), *in vivo* activity, and reintroducing efficiency should also be evaluated. Thus, it is worthwhile to assess the feasibility of these new methods and search for new directions that can improve the sustainability of the F&V industry.

3.4.3 TRENDS AND APPLICATIONS

This section aims to take the readers to the application areas for the main challenges in F&V processing manufacturing.

3.4.3.1 Intelligent Manufacturing

At the center of Industry 4.0 are robots, while robots in Industry 5.0 will be secondary in terms of artificial intelligence, but they remain a key component. Although the core of Industry 5.0 is human mass customization and personalization, this can only be achieved with the help of advanced robotics features. F&V processing plant architecture in Industry 5.0 is shown in Figure 3.4.1. In Industry 5.0, intelligent manufacturing represents the deep integration of new-generation artificial intelligence (AI) technology and advanced manufacturing technology. It runs through every link of the entire F&V life cycle in design, production, products, and services. The concept also involves the optimization and integration of corresponding systems. Continuously improve the product quality, performance and service level of F&V enterprises, and reduce resource consumption and increase the

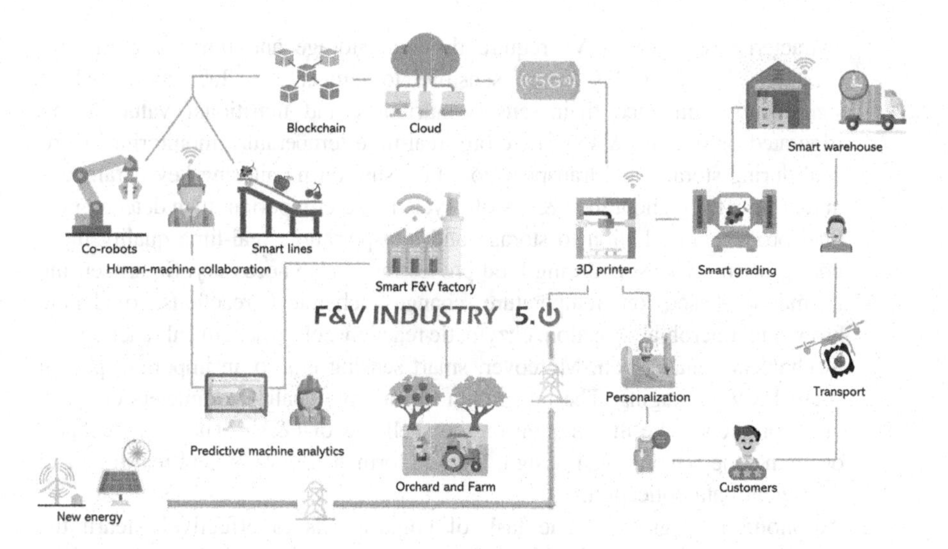

FIGURE 3.4.1 Schematic diagram of the future fruit and vegetable smart factory.

use of by-products, which promoting innovation, green, coordinated, open, and shared development of the F&V manufacturing industry. The new generation of smart factories further highlights the centrality of humanity. It is a magnificent integrated system that coordinates human, networks, and physical systems. This is a huge system, including advanced artificial intelligence, big data intelligence, human-machine hybrid enhanced intelligence, crowd intelligence, cross-media intelligence, high-tech sensors, cloud computing, the Internet of Things, and other advanced technologies. The integrated intelligent system is composed of intelligent equipment and human experts. It conducts intelligent activities in the manufacturing process, such as analysis, reasoning, judgment, conception, and decision making. It is expanded and extended through the joint efforts of people and intelligent equipment. And partly replace human labor in the manufacturing process. It extends the concept of manufacturing automation to flexible, intelligent, and highly integrated. Compared with traditional manufacturing, intelligent production has the characteristics of self-organization and ultra-flexibility, self-discipline, self-learning and self-maintenance, human-machine integration, and virtual reality. The core intelligent technologies of F&V smart factories are mainly divided into the following four categories: intelligent sensing, autonomous cognition, intelligent decision making, and intelligent control (Zhou et al. 2019).

1. Intelligent sensing. Perception, including the acquisition, transmission, and processing of information, is the foundation and prerequisite for cognitive learning, decision making, and control. Here, the core task is to effectively obtain the key parameters of real-time F&V processing, such as temperature, color, and pH (Gao et al. 2020). F&V industry depends on cold chain distribution to maintain the safety and quality of fresh F&V, which stable and effective storage/transportation management is essential. Due to showing different physiological

characteristics, fresh F&Vs require different storage and transportation temperatures. However, F&Vs are sensitive to temperature fluctuations, which significantly influence their sensory attributes and nutritional value of refrigerated or frozen F&Vs. Therefore, real-time temperature monitoring is critical during storage and transportation. Focusing on monitoring key parameters in real-time throughout the F&V's life cycle is more important than detecting the final product. In addition to storage and transportation, real-time quality monitoring of smart sensors during food processing is also necessary. Smart sensing is mainly based on temperature changes, chemical reactions, oxidation, browning, microbial detection, enzymatic reactions, electrochemical reactions, or mechanical denaturation. Moreover, smart sensing is also an important part of smart F&V packaging. The integration of multiple quality parameters can provide comprehensive information on the shelf life of F&Vs. Their key technologies include sensing plan design, high-performance sensors, and real-time and intelligent data collection.

2. Autonomous cognition. The task of cognition is to effectively learn the specific knowledge required, which is the key to effective decision making and control. This is usually done based on the collaboration between network systems and humans, so the autonomous cognition of intelligent machines and human collaboration are needed. The core task of autonomous recognition of intelligent machines is system modeling (including parameter identification). Key technologies include deep learning of model structure and model parameters, model evaluation, and optimization. Industry 5.0 will optimally combine the high speed and accuracy of industrial automation with the cognitive and critical thinking skills of employees. Therefore, it would actually enhance their role in manufacturing rather than replacing technology to replace people. Responsibility for repetitive tasks, such as packaging or data entry, rests on automated collaborative systems. Employees could assume a higher level of responsibility when overseeing these systems, making real-time decisions, and looking for opportunities to improve quality and production processes.
3. Intelligent decision making. The task of intelligent decision making is to assess the state of the system and determine the best action. Key intelligent decision-making technologies include an accurate assessment of the state of fruit and vegetable processing systems, optimization of decision models, and predictive analysis of decision risks. In Industry 5.0, various types of data collection are further automated through robotic systems and Internet-connected devices. Smart factory workers will use the same charts and dashboards from quality smart solutions to monitor the future factory. Quickly and intelligently make decisions about how to optimize machines and processes prior to occur problems. If the robot suddenly stops working or the F&V processing line needs to be adjusted to correct substandard products, an automatic alert from the same system will immediately notify the relevant staff.
4. Intelligent control. Intelligent robots incorporated with a high-tech image processing system are turning out to be increasingly smart, having the option to "see" and respond to various circumstances dependent on plainly characterized

parameters. This incorporates distinguishing diverse F&V on the same processing line and then performing various assignments in a split second. Advanced digital image processing coordinated into the robots incorporates a progression of procedures that start with catching non-contact constant pictures, visual portrayal in a PC, automatic analysis, and generation of results or measurement readings based on control commands. This is particularly beneficial for F&V quality checks, such as confirming labeling accuracy, colors, and height or volume. Using a smart camera or other visual inspection systems can provide a variety of real-time data, including shape, size, color, weight, or foreign objects such as glass fragments and plastic. Analytical monitoring activates necessary adjustments based on deviations detected in the process. This can ensure that the required quality and safety standards for F&V are met, and defects can be detected early, thereby reducing their waste and high recall costs. In essence, this technology addresses limitations due to human factors. Meanwhile, the technology can automatically store data and upload it to the cloud for later use, e.g., evidence in the event of customer complaints.

3.4.3.2 Smart Grading and Assessment Systems

Quality grading of F&V prior to sales can improve their market value. Consumers' attention to the quality of F&V is not limited to external attributes but also future changes in internal quality. External attributes involve shape, size, color, texture, defects and bruises, and foreign materials, such as soil and insects, etc. The internal quality including maturity, sugar content, firmness, acidity, soluble solids content, browning, chilling injury, water core, nutritional content, and chemical contaminants, e.g., pesticides and antibiotics. Traditional F&V quality inspection and grading are highly dependent on manual operations or destructive sampling inspections, which are laborious, time-consuming, costly, and subjective. Industry 5.0 will apply a highly accurate, efficient, objective, non-contact, and robotic grading system. The optical-based inspection system eliminates the subjectivity and inconsistencies of manual labor while maintaining accuracy and reliability, and plays an indispensable role in the quality evaluation of F&V (Zhang et al. 2018). Moreover, a combination of spectroscopic methods (near-infrared, hyperspectral, multispectral imaging systems technology, and magnetic resonance imaging spectroscopy), thermal imaging, x-ray computed tomography imaging, odor imaging, computed tomography, 3D imaging, terahertz imaging, and non-destructive mechanical methods (acoustic, impact, ultrasonic, and vibration) can be widely used in non-destructive quality inspection and sorting of F&V classifiers (Cakmak 2019). Combined with deep learning and multi-source data fusion, including RGB images, spectrum, smell, taste, etc., will be used for a more comprehensive and accurate assessment of fruit and vegetable quality and safety (Zhou et al. 2019).

Mobile harvesting and grading platforms/robots for F&V will become a potential trend. The integrated combination of machines provides simultaneous harvesting and grading of F&V in an orchard or greenhouse. Impact prevention solutions and flexible mechanical structures will also be considered. F&Vs are flexible products that are easily damaged. Reducing heavy blows protects them from mechanical damage and ensures their quality. Higher levels of automation in feeding, washing, waxing, shipping, inspection, sorting, labeling, and packing are applied.

3.4.3.3 Traceability and Authenticity Systems

Intelligent F&V products are identified through a unique form, can be located at any time and can know their own history, current status, and alternative routes to achieve their target status. Historically, analytical methods have been used to detect authenticity problems, but these methods have disadvantages in terms of cost and practicality, and most of these applications have been performed after food fraud incidents. Traceability is defined as the ability to locate F&V commodities or ingredients and track their history (from source to consumer) or backward (from consumer to source) in the supply chain through recorded identification. As the complexity of the value chain increases, the traceability process becomes expensive and inefficient. Complexity can be associated with the unique characteristics of raw materials for F&V. Individual F&V have undergone a dynamic transformation from orchard or farm, picking, processing, and transportation to commodities. Another challenge is that F&V processing is mainly operated by humans, which can be difficult to monitor. New initiatives include big data-driven systems that predict risks in the F&V processing chain, as well as non-targeted analysis methods that have a wider range of applications than traditional technologies. Sensing technology for continuous online monitoring of pollutants in F&V processing. Multi-criteria evaluation of a blockchain-based supply chain traceability system. Sensor technology will give a huge contribution to Industry 5.0. There are many types of intelligent identification systems for better traceability. Quick response (QR) codes or radio frequency identification (RFID) tags have been systematically and effectively tracked F&V from planting, harvesting, transportation, processing, and packaging to the final product entering the market to be able to track the origin of the goods and monitor the entire process.

3.4.3.4 Personalization

Industry 5.0 will develop new business models and cooperation models that can meet the needs of those personalized and changing customers. Customers with special product characteristics require direct participation in all stages of product design, construction, booking, planning, production, operation, and recycling. What's more, if there is a temporary change in demand immediately before or during the production process, Industry 5.0 can immediately make it possible. Of course, this will still make money from producing unique products or small batches.

Human psychology determines the direction of technology. Generally, consumers want to stand out and be considered unique. One way is to choose (including purchase choices) to express the uniqueness of the individual. In Industry 5.0, people can use technology to produce personalized products to express themselves. Not only are the products that the super-rich can afford, but people with low incomes can also buy them. The desire for large-scale personalization has formed the psychological and cultural driving force behind Industry 5.0, which involves using technology to return human-added value to manufacturing. It needs to be clear that no one wants a wide range of personalized products, which is the perfect choice for Industry 4.0 settings and their traditional industrial robots. Namely, no one wants a personalized juicer blade, glass, or beverage cap. Everyone benefits if these products can be produced at the lower cost in the smart factory (Østergaard 2016).

Additive manufacturing (AM) may be considered one of the most important emerging technologies, completely renewing the possibilities of future F&V and its processing, especially AM based on 3D printing. Using the mixture of multiple plant food ingredients and multiple printing processes, hundreds of innovative plant foods in shape, size, consistency, microstructure, color, taste, flavor, etc. can be obtained. 3D printing technology can be applied in specific food printing fields, such as military foods, space foods, and culinary uses. F&V packages need to be individually customized for the army, and this ingredient needs to be compact enough to reduce the burden on soldiers with high fill rates. For long-term exploration missions, F&V is important to space foods, it requires safety, acceptability, diversity, and nutritional stability and long-term freshness. Current food processing systems cannot meet the shelf-life and nutritional needs of long-term tasks. "Printing" machines in additive-based spacecraft can print various geometries, from astronaut food ingredients to "reconstituted" food. These "reconstructed" foods can be made by designing shapes or scanning models of conventional foods, which reduce the long-term space life annoyance of astronauts. Moreover, 3D printing technology in food processing ranges from meeting necessities to high-end cooking and gourmet cuisine, which creates a special experience for guests. Not everyone can make beautiful cakes, which can take years of experience, but printers can make it easy.

Similarly, consumers' choice of food depends on taste, shape, cost, experience, convenience, and nutrition. Plant-based 3D food printing can meet all of these criteria to produce personalized/customized foods for specific consumer groups (children, seniors, pregnant women, vegetarians, adolescents, athletes, etc.) in terms of sensory and nutritional properties. Official dietary guidelines encourage the consumption of five portions of F&V, which are a key factor in preventing many diseases, especially for children and adolescents, but a large proportion does not meet the recommendation. In this case, 3D printing technology can be used to obtain nutritious personalized snacks for children based on F&V-based formulas (Derossi et al. 2018). European project PERFORMANCE-Personalized Food using fast-producing for the seniors, and even started using 3D printing to develop or attract new foods for the elderly consumers (Portanguen et al. 2019). Food design through 3D printing can make it easier for elderly people who have difficulty swallowing to consume foods that do not need to be mashed into a pulp, such as puree. Vegetarian meat products printed with F&V materials can help vegetarians make alternative animal foods (Vialva 2018).

For various F&V products on the shelf, they can also be classified based on the degree of processing, which is convenient for consumers to choose personally. First, scientifically classify F&V based on their processing levels. Custom mixes of purees or juices are delivered to customers on their labels. Second, establish an evaluation platform that can analyze any F&V from its ingredients and nutrition labels. Finally, the establishment of food labels allows consumers to choose the most natural and healthy F&V products on the shelves of the same supermarket.

3.4.3.5 Bioeconomy

Another vision for Industry 5.0 is the bioeconomy. The effective and full use of biological resources for industrial purposes will help to achieve a balance between ecology, industry, and economy (Demir, Döven, and Sezen 2019). F&V losses and wastes pose serious economic and environmental problems. However, these by-products have large amounts of dietary fiber and bioactive compounds. F&V processing wastes can be incorporated into other foods such as animals, dairy products, beverages, and baked goods (Trigo et al. 2020). A variety of edible F&V materials, including purees, pomace, extracts, and juices, have matrix-forming properties and can be further used to produce edible packaging materials (Kadzińska et al. 2019). This application of F&Vs is due to the presence of matrix-forming polysaccharides and proteins in their composition, while the presence of bioactive compounds such as vitamins, polyphenols, and carotenoids may confer antioxidant and antibacterial properties to active packaging materials.

With the improvement of living standards, consumers tend to have a healthier lifestyle. Consumers, comparing product labels, are more willing to buy natural foods rather than low-processed foods containing artificial color additives and preservatives. This trend has forced food designers to introduce more foods containing natural additives. Properly processed F&V by-products can be used as natural additives to improve the food quality, and to make other innovative food and edible food packaging. Pomace-derived compounds are also used in biofuels, biochemicals (green chemistry), cosmetics, artificial flavors and flavor enhancers, which can reduce environmental pollution. However, the contribution of traditional methods to F&V processing by-products is still far from the modern industry level. Therefore, the use of advanced technology and personalized analysis in Industry 5.0 could better develop these by-products on an industrial scale. The use of the new methods and human psychology can not only further upgrade and innovate the F&V processing industry, but also help maximize waste-free production to reduce environmental pollution around the factory (Majerska, Michalska, and Figiel 2019). Future F&V factories should also consider the design of the space and infrastructure for the pretreatment of the pomace. Similarly, according to various existing research results and data accumulation during processing, appropriate processing methods, parameters, and F&V are selected. Examples will be explained in detail below:

Brazilian fruit jabuticaba (*Myrciaria cauliflora* Mart) has medicinal properties e.g., it has significant effects on asthma, diarrhea, stomach, and bowel diseases, so its pomace can be successfully used as a nutraceutical. The production of bacterial nanocellulose from citrus pomace has strong texture and high purity characteristics, which makes it very suitable for use as a wound dressing ingredient in medicine and facilitates natural artificial materials research. Because dairy products should not be consumed by lactose-intolerant patients, some food scientists are considering using passion fruit pomace (high in vitamins, minerals, and antioxidants, and lacks dairy allergens) as a carrier for probiotic foods. Chokeberry pomace is a good source of anthocyanins with strong antioxidant properties; its pomace can be used in the production of natural food colorants. According to the processing time and method, fresh grapes and apple pomace are fermented to make the wine leading different taste characteristics. The addition of white grape pomace to seafood products can significantly improve its water retention capacity and inhibit lipid oxidation, making it softer, less elastic, and enhancing its sensory characteristics. Plum pomace has a high antioxidant capacity, and its extract can be applied to meat products, which can extend the shelf-life of meat products. Another popular method of F&V residue is to add it to livestock feed. The chemical composition of the pomace obtained from an F&V variety depends on the cultivar, climate, growing location, and processing method. These characteristics can guide its industrial use or design novel and innovative personalized food based on pomace.

Food processing involves a variety of processing methods and parameters, but usually reduces the content of polyphenols in F&Vs, which results in reduction of product quality. The use of artificial intelligence and machine learning in Industry 5.0 allows combining optimal processing methods, carefully designed processes, or selecting appropriate processing parameters to retain higher levels of biologically active substances in food and actively shape the best quality of the final product.

3.4.4 CONCLUSIONS

With aids of the tools such as collaborative robots, by relocating people to the center of industrial production, Industry 5.0 not only provides consumers with the products they want today, but also provides workers with more meaningful work than factory work. Although Industry 5.0 is still out of reach, it will bring major changes to the F&V processing industry. Collaborating with machines, not conflicts, humans must improve their creativity to maintain the correct "machine master" status. The role of humans will evolve with the role of machines to shape the future together. Humans will also have greater responsibilities and will have a more spacious, easier, and safer working environment. The most important thing is not to worry about machines replacing humans, because superb craftsmanship and imagination are unique to humans, and even the smartest machines cannot be copied. In addition, Industry 5.0 should develop in a green, intelligent, and ecological direction. The future scientific and technological revolution will focus on the restoration and protection of the ecological environment and the rational use of natural resources.

REFERENCES

Albrecht, Stefan, Peter Brandstetter, Tabea Beck, Pere Fullana-I-Palmer, Kaisa Grönman, Martin Baitz, Sabine Deimling, Julie Sandilands, and Matthias Fischer. 2013. "An extended life cycle analysis of packaging systems for fruit and vegetable transport in Europe." *International Journal of Life Cycle Assessment* 18 (8): 1549–1567. https://doi.org/10.1007/s11367-013-0590-4.

Alexandre, Elisabete M.C., Silvia A. Moreira, Luís M.G. Castro, Manuela Pintado, and Jorge A. Saraiva. 2018. "Emerging technologies to extract high added value compounds from fruit residues: Sub/supercritical, ultrasound-, and enzyme-assisted extractions." *Food Reviews International* 34 (6): 581–612. https://doi.org/10.1080/87559129.2017.1359842.

Balasooriya, Himali N., Kithsiri B Dassanayake, and Said Ajlouni. 2019. "The impact of elevated CO_2 and high temperature on the nutritional quality of fruits – A short review."

American Journal of Agricultural Research 4 (26): 1–9. https://doi.org/10.28933/ajar-2018-12-1608.

Birje, Anand. 2020. "A vision for Industry 5.0: Humans augmented with cobots and connectivity." https://www.logisticsit.com/articles/2020/01/21/a-vision-for-industry-5.0-humans-augmented-with-cobots-and-connectivity.

Boye, Joyce I., and Yves Arcand. 2013. "Current trends in green technologies in food production and processing." *Food Engineering Reviews* 5 (1): 1–17. https://doi.org/10.1007/s12393-012-9062-z.

Cakmak, Hulya. 2019. *Assessment of Fresh Fruit and Vegetable Quality with Non-Destructive Methods. Food Quality and Shelf Life*. Elsevier Inc. https://doi.org/10.1016/b978-0-12-817190-5.00010-0.

Craufurd, P.Q., and T.R. Wheeler. 2009. "Climate change and the flowering time of annual crops." *Journal of Experimental Botany* 60 (9): 2529–2539. https://doi.org/10.1093/jxb/erp196.

Demir, K.A., Kadir Alpaslan, and Halil Cicibaş. 2018. "The next industrial revolution: Industry 5.0 and discussions on Industry 4.0." In *Industry 4.0 From the Management Information Systems Perspectives*. Peter Lang GmbH, Internationaler Verlag der Wissenschaften, Bern, Switzerland. https://doi.org/10.3726/b15120

Demir, Kadir Alpaslan, Gözde Döven, and Bülent Sezen. 2019. "Industry 5.0 and human-robot co-working." *Procedia Computer Science* 158: 688–695. https://doi.org/10.1016/j.procs.2019.09.104.

Derossi, A., R. Caporizzi, D. Azzollini, and C. Severini. 2018. "Application of 3D printing for customized food. A case on the development of a fruit-based snack for children." *Journal of Food Engineering* 220: 65–75. https://doi.org/10.1016/j.jfoodeng.2017.05.015.

Gao, Tingting, You Tian, Zhiwei Zhu, and Da Wen Sun. 2020. "Modelling, responses and applications of time-temperature indicators (TTIs) in monitoring fresh food quality." *Trends in Food Science and Technology* 99: 311–322. https://doi.org/10.1016/j.tifs.2020.02.019.

Grabowski, J.A., V.D. Truong, and C.R. Daubert. 2008. "Nutritional and rheological characterization of spray dried sweetpotato powder." *LWT - Food Science and Technology* 41 (2): 206–216. https://doi.org/10.1016/j.lwt.2007.02.019.

Haokip, Songthat William, Kripa Shankar, and Jonathan Lalrinngheta. 2020. "Climate change and its impact on fruit crops." *Journal of Pharmacognosy and Phytochemistry* 9 (1): 435–438. http://www.bmet.org.bd/BMET/resources/StaticPDFandDOC/publication/BriefonClimateChange-ImpactonBangladesh.pdf.

Hoegh-Guldberg, O., D. Jacob, M. Taylor, M. Bindi, S. Brown, I. Camilloni, A. Diedhiou, et al. 2018. Impacts of 1.5 °C Global Warming on Natural and Human Systems. An IPCC Special Report on the Impacts of Global Warming of 1.5 °C. In Global Warming of 1.5 °C. An IPCC Special Report on the impacts of global warming of 1.5 °C above pre-industrial levels and related global greenhouse gas emission pathways, in the context of strengthening the global response to the threat of climate change, edited by V. Masson-Delmotte, P. Zhai, H.-O. Pörtner, D. Roberts, J. Skea, and P. R. Shukla, 175–311. World Meteorological Organization Technical Document, Geneva, Switzerland. https://doi.org/10.1002/ejoc.201200111

Kadir, Sorkel, Gaganpreet Sidhu, and Kassim Al-Khatib. 2006. "Strawberry (*Fragaria xa-nanassa* Duch.) growth and productivity as affected by temperature." *HortScience* 41 (6): 1423–1430. https://doi.org/10.21273/hortsci.41.6.1423.

Kadzińska, Justyna, Monika Janowicz, Stanisław Kalisz, Joanna Bryś, and Andzej Lenart. 2019. "An overview of fruit and vegetable edible packaging materials." *Packaging Technology and Science* 32 (10): 483–495. https://doi.org/10.1002/pts.2440.

Kizildeniz, T., I. Mekni, H. Santesteban, I. Pascual, F. Morales, and J.J. Irigoyen. 2015. "Effects of climate change including elevated CO_2 concentration, temperature and water deficit on growth, water status, and yield quality of grapevine (*Vitis vinifera* L.) cultivars." *Agricultural Water Management* 159: 155–164. https://doi.org/10.1016/j.agwat.2015.06.015.

Korus, Jaroslaw, Dorota Gumul, and Kamila Czechowska. 2007. "Effect of extrusion on the phenolic composition and antioxidant activity of dry beans of *Phaseolus vulgaris* L." *Food Technology and Biotechnology* 45 (2): 139–146.

Lin-Wang, Kui, Diego Micheletti, John Palmer, Richard Volz, Lidia Lozano, Richard Espley, Roger P. Hellens, et al. 2011. "High temperature reduces apple fruit colour via modulation of the anthocyanin regulatory complex." *Plant, Cell and Environment* 34 (7): 1176–1190. https://doi.org/10.1111/j.1365-3040.2011.02316.x.

Lo-Iacono-Ferreira, Vanesa G., Rosario Viñoles-Cebolla, María José Bastante-Ceca, and Salvador F. Capuz-Rizo. 2020. "Transport of Spanish fruit and vegetables in cardboard boxes: A carbon footprint analysis." *Journal of Cleaner Production* 244: 118784. https://doi.org/10.1016/j.jclepro.2019.118784.

Majerska, Joanna, Anna Michalska, and Adam Figiel. 2019. "A review of new directions in managing fruit and vegetable processing by-products." *Trends in Food Science and Technology* 88: 207–219. https://doi.org/10.1016/j.tifs.2019.03.021.

Mattos, Leonora M., Celso L. Moretti, Sumira Jan, Steven A. Sargent, Carlos Eduardo P. Lima, and Mariana R. Fontenelle. 2014. *Climate Changes and Potential Impacts on Quality of Fruit and Vegetable Crops. Emerging Technologies and Management of Crop Stress Tolerance: Biological Techniques*. Vol. 1. Elsevier Inc. https://doi.org/10.1016/B978-0-12-800876-8.00019-9.

Mello Vasconcelos, Osvaldo Campelo de, Guilherme José Bolzani de Campos Ferreira, José de Castro Silva, Barbara Janet Teruel Mederos, and Sérgio Tonetto de Freitas. 2019. "Development of an artificial fruit prototype for monitoring mango skin and flesh temperatures during storage and transportation." *Postharvest Biology and Technology* 158: 110956. https://doi.org/10.1016/j.postharvbio.2019.110956.

Mercier, Samuel, Sebastien Villeneuve, Martin Mondor, and Ismail Uysal. 2017. "Time–temperature management along the food cold chain: A review of recent developments." *Comprehensive Reviews in Food Science and Food Safety* 16 (4): 647–667. https://doi.org/10.1111/1541-4337.12269.

Moretti, C.L., L.M. Mattos, A.G. Calbo, and S.A. Sargent. 2010. "Climate changes and potential impacts on postharvest quality of fruit and vegetable crops: A review." *Food Research International* 43 (7): 1824–1832. https://doi.org/10.1016/j.foodres.2009.10.013.

Nayak, Balunkeswar, Rui Hai Liu, and Juming Tang. 2015. "Effect of processing on phenolic antioxidants of fruits, vegetables, and grains—A review." *Critical Reviews in Food Science and Nutrition* 55 (7): 887–918. https://doi.org/10.1080/10408398.2011.654142.

Østergaard, Esben H. 2016. "Industry 5.0 - Return of the human touch." 2016. https://blog.universal-robots.com/industry-50-return-of-the-human-touch.

Parajuli, Ranjan, Greg Thoma, and Marty D. Matlock. 2019. "Environmental sustainability of fruit and vegetable production supply chains in the face of climate change: A review." *Science of the Total Environment* 650: 2863–2879. https://doi.org/10.1016/j.scitotenv.2018.10.019.

Portanguen, Stéphane, Pascal Tournayre, Jason Sicard, Thierry Astruc, and Pierre Sylvain Mirade. 2019. "Toward the design of functional foods and biobased products by 3D printing: A review." *Trends in Food Science and Technology* 86: 188–198. https://doi.org/10.1016/j.tifs.2019.02.023.

Priyadarshini, Anushree, Gaurav Rajauria, Colm P. O'Donnell, and Brijesh K. Tiwari. 2019. "Emerging food processing technologies and factors impacting their industrial adoption." *Critical Reviews in Food Science and Nutrition* 59 (19): 3082–3101. https://doi.org/10.1080/10408398.2018.1483890.

Sagar, Narashans Alok, Sunil Pareek, Sunil Sharma, Elhadi M. Yahia, and Maria Gloria Lobo. 2018. "Fruit and vegetable waste: Bioactive compounds, their extraction, and possible utilization." *Comprehensive Reviews in Food Science and Food Safety* 17 (3): 512–531. https://doi.org/10.1111/1541-4337.12330.

Sage, Rowan F., Danielle A. Way, and David S. Kubien. 2008. "Rubisco, rubisco activase, and global climate change." *Journal of Experimental Botany* 59 (7): 1581–1595. https://doi.org/10.1093/jxb/ern053.

Springer, C. J., and J. K. Ward. 2007. Flowering time and elevated atmospheric CO_2 *New Phytologist* 176 (2): 243–255.

Trigo, João P., Elisabete M.C. Alexandre, Jorge A. Saraiva, and Manuela E. Pintado. 2020. "High value-added compounds from fruit and vegetable by-products – Characterization, bioactivities, and application in the development of novel food products." *Critical Reviews in Food Science and Nutrition* 60 (8): 1388–1416. https://doi.org/10.1080/10408398.2019.1572588.

Vialva, T. 2018. "Novameat 3D prints vegetarian steak from plant-based proteins." https://3dprintingindustry.com/news/novameat-3d-prints-vegetarian-steak-from-plant-based-proteins-144722/.

Wang, Jingyu, Min Zhang, Zhongxue Gao, and Benu Adhikari. 2018. "Smart storage technologies applied to fresh foods: A review." *Critical Reviews in Food Science and Nutrition* 58 (16): 2689–2699. https://doi.org/10.1080/10408398.2017.1323722.

Zhang, Baohua, Baoxing Gu, Guangzhao Tian, Jun Zhou, Jichao Huang, and Yingjun Xiong. 2018. "Challenges and solutions of optical-based nondestructive quality inspection for robotic fruit and vegetable grading systems: A technical review." *Trends in Food Science and Technology* 81: 213–231. https://doi.org/10.1016/j.tifs.2018.09.018.

Zhou, Ji, Yanhong Zhou, Baicun Wang, and Jiyuan Zang. 2019. "Human–cyber–physical systems (HCPSs) in the context of new-generation intelligent manufacturing." *Engineering* 5 (4): 624–636. https://doi.org/10.1016/j.eng.2019.07.015.

3.5 Application of Industry 5.0 in the Production of Fine Chemicals and Biopolymers

Nurul Natasha binti Azhar, Kai Ling Yu,
Tau Chuan Ling, and Pau Loke Show

CONTENTS

3.5.1 INTRODUCTION

The Fourth Industrial Revolution shows the world the interconnection of devices and the vast network of data that connect and control each other to increase the efficiency of a task or a process. Now, at the brink of Fifth Industrial Revolution where we will begin to see an increase in the frequency of co-operation between man and machine as well as the personalization of products by the consumers. There is already an increasing trend in customization of various products (Yang et al. 2017), from luxury cars to high-end apparel, where customers can choose the desired colours, design, material and various other properties of the product to suit their tastes. Adidas, for example, has introduced 3D-printing and automated manufacturing in their Speedfactory that allows for a better quality and faster personalization in their final products (Vetter 2016). With the Fifth Industrial Revolution already within sights, the boundaries of "personalization" is stretched to other industries that are, conventionally, mass produced and impersonal. Manufacturing lines and processes will become more automated and mundane tasks will be handed over to robots and artificially intelligent systems, leaving humans to become more involved in the designing of the product itself. This is the main and crucial difference between IR 4.0 and IR 5.0, which is the fact that the Fifth Industrial Revolution brings human intelligence back into the manufacturing equation with the development of a cyber physical system that is centred around people, artificial intelligence and the interconnecting network of different systems through the internet (Pathak et al. 2019). The progression of industrial revolutions is shown in Figure 3.5.1.

Sensors and transmitters can be installed into or onto the product itself to record data on how the product is being used in the field by the consumers. Such data would then be transmitted directly to the designers or engineers to further improve the manufacturing process for seamless data acquisition from the field to the manufacturing line (Rossi 2018). In doing so, there would be a greater freedom of design and begin to stretch the boundaries of physics on the design of the product. This idea has been implemented in a few companies such as Rolls Royce, whose aviation division has been able to obtain field data of their engines in real-time and analyze it to further improve their manufacturing process (Rolls-Royce Plc 2015). While it is easy to see Industry 5.0 happening in the world of electronics, it is forecasted that the biochemical engineering will also play a role in this industrial revolution.

Biochemical engineering is a field that has the discipline of chemical engineering at its core but adopts the concepts of biochemistry, bioorganic and bioinorganic chemistry as well as cell and molecular biology (Clark and Blanch 1997). In layman terms, biochemical engineering uses living organisms, or the chemical products that they produce such as enzymes, to develop new processes that produce chemical or biological materials (Clark and Blanch 1997). Early applications of biochemical

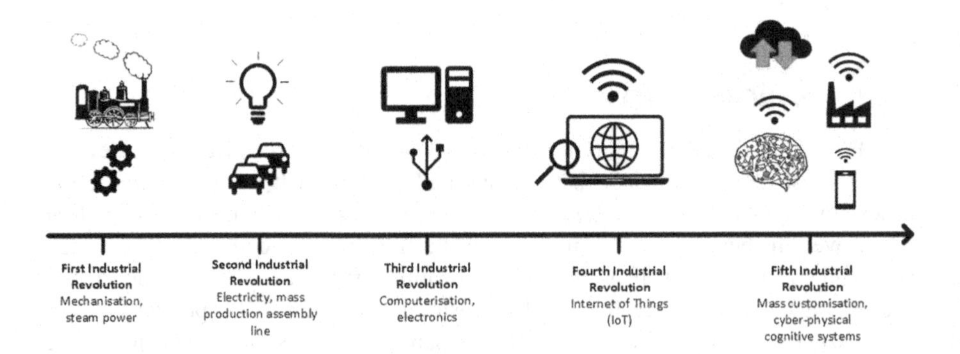

FIGURE 3.5.1 Progression of industrial revolutions.

engineering began when humans used yeast and fungi to make bread, wine, cheese and beer (Clark and Blanch 1997). Recent decades show that biochemical engineering has progressed to create biodegradable plastic containers from microbes (Philbrook, Alissandratos, and Easton 2013) as well as antibiotics (Najafpour 2015) and electrodes from fungi (Ludwig et al. 2013). One of the key environmental advantages of applying biochemical engineering concepts in a process is the fact that the processes are able to produce complex polymers and chemical compounds that cannot be achieved through conventional chemical production processes while having mild operating conditions and minimum waste generated (Takors 2020). In doing so, the environmental impacts related to the waste management of the process can be significantly reduced (Takors 2020). The Fifth Industrial Revolution presents the concepts of mass personalization and the collaboration between man and artificial intelligence, which can present an opportunity for the field of biochemical engineering to take part in the new manufacturing revolution. Biochemical engineering can partake in IR 5.0 through the advances and the applications of different fields such as white biotechnology, synthetic biology and evolutionary algorithms in the production process to create processes with higher flexibility at a lower environmental and economic cost. The concepts developed from the combination of the abovementioned fields with biochemical engineering can then be applied in the production processes of various manufactured goods including fine chemicals and biopolymers.

Fine chemicals fall into the category of chemicals that have a high purity and complexity in their structures (Sarah Delooze 2017). Compounds such as glycols (W. Song et al. 2019) and mono-aromatic compounds (Munick de Albuquerque Fragoso et al. 2020) are considered as fine chemicals and are essential to produce our everyday items such as pharmaceutical products, fragrances and food additives (Sarah Delooze 2017). However, fine chemicals are produced in small amounts of <1,000 metric tonnes per annum as compared to bulk chemicals due to the high cost and complexity of their production process that are usually batch processes or use biotechnological manufacturing processes (Sarah Delooze 2017). The main differences between fine chemicals and bulk chemicals are presented in Table 3.5.1.

TABLE 3.5.1
Main Differences between Fine Chemicals and Bulk Chemicals (Pollak 2007)

	Bulk Chemicals	Fine Chemicals
Chemical complexity	• Low to intermediate	• Usually high
Complexity of process	• Simple and economic	• Complex and expensive
Production rate	• >1,000 tonnes per year	• <1,000 tonnes per year
Price	• <$10/kg (low)	• >$10/kg (high)
Examples	• Petrochemicals, alcohols, benzenes, plastics	• Glycols, pharmaceutical active ingredients, food additives, catalysts

From proteins and gluten in our food to plastic and Styrofoam, polymers exist in our everyday lives and the application of these materials for millennia and even more so since the mid-20th century. Inorganic polymers, in particular, plastics are used in a wide range of applications due to their durability, optical properties and cheap production processes (Bajracharya et al. 2014). However, its high durability means that it has an incredibly long half-life and, hence, non-biodegradable, which causes severe negative impacts on the natural environment. Hence, researchers and manufacturers have turned to biopolymers which are a group of polymers which are manufactured from natural compounds that were either chemically produced from a bio-based material or entirely bio-synthesized by living organisms (Smith, Moxon, and Morris 2016). This category encompasses the natural polymers such as polysaccharides, proteins and cellulose as well as the synthetic biopolymers such as polyhydroxyalkanoates (PHAs) that have been developed for biodegradable packaging, medical applications and smart materials (G. Q. Chen, Zhang, and Wang 2015).

Twenty years ago, we would not have dreamt of holding computers in the palms of our hands that connected us to a multitude of other devices and a network of that provided information on almost anything that has ever been thought of, but now with the ability to design apparel, accessories and various other items from the comfort of our homes, IR 5.0 expands the field of consumer personalization to other products that were previously mass produced and detached such as medicine and packaging materials. With the rapid progress that is being made in the fields of synthetic biology and biotechnology, there is an increase in the variety of products that would be made available to consumers, thereby granting them a larger number of choices to choose from. Complex production processes that have multiple objectives can also be optimized and be made more affordable in IR 5.0 through an increase in the use of evolutionary algorithms in process optimization. This chapter will elaborate more on the advances being made in these fields, the roles that they play in the production of fine chemicals and biopolymers as well as how they correlate to the advent of the Fifth Industrial Revolution.

3.5.2 PROGRESSION AND DEVELOPMENTS

The rate of technological change has been accelerating at an exponential rate and it is proven by the fact that the technology nowadays is wildly different to what it was a few decades ago (Butler 2016). Progress and development are happening in all fields of technology and all would contribute towards the Fifth Industrial Revolution. In the case of bio-based products such as biopolymers and fine chemicals, there is a high possibility that white biotechnology, evolutionary algorithms and synthetic biology would play central roles in making the concepts and themes of IR 5.0 a reality.

3.5.2.1 WHITE BIOTECHNOLOGY

Biotechnology has been rapidly gaining attention over recent years as the general public becomes more aware of the environmental impacts of the everyday products usage. Products such as fertilizers, pesticides and detergents have long histories of having production processes and downstream effects that cause severe impacts towards the human health and the environment. For example, conventional household detergents and cleaning products contain volatile organic compounds (VOCs) that could not be entirely removed in wastewater treatment plants. These contaminants can cause eutrophication of the waterways and can lead to accumulation of the VOCs in the organisms of the local ecosystem. Now, there is an increase in "eco-friendly" cleaning products that use natural and non-toxic ingredients and enzymes that are biodegradable and have a lower environmental impact in their life cycle in comparison to the conventional products. These eco-friendly manufactured goods, which are not limited to cleaning products, are becoming more popular among the general public and they are willing to spend more on these products that are labelled as organic, eco-friendly or fair trade (Packaged Facts 2008). This market niche only started booming at the turn of the century and is forecasted to reach $150.1 billion in 2021 (Gelski 2019). The market for eco-friendly goods owes its growth to the advancements of white biotechnology or industrial biotechnology to produce naturally derived products through sustainable production processes (Gelski 2019).

White biotechnology is the branch of biotechnology that is devoted to developing and designing industrial processes using the naturally existing biodiversity such as yeast, bacteria, fungi and plants as well as natural enzymes to manufacture biodegradable products at a lower energy and resource consumption rate (Sachsenmeier 2016; Frazzetto 2003). In doing so, white biotechnology is inherently a technological field that uses organisms and bio-based chemicals to reduce greenhouse gas emissions and the volume of waste generated by industrial processes (Fasciotti 2017). Although "industrial biotechnology" is a modern term, the concepts of using biotechnology for industrial purposes has been around since humans started using yeast to make bread and wine. The most recent trend in white biotechnology is to produce biodegradable plastics to replace the petroleum-based polymers. Polymers such as high-density polyethylene (HDPE), polyethylene terephthalate (PET), polyester and polycarbonates are a few of the types of plastics that play a major role in our everyday lives from being used as water containers to the shirts on our backs. The optical properties, durability and low cost of plastics make them highly attractive for everyday use but these plastics impose severe negative environmental impacts throughout the life cycle as they are petroleum-based and have long half-lives in any natural ecosystem. This is the driving force behind the research and development being done to replace these polymers with a more eco-friendly substitute, biopolymers or bioplastics. These biopolymers are recognized for their biodegradability and their lower impacts towards the environment in their life cycle. Similar to the production of inorganic polymers, some fine chemicals such as aromatic compounds and higher alcohols also tend to cause negative impacts towards the environment throughout their life cycles. Through the application of white biotechnology, major companies are now producing bio-based fine chemicals not only for physiologically active compounds used in the healthcare industry but also for the production of additives for food, feed and fertilizers in a more environmentally sustainable manner (Hara et al. 2014). This advancement towards the design of more sustainable processes for the production of fine chemicals and biopolymers means that we are beginning to explore and stretch the conventional design boundaries that can, perhaps, allow for a wider variety of eco-friendly goods to be available for consumer personalization in the future.

To date, biopolymers have become increasingly popular due to its status as being a more non-toxic, biodegradable and sustainable option in comparison to their petroleum-based counterparts. In the packaging industry, there have been significant advances being made in the development of biopolymers that have features that are on par with conventional inorganic polymers. PET is predominantly used for producing plastic bottles, but its ecological consequences are becoming one of the most pressing issues for our environment today. In order to address this issue, there are companies that have been developing biopolymers for packaging purposes. The chemical company Avantium, for example, has developed polyethylene furanoate (PEF), a biopolymer made from vegetable-derived fructose that has shown thermal and mechanical properties that are on par with PET (Isikgor and Becer, 2015). Another chemical producing company known as Arkema, on the other hand, has recently developed a biopolymer from castor oil known as polyphthalamide (PPA), which is a thermoplastic with a high chemical and thermal resistance and can be used as a substitute for metal and rubber to produce under-hood equipment such as fuel and hydraulic lines (Arkema 2019). The rapid progress of biopolymers has also spurred the development of biopolymer-based products in the medical field. In medicine, biopolymers are used as surgical adhesives as biodegradable sutures, clamps, scaffolds and drug delivery systems (Cernadas et al. 2019). However, a long list of criteria must be fulfilled by these biopolymers before being used for medical applications such as having good adhesion while being non-toxic, able to cure fast and degrade after the right span of time under physiological conditions (Cernadas et al. 2019). Currently, materials such as cyanoacrylate glue, fibrin glue and glutaraldehyde glues have been approved of as surgical adhesives (Bhagat and Becker 2017). However, these conventional adhesives are subject to certain drawbacks as they are difficult to degrade in the human body, have poor biocompatibility and leach metallic ions when it decomposes (Bhagat and Becker 2017). In order to provide better options, there has been an increasing interest in nature-inspired biomimetic tissue adhesives (Bhagat and Becker 2017). These biomimetic tissue adhesives attempt to copy or mimic either the adhesion mechanisms of certain animals, such as frogs and geckos, or the biochemical secretion of certain marine organisms (Bré et al. 2013). For example, Gill et al. (2017) synthesized tuneable zinc-free denture adhesives from the protein glue secreted by marine mussels. This presents a safer option compared to the conventional adhesives as the risk of developing a neurological disease is increased when an excessive amount of zinc is ingested through the degradation of the adhesive (Gill et al. 2017). On a side note, Gill et al. (2017) found that by manipulating the pH of the formulation, the colour of the adhesives can be controlled for aesthetic purposes. This shows that by applying the concepts of white biotechnology, it becomes possible to find solutions for producing packaging options for the food and beverage industry in a more environmentally sustainable manner while being functional and practical at the same time. The healthcare industry also benefits with such advances by being able to produce surgical adhesives that are more biocompatible with the human body. Surgical adhesives and biodegradable packaging are the few of the diverse range of biopolymers that apply the concepts of white biotechnology in their production processes. Other biopolymers such as polylactic acid (PLA) and poly-glycolic acid (PGLA) are being used to produce pharmaceutical supplies (George et al. 2020) whereas bio-based nylon can be used for producing glass-fibre reinforced compounds for energy-efficient transportation vehicles (Kind et al. 2014). This shows that the concepts of white biotechnology can be used to reduce the environmental impacts of various products throughout its lifetime while having additional advantages unique to the chemical structure of the biopolymer. Industry 5.0 can take this a step further and incorporate seamless data acquisition by applying sensors in the products and relaying it back to the design team in the manufacturing line to improve the product design. For example, in the case of the surgical adhesives, sensors could obtain accurate physiological data of the patient prior to the surgery to enable the surgeon to correctly select or modify the surgical adhesive to better suit the patient. In terms of food and beverage packaging options, end-users can choose varying qualities and properties of biopolymer for their own applications and have it delivered to their doorstep. Perhaps this could be further extended using additive manufacturing, whereby biopolymer filaments can be sold to the consumer for them to 3D print their own products at home according to their unique aesthetics.

Although the production rate is much lower and more complex in comparison to bulk chemicals (Pollak 2007), fine chemicals are nonetheless essential for the chemical functions of various manufactured goods, especially in the production of pharmaceutical products and food additives. Due to the high complexity of their production process, nanomaterials can be considered to be fine chemicals and their applications have stretched from being used as industrial catalysts to potential drug delivery systems in the medical field. Silver nanomaterials are actively being used in the field of medicine and as pharmaceutical products for their antibacterial properties. However, the conventional methods of producing metallic nanomaterials can render the final products to be non-biocompatible and, hence, unsuitable for medical applications. Despite this, there is a growing effort in the scientific community to utilize biopolymers and apply concepts of biotechnology to manufacture nanomaterials as Susilowati et al. (2015) did by using glucose as a reducing agent to prepare silver-chitosan nanocomposites for medical applications. Similar to silver nanomaterials, short chains of amino acids known as peptides have both antimicrobial and anticancer properties that make them highly valuable compounds in the pharmaceutical industry (Kokel and Török 2018). The high antimicrobial activity of peptides also shows their potential as a substitute for synthetic preservatives (Przybylski et al. 2016). Przybylski et al. (2016) synthesized antimicrobial peptides through the valorization of bovine blood, which is a waste product from slaughterhouses. Other sources of peptides include snake (Ebrahim et al. 2016) and bee venom (K. S. Lee et al. 2016) which are used to synthesize anticancer drugs. The application of peptides as anti-cancer drugs is due to the fact that peptides are highly selective and sensitive towards their target molecules (Braun et al. 2018). This also makes peptides a highly attractive choice as biosorbents for extracting heavy metals, such as cobalt and nickel, in wastewater as was found by Braun et al. (2018). Waste-based organic materials such as rice husk ash (Jagaba et al. 2020), banana peels (Fabre et al. 2020) and waste mixtures (Silva et al. 2020) have also been investigated as potential biosorbents to replace synthetic commercial adsorbents for wastewater treatment purposes. Nanomaterials, peptides and biosorbents are a few of the wide range of compounds that make up the category of fine chemicals synthesized by using industrial biotechnology production processes. With the application of the concepts of white biotechnology and IR 5.0, it would be possible to challenge the conventional boundaries of chemical design to produce compounds that are tailored for a specific purpose but at a lower cost. One of the themes of IR 5.0 is the seamless data acquisition from the field to the design and manufacturing processes. For example, the real-time chemical composition data of the final discharge from a wastewater treatment plant can be sent to the engineers who are responsible for the production of biosorbents and tune the cocktail of biosorbents accordingly to ensure that the discharge limit is met and the complete reaction is achieved to ensure minimum wastage of the biosorbents.

3.5.2.2 Evolutionary Algorithms

The term "evolutionary algorithm" refers to heuristic optimization methods inspired by nature (Maesani, Fernando, and Floreano 2014). The word "evolution" is defined as the development of new species through natural selection, genetic mutation and hybridization of the pre-existing forms over successive generations (Wilkins 2008). In the context of evolutionary algorithms, it is the results that undergo evolution over multiple iterations (Maesani, Fernando, and Floreano 2014). These algorithms would then operate through the selection, reproduction and mutation of the genotypes (Manning, Sleator, and Walsh 2013). The basic structure of an evolutionary algorithm is shown as Figure 3.5.2. In this case, the genotypes are the set of parameters that identifies the proposed solution of the problem given to the algorithm (Manning, Sleator, and Walsh 2013). Each of these proposed solutions would then be identified as an "individual" and a group of these solutions would be known as the "population" (Gad 2018). In accordance to the old adage of "survival of the fittest", each of these individual solutions has a fitness value that is determined using a fitness function and it represents the quality of the solution, where a higher fitness value corresponds to a higher quality of the solution (Gad 2018). The individual solutions with higher quality are selected to generate a "mating pool" and these individuals would be known as the "parents" (Gad 2018). A pair of parents selected from the mating pool would produce two "children" and by coupling high-quality individuals, the offspring is expected to have a better quality than its parents and the "bad" individuals would be eliminated to ensure the highest quality solution would be obtained (Gad 2018). This allows for a selective breeding of solutions that has a higher probability of maintaining the good properties of the solutions while excluding the bad ones (Gad 2018). However, if this process repeats itself, the offspring would have the same disadvantages as their parents (Gad 2018). In order to overcome this obstacle, certain changes or "mutations" would be made to the offspring to create new and different individuals (Gad 2018). This new set of

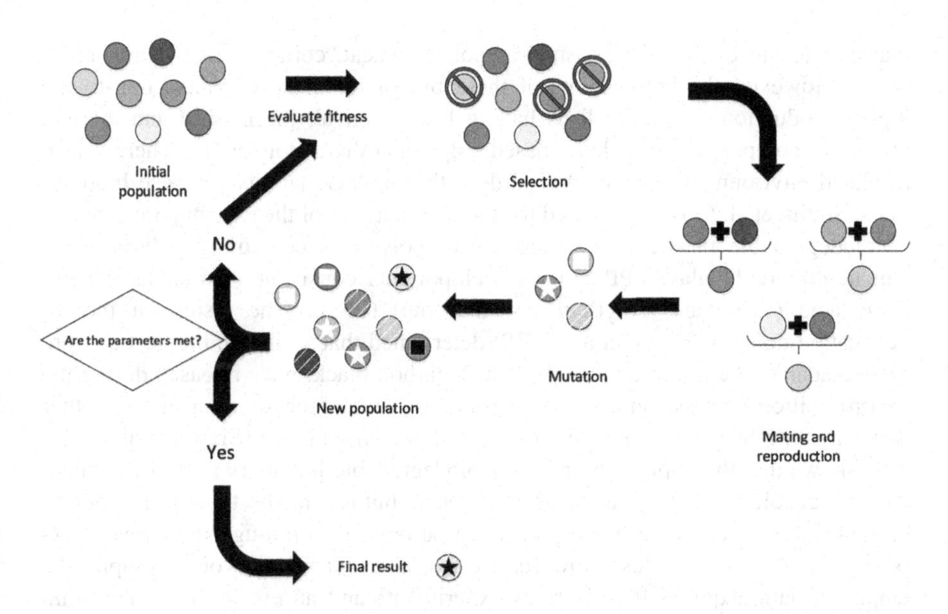

FIGURE 3.5.2 Basic structure of an evolutionary algorithm.

individuals would represent the new population that supersedes the old population and each of these newly generated populations is called a "generation" (Gad 2018). The process of selection, reproduction and mutation of the solutions would be repeated until the optimal solution is achieved (Gad 2018). Evolutionary algorithms are now being widely investigated as a method for solving multi-objective optimization problems, constructing regularization and constraint processing strategies as well as many other potential applications due to the dynamic nature of the algorithm (G. Chen et al. 2020). Production processes, regardless of whether manufacturing lines or chemical or biochemical processing plants, are required to fulfil various interrelated parameters in order to deliver the product at the required quality while maximizing profit and minimizing loss in the plant. Other fluctuating variables such as potential emissions, raw material availability, energy consumption and process safety are the few of the many points that must be taken into consideration as well. Hence, by applying these dynamic algorithms to optimize production processes, it would be possible to make the process more flexible while minimizing wastage of energy and resources that would benefit the manufacturer, consumer and the environment.

The development of evolutionary algorithms encroaches onto the field of artificial intelligence (AI), where mundane and iterative tasks become increasingly managed by AI and robots, thereby allowing the human designers to focus on setting the desired parameters of the product (Rossi 2018). This is highly applicable in the field of biopolymers where, not only is there a diverse range of biopolymers, but also an even larger range of applications of each type of biopolymer. For example, some biopolymers, such as polylactic acid, that are being used as biodegradable substitutes for single-use packaging are usually synthesized from crops that are rich in carbohydrates, such as potato, wheat, corn and rice (Kabir et al. 2020). However, the applications of these biopolymers are restricted due to the higher production cost as well as having lower optical, mechanical and thermal properties compared to petroleum-based polymers (Viera et al. 2020). There is also a related environmental concern regarding the biodegradability of these biopolymers. Sintim et al. (2019) evaluated the biodegradability of the two major categories of biodegradable plastics which are the co-polyesters containing poly(butylene adipate-co-terephthalate) (PBAT) and a biopolymer consisting of a blend of polylactic acid (PLA) and poly(hydroxy-alkanoate) (PHA). The results of the investigation done by Sintim et al. (2019) determined that while the bioplastics were biodegradable, the minor additives, such as carbon black, were released during the decomposition process and its toxicity to soil micro- and macroorganisms and other downstream effects of these additives are still not fully known (Sintim et al. 2019). This shows that the application of these biodegradable polymers is far from being the perfect solution to the plastic waste problem, but it is the best available solution currently. However, these biopolymers can be optimized through iterations of experiments. As moving closer towards IR 5.0, a software that would compile the empirical data acquired from various experiments and an evolutionary algorithm that would be able to utilize this data as a starting population. Designers and engineers would then be able to utilize this algorithm to determine the optimum solution based on the desired parameters. There are already several types of evolutionary algorithms that have been developed worldwide to solve engineering problems such as the Black Widow Optimization algorithm (Hayyolalam and Pourhaji Kazem 2020), the Barnacles Mating Optimizer algorithm (Sulaiman et al. 2020) and the Particle Swarm Optimization algorithm (Katoch et al. 2019). These algorithms are expected to be used for industrial applications and implemented in designing software for real-world optimization purposes. As an example, engineers and designers would be able to choose the mechanical and thermal properties of the biodegradable plastics while lowering its production costs and ensuring its environmental footprint throughout its entire lifecycle is kept to a minimum or eliminated entirely.

Similar to biopolymers, the category of fine chemicals covers a wide range of complex and single compounds that can either have a highly specific application or be used to synthesize various products (Bennett 2013). Penicillin, for example, would be considered a fine chemical as it has a lower production rate compared to commodity chemicals and it is specifically administered as a pharmaceutical drug to treat bacterial infections (Sinha 2018). On the other hand, pyridine is also considered to be a fine chemical (Pollak 2007) but it is used in the production of various products such as medicine, food flavourings, paints, dyes and adhesives (National Center for Biotechnology Information 2019). Other characteristics that define fine chemicals are the high complexity of the production processes and the high purity of the end product, which significantly increases its retail price per unit weight compared to bulk chemicals. As was mentioned in the earlier section, one of the usual applications of fine chemicals is in the healthcare industry for producing the active ingredients used in pharmaceutical drugs. For example, Vincristine is a chemotherapeutic drug that is administered to treat lymphomas, leukaemia, brain tumours and other solid cancers (F. Liu, Huang, and Liu 2019). Vincristine itself is a vinca alkaloid derived from the plant *Catharanthus roseus*, also known as the Madagascar periwinkle, that requires extensive processing to extract the active ingredient (Karimi and Raofie 2019). Recently, there have been reports that certain cancer lines did not have the ability to absorb Vincristine due to the low solubility of the compound since it has a large particle size (Karimi and Raofie 2019). Hence, there have been a number of methods that have been used to reduce the particle size such as spray drying, milling and crushing (Karimi and Raofie 2019). However, these conventional methods induce thermal and chemical degradation of the active ingredient, produce a final product that has a broad particle size distribution and consume a large amount of energy and solvent (Karimi and Raofie 2019). The high consumption of energy and resources likely contribute to the high cost of Vincristine with a price tag of 14.25 USD/mL (Drugs.com 2020) and with the reported number of new cases of leukaemia being over 437,000 worldwide in 2018 alone (American Cancer Society 2018). It is clear that there is a demand for chemotherapeutic drugs such as Vincristine. However, cancer disregards the financial status of the patient and not all patients are able to afford the high costs of the treatment. One potential solution for this is through the optimization of the production process of chemotherapeutic drugs and pharmaceutical products, and other fine chemicals as well. A compilation of an archive of the various empirical data and the implementation of evolutionary algorithms in the production process could potentially produce a high-quality product while reducing the consumption of energy and resources, thereby reducing the overall cost of the product. By using evolutionary algorithms and with sufficient data acquisition, compounds and active ingredients used in the pharmaceutical industry could also be tailored to each patient's needs by adjusting the parameters of the production process. Fine chemicals are also used as food additives, agrichemicals and catalysts, such as enzymes and zeolites, for various industries. Since production of fine chemicals is usually through batch processes, the customization of the products would also be simpler in comparison to bulk chemicals and with algorithms that could take into account the multiple objectives, it would be possible to be able to produce in smaller bespoke quantities while reducing the start-up and shutdown costs of the plant.

3.5.2.3 Synthetic Biology

Synthetic biology is the scientific field that entails the reprogramming of the genome of organisms by modifying them to have controllable and functional properties (National Human Genome Research Institute USA 2019; H. H. Wang, Mee, and Church 2013). Since it is a relatively new field, the exact definition of synthetic biology is still ambiguous but the general consensus is that synthetic biology re-designs and re-constructs the genome of existing biological systems for an entirely new purpose (Jin et al. 2019). On that note, synthetic biology seems to be similar to genome editing or genetic modification but the National Human Genome Research Institute USA (2019), draws the line between synthetic biology and genome editing based on how the changes are made. Genome editing typically involves cutting out a section of an organism's genetic codes to make small changes in the DNA (National Human Genome Research Institute USA 2019). Synthetic biology involves weaving and stitching the genes of various other organisms or entirely new genes to create a synthetic DNA that does not exist in nature as shown in Figure 3.5.3 (National Human Genome Research Institute USA 2019). This cutting, stitching and manipulating of biological components means that this scientific field is a fusion of biology with chemistry, computer science, mathematics and engineering (F. Wang and Zhang 2019). The rapid advances being made in these respective fields have a direct effect on the progress being made in synthetic biology (F. Wang and Zhang 2019). One of the first achievements of synthetic biology was the creation of an engineered yeast that produces the precursor of the antimalarial drug, artemisinin (Ro et al. 2006). Ro et al. (2006) re-designed the common baker's yeast, *Saccharomyces cerevisiae* to produce artemisinic acid, which is the immediate precursor of artemisinin and the result was a high quality and reliable source of the antimalarial drug produced in a cost-effective manner with minimum environmental impacts. A process that produces high-quality products while being profitable and environmentally friendly is what process design engineers strive for and applying synthetic biology within the process line could help achieve that. Employing the concepts of synthetic biology does not have to come in the form of directly fitting in a bioreactor into the process, but in the form of producing the catalyst or the intermediate chemical as these tend to be the most expensive raw materials used in the process. There is already a database of the genetic information of various species of microorganisms and by integrating an

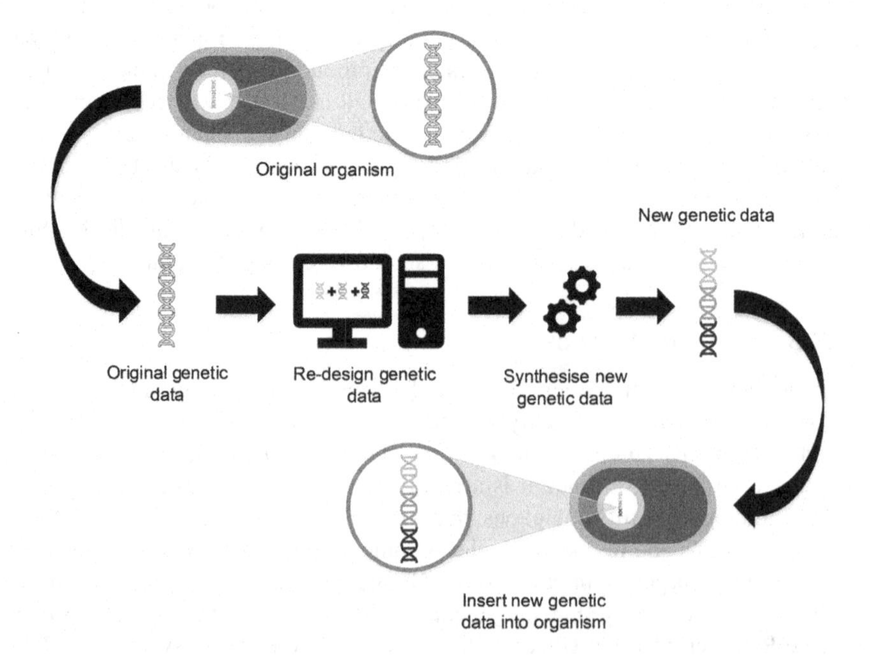

FIGURE 3.5.3 Synthetic biology involves weaving and stitching the genes of various other organisms or entirely new genes to create a new synthetic DNA.

evolutionary algorithm and machine learning with the database, there is a high possibility of synthetic biology being implemented for other industrial applications (Presnell and Alper 2019). With the highly anticipated IR 5.0 happening in the near future, there will be a challenge to the conventional boundaries of nature with the advances being made in synthetic biology. The application of the concepts of synthetic biology in various products such as biopolymers and fine chemicals is only the beginning.

The advances being made in synthetic biology opens new doorways into the modification of various micro-consortia and has the potential of being applied in the production of biopolymer. For some, the term biopolymer is synonymous to biodegradable packaging, academics have focused on modifying the production process of these biodegradable polymers through the application of industrial biotechnology. However, there have been several researchers that have looked towards synthetic biology as a solution, and recently, Heras (2017) succeeded in using synthetic biology to reprogram the metabolism of *S. cerevisiae* to produce the biodegradable plastic (PHB). Investigations done by Tripathi et al. (2013) and Arias et al. (2013) yielded successful results in producing PHAs using *Pseudomonas putida*. Controlling the production of the biopolymers is also essential in order to ensure that the productivity and yield of the final product. Hence, Durante-Rodríguez, De Lorenzo, and Nikel (2018) have re-engineered a protein by constructing a novel set of plasmids that acts as a metabolic switch for the PHA-producing *Escherichia coli* to cease producing PHA at a set level. Synthetic biology can also be suitably applied in producing biopolymers for medical purposes. For example, hydrogels are commonly used as dressings for moist wound management (Leveriza-Oh and Phillips 2012) but it must be replaced frequently to minimize risks of infection. Azam et al. (2016) synthesized biopolymer-forming proteins that can be integrated into *Salmonella enterica* to produce protein-based customizable antimicrobial hydrogels at a sufficiently high yield and productivity rate and replicable rheological properties. Hydrogels can also be formed from alginates, which are considered to be a subset of polysaccharides and are commonly used as stabilisers and gelling agents in food, cosmetics and pharmaceutical products (Anderson, Islam, and Prather 2018). Due to the continuing high demand for alginates, Maleki et al. (2015) analyzed the effects of re-programming the enzyme producing genes of *Pseudomonas fluorescens* and determined that the engineered strain had an increased production of alginate compared to the other strains of *Pseudomonas* spp. that they investigated. The high volume of research in the field of synthetic biology shows diverse material design options that can be applied in various industries and opens new avenues to the production of novel materials tailored to the needs of the consumer or client (Anderson, Islam, and Prather 2018) as proven by Azam et al. (2016). In the packaging industry, for example, it would be possible that the bioplastics could be customized without adding plasticisers and colourants during the manufacturing process. Instead, the properties of the bioplastics could be manipulated at the cellular level, whereby synthetic biology is used to modify the genetic makeup of the microorganism according to the desired qualities and aesthetics of the consumer to minimize downstream waste and any associated environmental impacts. This technology could perhaps be made available to the general public, where people can easily modify the genes of the microorganisms to produce the bioplastics at home and integrate it with a 3D printer to print their own packaging.

Several categories of fine chemicals, such as pharmaceutical drugs and food additives, are already being synthesized using industrial biotechnology. These processes, however, have low production rates and high costs due to the high complexity of the process. By implementing synthetic biology to re-engineer microorganisms to produce these chemicals prior to the process, it would be possible to significantly reduce the production cost while minimizing the environmental impacts of the process as was proven by Ro et al. (2006). The flavonoid naringenin, for example, is commonly found in some fruits, such as the citrus family, bergamot and tomatoes (Salehi et al. 2019). The high potential of this flavonoid in the pharmaceutical industry is likely due to the panoply of pharmacological benefits such as being an antioxidant as well as having anticancer, antiviral, antimicrobial and anti-inflammatory activities (Salehi et al. 2019). Owing to the complex extraction and high resource consumption of the process itself, this compound has been experiencing a low growth rate (Koopman et al. 2012). Koopman et al. (2012) succeeded in improving the production rate of the flavonoid by re-engineering *S. cerevisiae* to produce naringenin by co-expressing the naringenin-producing genes from *Arabidopsis thaliana*, which is a small flowering plant that originates from Eurasia and Africa. Producing flavonoids is but one of the many applications of synthetic biology. Liu et al. (2013) reviewed the development *Bacillus spp.* for producing enzymes and industrial biochemicals. One of the enzymes listed in the review written by Liu et al. (2013) is the enzyme α-amylase, which is widely used in the paper, food and textile industries to break down starch and other types of oligosaccharides. As the paper, food and textile industries play a major role in developing consumer goods there have been several researchers that have built upon the idea of using *Bacillus spp.* to increase the production of this enzyme. For example, Song et al. (2016) evaluated 84 different protein candidates that can be used as components to be integrated into the *Bacillus subtilis* to enhance the production of the α-amylase enzyme. These proteins exhibit characteristics such as having resistance to heat-shock and toxic metals as well as good stress response that can promote the *B. subtilis* to express these traits to increase the productivity of the microbes under industrial conditions (Y. Song et al. 2016). With many of the world's fossil fuel resources already reaching or surpassed its peak production rate, synthesizing fine chemicals through a more sustainable, bio-based route presents an attractive alternative. As the research and development being done in the field of synthetic biology continues to advance rapidly, the option for an eco-friendly production method could become the mainstream in the future with an increasing number of people becoming more conscious about the environmental impacts of the products they are using (Barbarossa and De Pelsmacker, 2016). The database of genetic information and components is already available in the form of BioBricks™, which is a standard of interchangeable parts of biological information that can be used to build biological systems in living cells (IGEM 2015). In other words, BioBricks™ is like a box of building blocks, where it is possible to build an entirely new biological system with synthetically derived foreign traits or characteristics of different organisms and insert them into a living cell, such as the *E. coli*. BioBricks™ is one of the many databases that can be used to reprogram organisms using synthetic biology. As synthetic biology progresses, the future prospects of these databases could be where both the software and the hardware are available to be safely used by the general public and industries to allow for the customization of the organisms to improve productivity. It could be possible to produce new types of flavonoids or enzymes that can be applied in the food and beverage industry to produce customizable goods. Another potential would be pharmaceutical drugs that can be tailored according to the physiological conditions of the patient.

3.5.3 ADVANTAGES OF IR 5.0 IN THE PRODUCTION OF FINE CHEMICALS AND BIOPOLYMERS

Section 3.5.2 is a list of three fields among many others that have a high potential in playing a major role in the Fifth Industrial Revolution. With the main themes of IR 5.0 being the mass customization of products and an increased cooperation between man and machine, there is much that can be achieved and even more that can be of significant benefit to the general public. Section 3.5.3 will focus on the advantages of the technological advancements that could potentially be made in IR 5.0 and how it can benefit the production of fine chemicals and biopolymers.

3.5.3.1 Data Sensor Network

The implementation of cloud storage and the interlinking network of digital devices that is happening right now is the foundation that could be built upon for the future network of data sensors. Rather than the sensors that are directly installed into the production line, it can be sensors that are installed at the department stores or supermarkets themselves (Nahavandi 2019). These sensors would allow for real-time tracking of the products that can help develop an online process optimization of the production line for both biopolymers and fine chemicals (Nahavandi 2019). The sales orders from customers can be linked to the production orders, which would lead to an increase in the efficiency of resource management and minimize waste generation (Nahavandi 2019). Various companies have already developed an array of intelligent packaging that exhibit various purposes from showing the chemical changes of the product within to indicating the integrity of the entire distribution chain (Realini and Marcos 2014). Lee and Rahman (2013) reviewed the potential of using radiofrequency identification (RFID) tags to store and communicate real-time data of the product. In doing so, the tags would allow for the product to be automatically identified and traced for various purposes (Realini and Marcos 2014). Hence, adapting tracking tags into products such as biodegradable packaging is a potential goal that can be set by researchers and manufacturers. The sensors would not only allow for identification and traceability, but also other information such as the product is being used, the chemical status of the contents and the quantity of the goods. Transponders that are synchronized with these sensors would be able to transmit to the real-time data to the design engineers to optimize both the design of the product and the production process itself. Sensors in biodegradable bottles, for example, could record the intensity of mechanical and thermal stress data throughout its lifetime as well as the span of its lifetime. The collective information from various consumers would be transmitted back to the designers for them to enhance the usability of the product and at the same time optimize the process by omitting any unnecessary raw materials for better resource management.

RFID sensors are just one of the many types of indicators that are currently being developed and for a multitude of applications. One of the categories of this emerging field is biosensors. The idea of biosensors was first conceived in the 1960s by Clark and Lyons, whereby the biosensors would convert biological responses into electrical signals and can be applied in various industries from the food and beverage industry (Mehrotra 2016) to wastewater treatment plants (Ejeian et al. 2018). In the field of medicine, biosensors are already being used to diagnose infectious diseases, diabetes and cardiovascular conditions (Mehrotra 2016). At the rate of technological advances that we are experiencing now, these biosensors could be used to minimize the occurrence of misdiagnosis and prescribe customized doses of medicine for each patient. Currently, the doses of prescription drugs are calculated using simple formulas that are based on the manufacturer's instructions (Toney-Butler and Wilcox 2019). Each human is, however, physiologically unique. Biosensors could be used to determine the various factors, such as the patient's metabolism and the presence of various hormones, that can affect the drug efficacy of a patient and transmit the data to the doctors for an improved treatment process. In that sense, installing biosensors in the patient could benefit the production of fine chemicals used in pharmaceutical products. For instance, once the patient finishes the treatment course, the data on the drug's efficacy can be sent back to the research and development department of the pharmaceutical company to further improve the chemical composition and delivery methods of the drug itself. This would potentially optimize the production process as any ingredients that were found to be unnecessary in the drug itself can be eliminated for a better resource management.

3.5.3.2 VISUALIZATION AND MODELLING OF PRODUCTION LINE

Virtual reality (VR) was an idea that began in 1987 (Berkman 2018) but has been gaining ground at an increasing within the past decade or so and Sulema (2018) presented the idea of building a virtual model of a process. This concept would be beneficial for management and personalization of both the products and production lines and could fundamentally optimize the production process (Nahavandi 2019). Application of VR would be advantageous in both the production of biopolymers and fine chemicals. For example, biopolymers and bio-based fine chemicals require careful control of the bioreactors to ensure the productivity of the microbial consortia and the yield as well as the quality of the final product. By creating a realistic virtual model of the bioreactor, which would essentially be its digital twin, the plant operators could monitor the most crucial step of the process more carefully to minimize downtime and improve risk management of the production line

(Nahavandi 2019). Ciortea, Mayer, and Michahelles (2018), for example, have successfully created a functional prototype of a production cell that integrates two industry-grade robots and an augmented reality (AR) interface for the human workers. The system can be modified and repurposed on-the-go by the engineers through an intuitive web user interface that was designed to facilitate seamless integration of the geographical positions of the production cells (Ciortea, Mayer, and Michahelles 2018). Virtual models of the process could be coupled with an evolutionary algorithm to create, model and assess different operating conditions to account for uncertainties that could arise during the production (Nahavandi 2019). In doing so, any scenarios where issues such as shock loading and safety hazards that could happen can be thoroughly evaluated and addressed prior to its occurrence. This can minimize the downtime required for the plant and, hence, minimize the production costs of the product while maintaining its profitability. Since one of the drawbacks of fine chemicals and biodegradable packaging is its high cost, this would be highly advantageous for both products. Ciortea, Mayer, and Michahelles (2018) also designed their prototype system to have an improved flexibility and adaptability, which allowed the engineers to customize the products easily using the web-based AR interface. This demonstrates the possibility of extending the capability of product customization beyond the factory, whereby consumers can customize large products such as biopolymer-based furniture, accessories and ornaments from home and have the data directly transferred to the manufacturing line. By employing a web-based AR interface, the customer would also be able to gauge the actual size and appearance of the product before purchase, which would save time, effort and travelling costs of the customer.

3.5.3.3 Intelligent Autonomous Systems for Manufacturing Lines

As the Fourth Industrial Revolution gains momentum, the technological advances being made in the field of artificial intelligence (AI) follows suit with the development of intelligent and reconfigurable manufacturing systems (Li et al. 2017; Renzi et al. 2014). Currently, researchers are looking to integrate AI with the technologies of IR 4.0 such as Internet of Things (IoT), big data analytics, cloud computing and cyber physical systems to meet the current market demands (J. Lee et al. 2018). With the increasing demands for eco-friendly products (Gelski 2019), there is a high possibility that AI technologies would be integrated into the production of fine chemicals and biopolymers. For example, evolutionary algorithms, which is considered to be a sub-category of AI (Larrañaga et al. 2013) could play a role in the development of self-learning systems that can evolve and provide solutions for optimizing a production line to meet the standards and parameters that are set by the design engineers. Taking a step further, concepts and ideas of AI applied to the software of the production lines would allow the manufacturing units to learn and execute the desired tasks autonomously (Nahavandi 2019). An autonomous manufacturing line would also be inherently safer and become more efficient by minimizing human error and manual labour on-site as the menial tasks would be taken over by the machines themselves. In doing so, there would be an increase in the productivity of the production line while providing social benefits by increasing earnings and the demand for labour in new employment categories (Autor 2015).

3.5.4 CHALLENGES, PERSPECTIVES AND FUTURE PROSPECTS

We are currently in the Fifth Industrial Revolution and are becoming more aware of the importance of sustainability in, not only the environmental perspective, but also economic and social aspects as well. The Fifth Industrial Revolution has the potential to achieve the goal of increasing production rates while fulfilling the three Pillars of Sustainable Development of environmental, economic and social sustainability (United Nations Economic and Social Council 2015) through more advanced and rigorous applications of technologies such as AI, industrial biotechnology and biochemical engineering. In doing so, it is possible for the industry to satisfy the dynamic demands of the consumers while improving the livelihood of the employees and minimizing environmental impacts of the production process. Yet, these statements warrant a certain level of speculation in the eyes of the public, industry and policymakers in terms of employability, ethics and finance.

3.5.4.1 Societal Challenges

There have always been oppositions and negative pre-conceived notions that new technology and automation will cause a significant drop in the number of middle-class jobs (Autor 2015). One of the best-known examples is the Luddite movement that happened during the First Industrial Revolution, whereby a group of English textile artisans sought to sabotage the textile production machines and protest against the automation of the textile industry (Autor 2015). As the world adjusts to the new workplace environment of IR 4.0, there is an inherent concern from the public regarding the risk of increasing the unemployment rate due to the increase in digitization and automation across all industries, which includes the biopolymer and fine chemicals manufacturing lines as well (Autor 2015). Following that trend, it is likely that anxieties about unemployment would be brought forward in IR 5.0 with an increase in the use of AI and autonomous machines both in the production line and the factory floor. However, IR 5.0 aims to provide a solution for the issue of unemployment by emphasizing the human-robot co-working relationship, whereby automation and new technologies complement the workers to improve productivity, increase income and the demand for new labour (Autor 2015). Autor (2015) established that while automation substitutes labour, it increases the reliability of certain steps in a process while reducing the overall cost of the production line, which increases the value of the human links in the manufacturing chain. As more production line employees have an improved livelihood, the rising income could create new demands for other fields of goods and services that are unrelated to the booming technology (Autor 2015).

Another potential concern that can emerge during IR 5.0 is cyber-security. The Fifth Industrial Revolution puts forth the concept for mass customization of products at a lower price, but it would mean an increased amount of data that has to be divulged by the consumers themselves. The use of the Internet is already not entirely anonymous with the extensive use of various social media platforms and there have been those who take advantage of this and misuse it for malicious purposes. IR 5.0 seeks to further advance the ideas that are currently being developed in the Fourth Industrial Revolution, which is centred around the accessibility and employment of large amounts of data through the increased interconnectivity of smart machines (Marr 2018). Mass customization would mean that larger amounts of personal data would be interspersed throughout the internet, thereby increasing the risk of cyber threat for consumers (Clim 2019). Online pharmacies, for example, offer a direct-to-consumer healthcare and an improved accessibility to the global supply of pharmaceutical products (Seneff 2016). A fraction of these online pharmacies, however, have been in violation of professional, legal and ethical principles as well as being subjected to cybersecurity threats due to inadequate protection for their online customers (Seneff 2016). In a hypothetical case of personalization of pharmaceutical fine chemicals, would require a certain amount of highly detailed medical data to be extracted to personalize the products in the first place and such sensitive information would then be wholly reliant on the cyber security of the system. Should the security system be inadequate, it would mean that the medical data could be stolen and the patient could be at risk of identity theft that could lead to the patient being the victim of extortion and tax fraud (Steger 2019). Financial distress of the consumer could be considered the worst-case scenario, but it would mean that if the Fifth Industrial Revolution aims to employ IoT for mass customization, improved cyber security must be made available for all at an affordable cost. Although this scenario appears to have a bleak outlook, the financial sector has been catching up with other industries and have started to employ AI to provide better service at a lower cost (Golić 2020). Golić (2020) also described that the use of AI could improve pattern recognition in the financial sector whereby the system can pinpoint anomalies in transactions for a better fraud prevention system to protect the customers against financial losses.

3.5.4.2 Challenges in Industrialization

The one aspect that all the previous industrial revolutions have in common is the fact that an industrial revolution brings about a disruption towards the pre-existing social, economic and industrial norms. The Fifth Industrial Revolution is no exception to this pattern, especially with its main themes being mass personalization and human-centred cyber physical systems (Pathak et al. 2019). Aside from the potential changes being made in employment opportunities, IR 5.0 would certainly cause significant changes within all industries, including the biopolymer and fine chemicals production sectors. With the increasing awareness regarding the depleting fossil fuels and the associated environmental impacts of petrochemicals, the demand for bio-based, eco-friendly products would increase dramatically in the future (Gelski 2019). This implies that the manufacturers of products such as biodegradable plastics and eco-friendly detergents would have to significantly increase the productivity of their manufacturing line. Moreover, the demand for mass customization of products at lower costs mean that the manufacturing line must be made modular and more adaptable to changes (Ivanov, Dolgui, and Sokolov 2019).

Increased productivity, modularity and adaptability will catalyze radical changes in the factory floor, supply chain and the logistics of product process organization (Ivanov, Dolgui, and Sokolov 2019). There are also added concerns of data security and more complex design and control of the production line (Ivanov, Dolgui, and Sokolov 2019). Catalysts are considered to be fine chemicals that tend to be the most expensive raw material in a process. There are various variables that can be manipulated, such as its material, porosity, geometry and chemical makeup, that can improve the rate of a reaction using the catalyst. If a company invests on developing an evolutionary algorithm that allows them to optimize and customize the characteristics of the catalyst for each industrial client, it will certainly disrupt the conventional supply chain and affect the original manufacturers of the compound. Hence, the managers, plant operators, engineers and logistics team of the production lines in IR 5.0 will have to adapt to the changes to ensure a smooth flow of the production line by conducting supply chain analysis and constructing contingency plans using the appropriate optimization and simulation models (Ivanov, Dolgui, and Sokolov 2019).

3.5.4.3 Future Prospects

One of the emerging concepts that is slowly gaining ground is sustainable development and IR 5.0 has the potential to make this concept a reality for the global environment. The energy sector, for example, has been working to increase the renewable energy shares in the current energy mix and, in turn, this has spurred the market for all technologies related to renewable energy. With an increasing market demand and technological advancements, the production costs of technologies such as solar cells have been reducing steadily over the past decade (Chandler 2018). However, one of the concerns regarding the use of solar cells is the use of minerals such as perovskite within the solar cells, which can have a negative impact on the environment during its life cycle (Espinosa et al. 2015). There have been several solutions that have been employed by the industry to remedy this issue and academics have been rigorously studying alternatives for solar cells with higher efficiency but at lower environmental and economic costs. Suresh et al. (2019), for example, fabricated a biodegradable photoelectrochemical cell that uses solar energy to generate power using cellulose-based electrodes that contain a photosynthetic protein. This is a potential technology that could be manufactured using industrial biotechnology and optimized using AI and evolutionary algorithms for an improved efficiency of the production line. The fact that they used a biopolymer-based electrode opens new avenues in applications of biopolymer. Perhaps, synthetic biology can be applied in this field further down the line to engineer new microbial consortia that could be used to absorb solar energy for energy conversion at an increased efficiency.

Another future prospect would be the widespread use of genetic circuits. Genetic circuits or synthetic regulation can be loosely defined as using a living cell to perform computation and can be grouped under the category of synthetic biology (Brophy and Voigt 2014; Mózsik et al. 2019). As IR 5.0 aims to increase the productivity of the biotechnology sector, genetic circuits can aid in improving existing processes and develop new applications for bio-based products (Brophy and Voigt 2014). Brophy and Voigt (2014) hypothesized that genetic circuits can be used to calibrate the gene expressions of the microorganism at different stages of fermentation or activate enzymes only when the specific conditions are met, which can provide a boost to the manufacturing process of bio-based chemicals. Further development of these genetic circuits would allow for more advanced algorithms to be used to enhance the biochemical production process (Brophy and Voigt 2014). Moreover, the synthetic regulation of living cells will play a central role in the development of natural products and novel classes of chemicals, which can aid in the demand for mass customization of fine chemicals and biopolymers (Brophy and Voigt 2014).

There are many other outcomes and possibilities in the development of the technologies for the production of fine chemicals and biopolymers. One other prospect that is likely to happen in the Fifth Industrial Revolution is the integration and combination of the various technologies mentioned in Section 3.5.2 in the development of bio-based products. Biopolymers and bio-based fine chemicals are already using industrial biotechnology to satisfy the demands for mass production of the products. By having white biotechnology as the core of the production line, it would be possible to adopt synthetic biology to develop novel chemicals and biopolymers by manipulating and re-engineering the genetic makeup of microorganisms as was proven by Azam et al. (2016). Song et al. (2016) successfully re-engineered the microorganisms to be more resistant to industrial conditions and ensure that the microorganisms remain productive under various conditions, whereas the integration of genetic circuits into the production line would help to boost the productivity of the biochemical production line (Brophy and Voigt 2014). Evolutionary algorithms and AI could be employed to optimize and improve the adaptability of the process as well as to establish the logistics of the supply chain and process organization (Ivanov, Dolgui, and Sokolov 2019).

3.5.5 CONCLUSIONS

The world is poised for the Fifth Industrial Revolution that is approaching with the rapid advancements being made in human-centred cyber physical systems and the increasing demand for mass customization of products. Autonomous manufacturing lines would become more common to put human creative intelligence back into the production process flow. The IoT would be used more in various industries to establish machine learning and to compile data for mass customization purposes by employing sensors and transmitters in the product itself. As we approach Industry 5.0, humans will begin to stretch the boundaries of physics in the product design. Combining biochemical engineering, white biotechnology, synthetic biology and evolutionary algorithms with the technological concepts of IR 5.0 would open new avenues in the design and development of bio-based products, including fine chemicals and biopolymers. Conventional biopolymers are mainly used for packaging purposes but with the combined application of the ideas of Industry 5.0 with white biotechnology, synthetic biology and evolutionary algorithms, it would be possible to expand the applications of biopolymers in other fields and allow for the mass customization of the products. For fine chemicals, integrating the concepts of IR 5.0 with synthetic biology and evolutionary algorithms would allow for the development of new biochemicals for mass customization and reduce the costs of the production process itself. However, there are a few potential challenges that must be overcome for a widespread implementation of the concepts of IR 5.0 in the production of biopolymers and fine chemicals such as concerns in the changes in employment and supply chain logistics, production process management as well as the privacy issues. In conclusion, the Fifth Industrial Revolution has the potential to improve the productivity of the manufacturing processes of fine chemicals and biopolymers with the applications of industrial biotechnology, synthetic biology and evolutionary algorithms. Adopting these branches of technology in the production line would also allow for the products to be manufactured in a sustainable manner while satisfying the demand for mass customization of the products.

REFERENCES

American Cancer Society. 2018. "Worldwide Cancer Data, World Cancer Research Fund." *Cancer Facts & Figures for African Americans 2016-2018.* https://www.wcrf.org/dietandcancer/cancer-trends/worldwide-cancer-data.

Anderson, Lisa A., M. Ahsanul Islam, and Kristala L.J. Prather. 2018. "Synthetic biology strategies for improving microbial synthesis of 'green' biopolymers." *Journal of Biological Chemistry.* doi:10.1074/jbc.TM117.000368.

Arias, Sagrario, Monica Bassas-Galia, Gabriella Molinari, and Kenneth N. Timmis. 2013. "Tight coupling of polymerization and depolymerization of polyhydroxyalkanoates ensures efficient management of carbon resources in *Pseudomonas putida.*" *Microbial Biotechnology* 6 (5): 551–563. doi:10.1111/1751-7915.12040.

Arkema. 2019. "Bio-based products – arkema.com." https://www.arkema.com/en/arkema-group/innovation/bio-based-products/.

Autor, David H. 2015. "Why are there still so many jobs? The history and future of workplace automation." *Journal of Economic Perspectives*, 29:3–30. doi:10.1257/jep.29.3.3.

Azam, Anum, Cheng Li, Kevin J. Metcalf, and Danielle Tullman-Ercek. 2016. "Type III secretion as a generalizable strategy for the production of full-length biopolymer-forming proteins." *Biotechnology and Bioengineering* 113 (11): 2313–2320. doi:10.1002/bit.25656.

Bajracharya, Rohan Muni, Allan C. Manalo, Warna Karunasena, and Kin tak Lau. 2014. "An overview of mechanical properties and durability of glass-fibre reinforced recycled mixed plastic waste composites." *Materials and Design.* doi:10.1016/j.matdes.2014.04.081.

Barbarossa, Camilla, and Patrick De Pelsmacker. 2016. "Positive and negative antecedents of purchasing eco-friendly products: A comparison between green and non-green consumers." *Journal of Business Ethics* 134 (2): 229–247. doi:10.1007/s10551-014-2425-z.

Bennett, Anthony. 2013. "Filtration and separation in the diverse fine chemical sectors." *Filtration and Separation* 50 (6): 30–33. doi:10.1016/S0015-1882(13)70240-4.

Berkman, Mehmet Ilker. 2018. "History of virtual reality." In *Encyclopedia of Computer Graphics and Games*: 1-9. doi:10.1007/978-3-319-08234-9_169-1.

Bhagat, Vrushali, and Matthew L. Becker. 2017. "Degradable adhesives for surgery and tissue engineering." *Biomacromolecules* 18 (10): 3009–3039. doi:10.1021/acs.biomac.7b00969.

Braun, Robert, Stefanie Bachmann, Nora Schönberger, Sabine Matys, Franziska Lederer, and Katrin Pollmann. 2018. "Peptides as biosorbents – promising tools for resource recovery." *Research in Microbiology* 169 (10): 649–658. doi:10.1016/j.resmic.2018.06.001.

Bré, Lígia Pereira, Yu Zheng, Ana Paula Pêgo, and Wenxin Wang. 2013. "Taking tissue adhesives to the future: From traditional synthetic to new biomimetic approaches." *Biomaterials Science*. doi:10.1039/c2bm00121g.

Brophy, Jennifer A. N., and Christopher A. Voigt. 2014. "Principles of genetic circuit design." *Nature Methods*. doi:10.1038/nmeth.2926.

Butler, Declan. 2016. "Tomorrow's world: Technological change is accelerating today at an unprecedented speed and could create a world we can barely begin to imagine." *Nature* 530: 399–401. doi:10.1111/j.0955-6419.2004.00334.x.

Cernadas, T.M., F.A.M.M. Gonçalves, P. Alves, S.P. Miguel, C. Cabral, I.J. Correia, and P. Ferreira. 2019. "Preparation of biodegradable functionalized polyesters aimed to be used as surgical adhesives." *European Polymer Journal* 117: 442–454. doi:10.1016/j.eurpolymj.2019.05.019.

Chandler, David. 2018. "Explaining the plummeting cost of solar power | MIT News." *MIT News Office*. http://news.mit.edu/2018/explaining-dropping-solar-cost-1120.

Chen, Guo Qiang, Juanyu Zhang, and Ying Wang. 2015. "White Biotechnology for Biopolymers: Hydroxyalkanoates and Polyhydroxyalkanoates: Production and Applications." In *Industrial Biorefineries and White Biotechnology*, 555–574. Elsevier. doi:10.1016/B978-0-444-63453-5.00018-5.

Chen, Guodong, Kai Zhang, Xiaoming Xue, Liming Zhang, Jun Yao, Hai Sun, Ling Fan, and Yongfei Yang. 2020. "Surrogate-assisted evolutionary algorithm with dimensionality reduction method for water flooding production optimization." *Journal of Petroleum Science and Engineering* 185: 106633. doi:10.1016/j.petrol.2019.106633.

Ciortea, Andrei, Simon Mayer, and Florian Michahelles. 2018. "Repurposing manufacturing lines on the fly with multi-agent systems for the web of things." In *Proceedings of the International Joint Conference on Autonomous Agents and Multiagent Systems, AAMAS*: 813–822.

Clark, Douglas S., and Harvey W. Blanch. 1997. *Biochemical Engineering*, 2nd edition. CRC Press, - Science.

Clim, Antonio. 2019. "Cyber security beyond the industry 4.0 era. A short review on a few technological promises." *Informatica Economica* 23 (2/2019): 34–44. doi:10.12948/issn14531305/23.2.2019.04.

Delooze, Sarah. 2017. "Bulk chemicals vs fine chemicals." *Syntor Fine Chemicals*. http://www.syntor.co.uk/bulk-chemicals/.

Drugs.com. 2020. "Vincristine prices, coupons & patient assistance programs – drugs.com." https://www.drugs.com/price-guide/vincristine.

Durante-Rodríguez, Gonzalo, Víctor De Lorenzo, and Pablo I. Nikel. 2018. "A post-translational metabolic switch enables complete decoupling of bacterial growth from biopolymer production in engineered *Escherichia coli*." *ACS Synthetic Biology* 7 (11): 2686–2697. doi:10.1021/acssynbio.8b00345.

Ebrahim, Karim, Hossein Vatanpour, Abbas Zare, Farshad H. Shirazi, and Mryam Nakhjavani. 2016. "Anticancer activity a of caspian cobra (Naja Naja Oxiana) snake venom in human cancer cell lines via induction of apoptosis." *Iranian Journal of Pharmaceutical Research* 15 (Suppl): 101–112. doi:10.22037/ijpr.2016.1811.

Ejeian, Fatemeh, Parisa Etedali, Hajar Alsadat Mansouri-Tehrani, Asieh Soozanipour, Ze Xian Low, Mohsen Asadnia, Asghar Taheri-Kafrani, and Amir Razmjou. 2018. "Biosensors for wastewater monitoring: A review." *Biosensors and Bioelectronics*. doi:10.1016/j.bios.2018.07.019.

Espinosa, Nieves, Lucía Serrano-Luján, Antonio Urbina, and Frederik C. Krebs. 2015. "Solution and vapour deposited lead perovskite solar cells: Ecotoxicity from a life cycle assessment perspective." *Solar Energy Materials and Solar Cells* 137: 303–310. doi:10.1016/j.solmat.2015.02.013.

Fabre, Elaine, Cláudia B. Lopes, Carlos Vale, Eduarda Pereira, and Carlos M. Silva. 2020. "Valuation of banana peels as an effective biosorbent for mercury removal under low environmental concentrations." *Science of the Total Environment* 709: 135883. doi:10.1016/j.scitotenv.2019.135883.

Fasciotti, Maíra. 2017. "Perspectives for the use of biotechnology in green chemistry applied to biopolymers, fuels and organic synthesis: From concepts to a critical point of view." *Sustainable Chemistry and Pharmacy*. doi:10.1016/j.scp.2017.09.002.

Frazzetto, Giovanni. 2003. "White biotechnology. The application of biotechnology to industrial production holds many promises for sustainable development, but many products still have to pass the test of economic viability." *EMBO Reports* 4 (9): 835–837. doi:10.1038/sj.embor.embor928.

Gad, Ahmed. 2018. "Introduction to optimization with genetic algorithm." https://towardsdatascience.com/introduction-to-optimization-with-genetic-algorithm-2f5001d9964b.

Gelski, Jeff. 2019. "Sustainable product market could hit $150 billion in U.S. by 2021 | 2019-01-10 | Food Business News." *Food Business News*. https://www.foodbusinessnews.net/articles/13133-sustainable-product-market-could-hit-150-billion-in-us-by-2021.

George, Ashish, M.R. Sanjay, Rapeeporn Sriusk, Jyotishkumar Parameswaranpillai, and Suchart Siengchin. 2020. "A comprehensive review on chemical properties and applications of biopolymers and their composites." *International Journal of Biological Macromolecules* 154: 329–338. doi:10.1016/j.ijbiomac.2020.03.120.

Gill, Simrone K., Nima Roohpour, Paul D. Topham, and Brian J. Tighe. 2017. "Tuneable denture adhesives using biomimetic principles for enhanced tissue adhesion in moist environments." *Acta Biomaterialia* 63: 326–335. doi:10.1016/j.actbio.2017.09.004.

Golić, Zorica. 2020. "Finance and artificial intelligence: The fifth industrial revolution and its impact on the financial sector." *Proceedings of the Faculty of Economics in East Sarajevo* 8 (19): 67. doi:10.7251/zrefis1919067g.

Hara, Kiyotaka Y., Michihiro Araki, Naoko Okai, Satoshi Wakai, Tomohisa Hasunuma, and Akihiko Kondo. 2014. "Development of bio-based fine chemical production through synthetic bioengineering." *Microbial Cell Factories*. doi:10.1186/s12934-014-0173-5.

Hayyolalam, Vahideh, and Ali Asghar Pourhaji Kazem. 2020. "Black widow optimization algorithm: A novel meta-heuristic approach for solving engineering optimization problems." *Engineering Applications of Artificial Intelligence* 87: 103249. doi:10.1016/j.engappai.2019.103249.

Heras, Alejandro Muñoz De Las. 2017. *Application of Synthetic Biology for Biopolymer Production Using Saccharomyces Cerevisiae*. Department of Chemistry, Lund University.

IGEM. 2015. "Help: An introduction to BioBricks – Parts.Igem.Org." https://parts.igem.org/Help:An_Introduction_to_BioBricks.

Isikgor, Furkan H., and C. Remzi Becer. 2015. "Lignocellulosic biomass: A sustainable platform for the production of bio-based chemicals and polymers." *Polymer Chemistry* 6 (25): 4497–4559. doi:10.1039/c5py00263j.

Ivanov, Dmitry, Alexandre Dolgui, and Boris Sokolov. 2019. "The impact of digital technology and industry 4.0 on the ripple effect and supply chain risk analytics." *International Journal of Production Research* 57 (3): 829–846. doi:10.1080/00207543.2018.1488086.

Jagaba, A.H., S.R.M. Kutty, S.G. Khaw, C.L. Lai, M.H. Isa, L. Baloo, I.M. Lawal, S. Abubakar, I. Umaru, and Z.U. Zango. 2020. "Derived hybrid biosorbent for Zinc(II) removal from aqueous solution by continuous-flow activated sludge system." *Journal of Water Process Engineering* 34: 101152. doi:10.1016/j.jwpe.2020.101152.

Jin, Shan, Beth Clark, Sharron Kuznesof, Xuan Lin, and Lynn J. Frewer. 2019. "Synthetic biology applied in the agrifood sector: Public perceptions, attitudes and implications for future studies." *Trends in Food Science and Technology*. doi:10.1016/j.tifs.2019.07.025.

Kabir, Ehsanul, Rajnish Kaur, Jechan Lee, Ki-Hyun Kim, and Eilhann E. Kwon. 2020. "Prospects of biopolymer technology as an alternative option for non-degradable plastics and sustainable management of plastic wastes." *Journal of Cleaner Production* 258: 120536. doi:10.1016/j.jclepro.2020.120536.

Karimi, Mehrnaz, and Farhad Raofie. 2019. "Micronization of vincristine extracted from *Catharanthus roseus* by expansion of supercritical fluid solution." *The Journal of Supercritical Fluids* 146: 172–179. doi: 10.1016/j.supflu.2019.01.021.

Katoch, Sanjeev, Rakesh Sehgal, Vishal Singh, Munish Kumar Gupta, Mozammel Mia, and Catalin Iulian Pruncu. 2019. "Improvement of tribological behavior of H-13 steel by optimizing the cryogenic-treatment process using evolutionary algorithms." *Tribology International* 140: 105895. doi:10.1016/j.triboint.2019.105895.

Kind, Stefanie, Steffi Neubauer, Judith Becker, Motonori Yamamoto, Martin Völkert, Gregory von Abendroth, Oskar Zelder, and Christoph Wittmann. 2014. "From zero to hero – Production of bio-based nylon from renewable resources using engineered *Corynebacterium glutamicum*." *Metabolic Engineering* 25: 113–123. doi:10.1016/j.ymben.2014.05.007.

Kokel, Anne, and Béla Török. 2018. "Sustainable production of fine chemicals and materials using nontoxic renewable sources." *Toxicological Sciences* 161 (2): 214–224. doi:10.1093/toxsci/kfx214.

Koopman, Frank, Jules Beekwilder, Barbara Crimi, Adele van Houwelingen, Robert D. Hall, Dirk Bosch, Antonius J.A. van Maris, Jack T. Pronk, and Jean Marc Daran. 2012. "De novo production of the flavonoid naringenin in engineered saccharomyces cerevisiae." *Microbial Cell Factories* 11 (1): 155. doi:10.1186/1475-2859-11-155.

Larrañaga, Pedro, Hossein Karshenas, Concha Bielza, and Roberto Santana. 2013. "A review on evolutionary algorithms in Bayesian network learning and inference tasks." *Information Sciences* 233: 109–125. doi:10.1016/j.ins.2012.12.051.

Lee, Jay, Hossein Davari, Jaskaran Singh, and Vibhor Pandhare. 2018. "Industrial artificial intelligence for industry 4.0-based manufacturing systems." *Manufacturing Letters* 18: 20–23. doi:10.1016/j.mfglet.2018.09.002.

Lee, Kwang Sik, Bo Yeon Kim, Hyung Joo Yoon, Yong Soo Choi, and Byung Rae Jin. 2016. "Secapin, a bee venom peptide, exhibits anti-fibrinolytic, anti-elastolytic, and anti-microbial activities." *Developmental and Comparative Immunology* 63: 27–35. doi:10.1016/j.dci.2016.05.011.

Lee, Seung Ju, and A.T.M. Mijanur Rahman. 2013. "Intelligent packaging for food products." In *Innovations in Food Packaging*. Second Edition, 171–209. Elsevier Ltd. doi:10.1016/B978-0-12-394601-0.00008-4.

Leveriza-Oh, May, and Tania J. Phillips. 2012. "Dressings and postoperative care." In *Lower Extremity Soft Tissue & Cutaneous Plastic Surgery*.Second Edition, 471–488. Elsevier Ltd. doi:10.1016/B978-0-7020-3136-6.00032-1.

Li, Bo hu, Bao cun Hou, Wen tao Yu, Xiao bing Lu, and Chun wei Yang. 2017. "Applications of artificial intelligence in intelligent manufacturing: A review." *Frontiers of Information Technology and Electronic Engineering*. Zhejiang University. doi:10.1631/FITEE.1601885.

Liu, Fangkun, Jing Huang, and Zhixiong Liu. 2019. "Vincristine impairs microtubules and causes neurotoxicity in cerebral organoids." *Neuroscience* 404: 530–540. doi:10.1016/j.neuroscience.2018.12.047.

Liu, Long, Yanfeng Liu, Hyun Dong Shin, Rachel R. Chen, Nam Sun Wang, Jianghua Li, Guocheng Du, and Jian Chen. 2013. "Developing Bacillus Spp. as a cell factory for production of microbial enzymes and industrially important biochemicals in the context of systems and synthetic biology." *Applied Microbiology and Biotechnology*. doi:10.1007/s00253-013-4960-4.

Ludwig, Roland, Roberto Ortiz, Christopher Schulz, Wolfgang Harreither, Christoph Sygmund, and Lo Gorton. 2013. "Cellobiose dehydrogenase modified electrodes: Advances by materials science and biochemical engineering." *Analytical and Bioanalytical Chemistry*. doi:10.1007/s00216-012-6627-x.

Maesani, Andrea, Pradeep Ruben Fernando, and Dario Floreano. 2014. "Artificial evolution by viability rather than competition." *PLoS One* 9 (1): e86831. doi:10.1371/journal.pone.0086831.

Maleki, Susan, Mali Mærk, Svein Valla, and Helga Ertesvåg. 2015. "Mutational analyses of glucose dehydrogenase and glucose-6-phosphate dehydrogenase genes in *Pseudomonas fluorescens* reveal their effects on growth and alginate production." *Applied and Environmental Microbiology* 81 (10): 3349–3356. doi:10.1128/AEM.03653-14.

Manning, Timmy, Roy D. Sleator, and Paul Walsh. 2013. "Naturally selecting solutions: The use of genetic algorithms in bioinformatics." *Bioengineered*. doi:10.4161/bioe.23041.

Marr, Bernard. 2018. "The fourth industrial revolution is here: Are you ready?" *Deloitte Insight*, 1–26.

Mehrotra, Parikha. 2016. "Biosensors and their applications – A review." *Journal of Oral Biology and Craniofacial Research*. Elsevier B.V. doi:10.1016/j.jobcr.2015.12.002.

Mózsik, László, Zsófia Büttel, Roel A.L. Bovenberg, Arnold J.M. Driessen, and Yvonne Nygård. 2019. "Synthetic control devices for gene regulation in *Penicillium chrysogenum*." *Microbial Cell Factories* 18 (1): 203. doi:10.1186/s12934-019-1253-3.

Munick de Albuquerque Fragoso, Danielle, Florent P. Bouxin, James R.D. Montgomery, Nicholas J. Westwood, and S. David Jackson. 2020. "Catalytic depolymerisation of isolated lignin to fine chemicals: Depolymerisation of kraft lignin." *Bioresource Technology Reports* 9: 100400. doi:10.1016/j.biteb.2020.100400.

Nahavandi, Saeid. 2019. "Industry 5.0 – A human-centric solution." *Sustainability (Switzerland)* 11 (16): 4371. doi: 10.3390/su11164371.

Najafpour, Ghasem D. 2015. "Chapter 1 – Industrial microbiology." In *Biochemical Engineering and Biotechnology*. Elsevier: 1–18. doi:10.1016/B978-0-444-63357-6.00001-8.

National Center for Biotechnology Information. 2019. "Pyridine | C5H5N – PubChem." *PubChem Database*. https://pubchem.ncbi.nlm.nih.gov/compound/Pyridine.

National Human Genome Research Institute USA. 2019. "Synthetic biology | NHGRI." https://www.genome.gov/about-genomics/policy-issues/Synthetic-Biology.

Packaged Facts. 2008. "Household Cleaning Products Go Green with a Dash of Upscale." *Focus on Surfactants* 2008 (3). Elsevier BV: 6–7. doi:10.1016/s1351-4210(08)70103-3.

Pathak, Pankaj, Parashu Ram Pal, Manish Shrivastava, and Priyanka Ora. 2019. "Fifth revolution: Applied AI & human intelligence with cyber physical systems." *International Journal of Engineering and Advanced Technology* 8(3):23–27.

Philbrook, Amy, Apostolos Alissandratos, and Christopher Easton. 2013. "Biochemical processes for generating fuels and commodity chemicals from lignocellulosic biomass." In *Environmental Biotechnology – New Approaches and Prospective Applications*. InTech. doi:10.5772/55309.

Pollak, Peter. 2007. *Fine Chemicals: The Industry and the Business*. Wiley-Interscience.

Presnell, Kristin V., and Hal S. Alper. 2019. "Systems metabolic engineering meets machine learning: A new era for data-Driven metabolic engineering." *Biotechnology Journal* 14 (9): 1800416. doi:10.1002/biot.201800416.

Przybylski, Rémi, Loubna Firdaous, Gabrielle Châtaigné, Pascal Dhulster, and Naïma Nedjar. 2016. "Production of an antimicrobial peptide derived from slaughterhouse by-product and its potential application on meat as preservative." *Food Chemistry* 211: 306–313. doi:10.1016/j.foodchem.2016.05.074.

Realini, Carolina E., and Begonya Marcos. 2014. "Active and intelligent packaging systems for a modern society." *Meat Science* 98 (3): 404–419. doi:10.1016/j.meatsci.2014.06.031.

Renzi, C., F. Leali, M. Cavazzuti, and A.O. Andrisano. 2014. "A review on artificial intelligence applications to the optimal design of dedicated and reconfigurable manufacturing systems." *International Journal of Advanced Manufacturing Technology* 72 (1–4): 403–418. doi:10.1007/s00170-014-5674-1.

Ro, Dae Kyun, Eric M. Paradise, Mario Quellet, Karl J. Fisher, Karyn L. Newman, John M. Ndungu, Kimberly A. Ho, et al. 2006. "Production of the antimalarial drug precursor artemisinic acid in engineered yeast." *Nature* 440 (7086): 940–943. doi:10.1038/nature04640.

Rolls-Royce Plc. 2015. "Civil Aerospace – Rolls-Royce." Rolls-Royce Website. https://www.rolls-royce.com/products-and-services/civil-aerospace.aspx#/IntelligentEngine.

Rossi, Ben. 2018. "Industry 5.0: What is it and what will it do for manufacturing?" Raconteur Media Ltd. https://www.raconteur.net/technology/manufacturing-gets-personal-industry-5-0.

Sachsenmeier, Peter. 2016. "Industry 5.0—The relevance and implications of bionics and synthetic biology." *Engineering* 2 (2): 225–229. doi:10.1016/J.ENG.2016.02.015.

Salehi, Bahare, Patrick Valere Tsouh Fokou, Mehdi Sharifi-Rad, Paolo Zucca, Raffaele Pezzani, Natália Martins, and Javad Sharifi-Rad. 2019. "The therapeutic potential of naringenin: A review of clinical trials." *Pharmaceuticals*. doi:10.3390/ph12010011.

Seneff, Stephanie. 2016. "Statins and myoglobin: How muscle pain and weakness progress to heart, lung and kidney failure." *British Medical Bulletin* 119 (1): 75. doi:10.1093/BMB.

Silva, Bruna, Mariana Martins, Mihaela Rosca, Verónica Rocha, Ana Lago, Isabel C. Neves, and Teresa Tavares. 2020. "Waste-based biosorbents as cost-effective alternatives to commercial adsorbents for the retention of fluoxetine from water." *Separation and Purification Technology* 235: 116139. doi:10.1016/j.seppur.2019.116139.

Sinha, Sanjai. 2018. "Penicillin uses, side effects & allergy warnings – Drugs.Com." https://www.drugs.com/penicillin.html.

Sintim, Henry Y., Andy I. Bary, Douglas G. Hayes, Marie E. English, Sean M. Schaeffer, Carol A. Miles, Alla Zelenyuk, Kaitlyn Suski, and Markus Flury. 2019. "Release of micro- and nanoparticles from biodegradable plastic during in situ composting." *Science of the Total Environment* 675: 686–693. doi:10.1016/j.scitotenv.2019.04.179.

Smith, A.M., S. Moxon, and G.A. Morris. 2016. "Biopolymers as wound healing materials." In *Wound Healing Biomaterials*, vol. 2. 261–287. Elsevier Inc. doi:10.1016/B978-1-78242-456-7.00013-1.

Song, Wei, Xiulai Chen, Jing Wu, Jianzhong Xu, Weiguo Zhang, Jia Liu, Jian Chen, and Liming Liu. 2019. "Biocatalytic derivatization of proteinogenic amino acids for fine chemicals." *Biotechnology Advances*. doi:10.1016/j.biotechadv.2019.107496.

Song, Yafeng, Jonas M. Nikoloff, Gang Fu, Jingqi Chen, Qinggang Li, Nengzhong Xie, Ping Zheng, Jibin Sun, and Dawei Zhang. 2016. "Promoter screening from *Bacillus subtilis* in various conditions hunting for synthetic biology and industrial applications." *PLoS One* 11 (7): e0158447. doi:10.1371/journal.pone.0158447.

Steger, Andrew. 2019. "Healthcare data breach: What happens to stolen healthcare data?" *HealthTech*. https://healthtechmagazine.net/article/2019/10/what-happens-stolen-healthcare-data-perfcon.

Sulaiman, Mohd Herwan, Zuriani Mustaffa, Mohd Mawardi Saari, and Hamdan Daniyal. 2020. "Barnacles mating optimizer: A new bio-inspired algorithm for solving engineering optimization problems." *Engineering Applications of Artificial Intelligence* 87: 103330. doi:10.1016/j.engappai.2019.103330.

Sulema, Yevgeniya. 2018. "ASAMPL: Programming language for mulsemedia data processing based on algebraic system of aggregates." *Advances in Intelligent Systems and Computing*. 431–442. doi:10.1007/978-3-319-75175-7_43.

Suresh, Lakshmi, Jayraj V. Vaghasiya, Michael R. Jones, and Swee Ching Tan. 2019. "Biodegradable protein-based photoelectrochemical cells with biopolymer composite electrodes that enable recovery of valuable metals." *ACS Sustainable Chemistry and Engineering* 7 (9): 8834–8841. doi:10.1021/acssuschemeng.9b00790.

Susilowati, Endang, Triyono, Sri Juari Santosa, and Indriana Kartini. 2015. "Synthesis of silver-chitosan nanocomposites colloidal by glucose as reducing agent." *Indonesian Journal of Chemistry* 15 (1): 29–35. doi:10.22146/ijc.21220.

Takors, Ralf. 2020. "Biochemical engineering provides mindset, tools and solutions for the driving questions of a sustainable future." *Engineering in Life Sciences* 20 (1–2): 5–6. doi:10.1002/elsc.201900150.

Toney-Butler, Tammy J., and Lance Wilcox. 2019. "Dose calculation (desired over have or formula)." *StatPearls*, StatPearls Publishing, 2–6. http://www.ncbi.nlm.nih.gov/pubmed/29630214.

Tripathi, Lakshmi, Lin Ping Wu, Meng Dechuan, Jinchun Chen, Qiong Wu, and Guo Qiang Chen. 2013. "*Pseudomonas putida* KT2442 as a platform for the biosynthesis of polyhydroxyalkanoates with adjustable monomer contents and compositions." *Bioresource Technology* 142: 225–231. doi:10.1016/j.biortech.2013.05.027.

United Nations Economic and Social Council. 2015. "Sustainable development | UNITED NATIONS ECONOMIC and SOCIAL COUNCIL." *Post-2015 Development Agenda*. https://www.un.org/ecosoc/en/sustainable-development.

Vetter, Phillip. 2016. "At Adidas, Shoes Now Come from the 3D Printer - WORLD." *Welt*. https://www.welt.de/wirtschaft/article155658067/Die-Speedfactory-ist-fuer-Adidas-eine-Revolution.html.

Viera, João S.C., Mônica R.C. Marques, Monick Cruz Nazareth, Paula Christine Jimenez, and Ítalo Braga Castro. 2020. "On replacing single-use plastic with so-called biodegradable ones: The case with straws." *Environmental Science and Policy* 106: 177–181. doi:10.1016/j.envsci.2020.02.007.

Wang, Fangzhong, and Weiwen Zhang. 2019. "Synthetic biology: Recent progress, biosafety and biosecurity concerns, and possible solutions." *Journal of Biosafety and Biosecurity* 1 (1): 22–30. doi:10.1016/j.jobb.2018.12.003.

Wang, Harris H., Michael T. Mee, and George M. Church. 2013. "Applications of engineered synthetic ecosystems." In *Synthetic Biology*, 317–325. Elsevier Inc. doi:10.1016/B978-0-12-394430-6.00017-0.

Wilkins, John. 2008. "Defining evolution | National Center for Science Education." *National Center for Science Education*. https://ncse.ngo/defining-evolution.

Yang, Chen, Shulin Lan, Weiming Shen, George Q. Huang, Xianbin Wang, and Tingyu Lin. 2017. "Towards product customization and personalization in IoT-enabled cloud manufacturing." *Cluster Computing* 20 (2): 1717–1730. doi:10.1007/s10586-017-0767-x.

4.1 State-of-the-Art Technologies in Industry 5.0

Yee Ho Chai, Guo Yong Yew, Suzana Yusup, and Pau Loke Show

CONTENTS

4.1.1 INTRODUCTION

To date, the human evolution had experienced four industrial revolutions that brought about drastic transformations to the ways of life today. The various stages of industrial revolutions were fuelled by a common objective – to enhance production outputs by means of technological advancements. Consequently, this single concept had initiated a series of chain reactions in innumerable industries and businesses to meet the everchanging supply and demands of the consumers. These drastic changes induced in society paved the way to how science and technology are perceived and advanced to relentlessly solve newer challenges posed. Inevitably, diversification and specialization of newer industries had emerged with each industrial revolution, from generation of steam power for locomotives in the First Industrial Revolution to the Internet of Things (IoT) in the Fourth Industrial

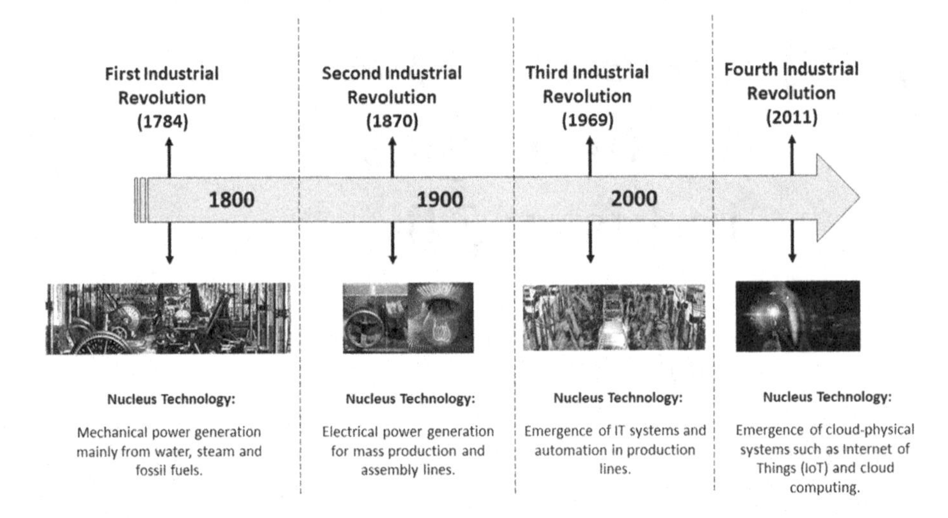

FIGURE 4.1.1 The timeline progress of industrial revolution.

Revolution, to cater for each society's needs. Figure 4.1.1 illustrates the timeline progression of each industrial revolution and its associated nucleus technologies.

The main objective of Fourth Industrial Revolution (Industry 4.0) was to integrate the core components between business leaders and manufacturing managers for a holistic overview of the entire business model to enhance its overall process efficiency by relying solely based on big data analytics to optimize the overall process (Nahavandi 2019). In this regard, the development of Digital Twin as a predictive tool for biomanufacturing industries is seen to benefit better analytical data methods of high-throughput data obtained from cell culture processes towards flexible manufacturing processes to counter unwarranted product quality and its associated costs in cell culture processes (Nargund and Guenther 2019). A survey conducted by Reinhardt et al. (2020) indicated adaptation of Industry 4.0 will principally optimize current production processes in the biomanufacturing industry.

However, the concept of Industry 4.0 lacked environmental considerations as well as high unemployment rates in the working sectors (Demir and Cicibas 2019). With this in mind, the alternative concept of Industry 5.0 by considering the elements of sustainability, bioeconomy and "human-robot co-working relationship" were proposed (Demir and Cicibas 2019). In essence, this gave rise to the emphasis of bioeconomy paradigm that bridges biotechnology, economy, science, technology and society into a singular helix that exploits and develops economic systems based on the sustainable utilization of biological resources (Aguilar et al. 2019). Thus, biotechnology, especially in biomanufacturing technologies, are expected to diversify based on existing technologies to further develop bioeconomy framework.

This chapter discusses the role of biomanufacturing in bioeconomy context and how the role and integration of supercritical fluid technology as well as algae biomass technology can be capitalized as a state-of-art technology soar to the peak in the field of biomanufacturing, specifically in biomaterials and bioenergy sectors, in Industry 5.0.

4.1.2 ROLE OF BIOMANUFACTURING IN BIOECONOMY

According to Food and Agriculture Organization of United Nations (FAO), bioeconomy can be defined as "the production, utilization and conservation of biological resources, including related knowledge, science, technology, and innovation, to provide information, products, processes and services across all economic sectors aiming towards a sustainable economy" (Von Braun 2018). Figure 4.1.2 illustrates the inter-relational elements of the bioeconomy concept. In this regard, the dependency and transition to bio-based resources from fossil fuel-based diminishes the overall damage rendered against climate and environment. In principle, valorization of biological resources into value-added products is highly emphasized in bioeconomy but efforts for sustainable management of food security and natural resource scarcity must be recognized as well (Von Braun 2018).

In addition, the roles and applications of biotechnology in biomanufacturing disciplines act as foundations to the positive progress of bioeconomy areas. Biomanufacturing is a type of manufacturing discipline that employs biological systems to commercially produce value-added bio-compounds for use in medicinal, food and beverage processing, and industrial applications (Heng et al. 2016). The early applications of biomanufacturing can be seen several thousand years ago in the preparation of wine from rice, honey and fruits (Mcgovern et al. 2004) by ancient Chinese as well as the preservation of pickles and cucumbers by pickling. The intrinsic mechanism of fermentation by microbes was not comprehended in the early days and it was only during the Second Industrial Revolution that biomanufacturing disciplines begin to emerge. The first biomanufacturing revolution (Biomanufacture 1.0) largely emphasized the fermentation production of acetone, butanol and ethanol (ABE) in the early 1910s. The second biomanufacturing

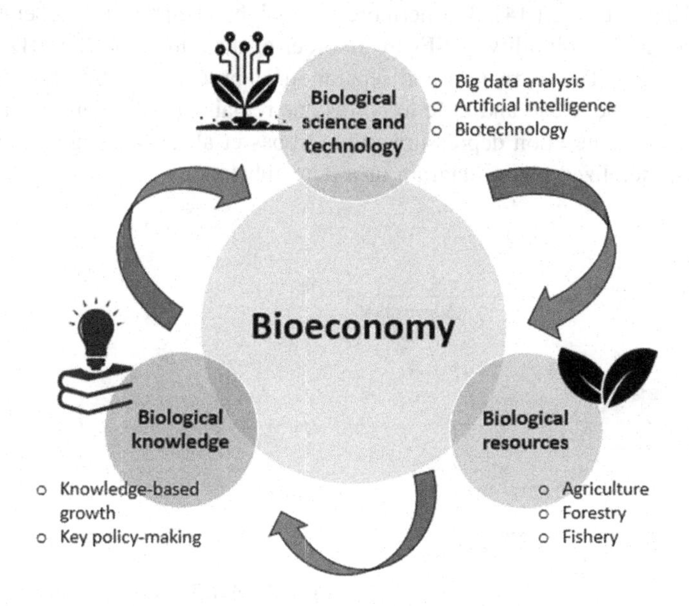

FIGURE 4.1.2 The inter-relational element of bioeconomy.

revolution (Biomanufacture 2.0) led with the production of secondary metabolites, especially penicillin fermentation in the 1940s while the third biomanufacturing revolution (Biomanufacture 3.0) involved efforts to produce proteins and fermentation of microbial cells as biocatalyst in life sciences. The emergence of the fourth biomanufacturing revolution (Biomanufacture 4.0) in the early 2000s explored deliverance of newer products such as regenerative medicine and artificial food, as well as competent biotechnologies for production of existing products with regards to productivity, scalability and sustainability (Heng et al. 2016). This sub-chapter reviews the potential technologies, namely supercritical fluid technology and algal biomass technology that should be capitalized for the emerging Industry 5.0 revolution.

4.1.3 SUPERCRITICAL FLUID TECHNOLOGY

In any industrial development processes, solvent substitution remains as an important process in delivering environmentally friendly and less hazardous by-products or wastes without compromising the end objective of the production line. The introduction of supercritical fluid (SF) technology is touted as a critical progress that propelled the boundaries of principles of green engineering even further towards safer and efficient industrial processes development. SFs are highly compressed fluids that co-exist beyond the fluid's critical points in both liquid and gaseous phases simultaneously. At supercritical state, the density properties of SFs are analogous to liquid-like while maintaining gaseous-like viscosity properties as well. The unique properties of SFs are the fluids' tunable physicochemical properties, namely diffusivity, viscosity, density and dielectric constants, that are easily influenced by the variation of temperature and pressure conditions in an enclosed system (Knez et al. 2014). Furthermore, the slight changes in temperature and pressure alters the solubility of SFs by an order of magnitude or more (Darani and Mozafari 2009). The extraction and separation of products by SF technology are easily recoverable, clean and little to no residue remained as SFs are reverted back to the gaseous state upon depressurization (Abbas et al. 2008). Figure 4.1.3 illustrates the generalized phase diagram of a pure substance.

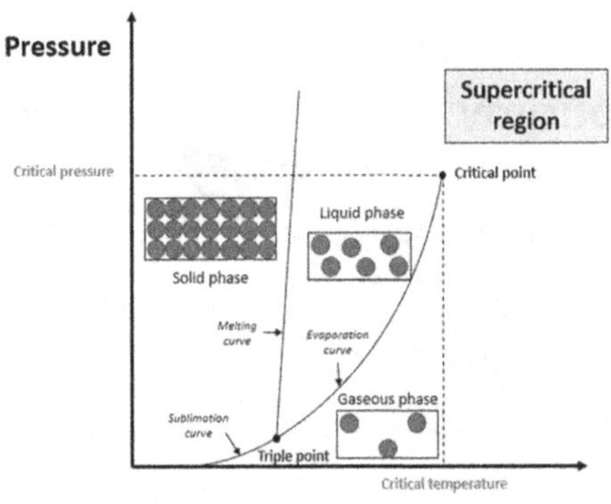

FIGURE 4.1.3 The generalized phase diagram of pure substance.

Carbon dioxide (CO_2) is often selected as the main solvent due to its cheap and abundant form in its pure state, as well as its non-toxicity and non-flammable properties (Ekinci and Gürü 2014). The low critical points of CO_2 at 304.25 K and 7.39 MPa were also positive features to conduct experimental works in laboratory and pilot scales in a safer manner. Furthermore, supercritical CO_2 solvents are substantially employed in supercritical fluid extraction (SFE) and considered to be carbon-neutral as CO_2 released by industrial emissions are taken advantage of instead of solely releasing it into the environment. Prior to this, chlorodifluoromethane ($CHClF_2$) and nitrous oxide (N_2O) were also suitable polar solvents as SFs. Due to the adverse properties of $CHClF_2$ that phased out chlorofluorocarbons (CFCs) detrimental to the ozone layer and potentially explosive oxidation reactions of N_2O in organic matters, both solvents were subsequently unfavourable for applications (Lang and Wai 2001; Raynie 1993). Furthermore, water is also widely considered as SF solvent in spite of its high thermodynamic critical points of 647.15 K and 22.1 MPa, where polarity of water shifts towards non-polar behaviour to be fully miscible with organic substances (Zhang et al. 2016). Under such circumstances, the practicality of supercritical water is focused eminently towards oxidation of organic matters in landfills although corrosion and precipitation of salts are some of the major challenges faced (Vadillo et al. 2013). In this sub-section, the applications of supercritical fluid technology are focused mainly on enzymatic pretreatment and activation, biological membrane synthesis and bioalcohol recovery.

4.1.4 ENZYMATIC PRETREATMENT AND ACTIVATION

As mentioned previously, the search for solvent substitutions in industrial processes in view of the current toxicity and environmental concerns based on the current utilization of organic chemical solvents revised technological generalizations in biotechnology disciplines, including enzymatic pretreatments. Apart from the versatile tunability properties possessed by dense SFs, the ease of integration of reaction-separation process designs are quickly becoming the new normal in future bioreactor designs.

Most of the literature studies have shown supercritical CO_2 to be the ideal candidate in enzymatic reactions due to its ideal operating temperature compatibility against enzymatic activities. Similar to other catalyst, enzyme functions akin to a biocatalyst and is heavily influenced by temperature in the reaction media. Furthermore, high mass transfer kinetics between reactants and enzymes for efficient conversion yields are expected owing to the high diffusivity properties of SFs (Oliveira and Oliveira 2000). Various studies for the extraction of esterification, transesterification and biodiesel production by lipase enzyme in the presence of supercritical CO_2 were carried out successfully (Badgujar et al. 2019; Folayan et al. 2019; Lee et al. 2017; Melgosa et al. 2019; Pollardo et al. 2017). The inhibition activity of α-amylase enzymes was carried out by Marillán and Uquiche (2020). Enzymatic hydrolysis in the presence of supercritical CO_2 for the pretreatment of agricultural residues was conducted as well (jiao Zhao et al. 2019; Nlandu et al. 2020; Putrino et al. 2020; Zhang et al. 2019).

Most literature findings indicated that pressure to have little effect on enzymatic activities in contrast to the dominant effects of temperature parameter. However, the presence of moisture content in biomass residues are often undesirable because of the possible conversion to carbonic acid in the presence of supercritical CO_2 (Knez et al. 2014). Depending on temperature and pressure, the study showed that supercritical CO_2 dissolved in 0.3–0.5 wt% of water (Caniaz and Erkey 2014) although excessive water content lead to acidification of the reaction media that disable enzymatic activity inadvertently. Furthermore, the use of high methanol concentration for transesterification of biodiesel also invokes enzyme deactivation due to methanol inhibition (Pollardo et al. 2017). Table 4.1.1 summarizes the current knowledge gaps and future perspectives for supercritical CO_2 technology in ezymatic reactions.

4.1.5 BIOLOGICAL MEMBRANE SYNTHESIS

Depending on the type of membrane, the applications of membrane can be distinguished into several types of operations such as pressure-driven types (ultrafiltration, reverse osmosis, etc.), concentration driven types (dialysis, artificial lung, gas separation, etc.), electrical-driven types (electrodialysis, fuel cell, etc.) and temperature-driven type (membrane distillation). The synthesis of membranes can be carried out via two routes: firstly, involving chemical reactions such as polymerization and functionalization, and secondly, involving non-chemical reactions such as organic solvent dissolution, solution castings and phase inversion evaporation processes. As such, membrane synthesis is commonly inevitable to not use toxic organic solvents, such as acetone, methanol, dimethylformamide (DMF), toluene, N-methyl-2-pyrrolidone and tetrahydrofuran, that are harmful to the environment and users.

The use of non-polar supercritical CO_2 in polymeric membrane formation circumvents some of the limitations of wet phase inversion techniques (Kim et al. 2013), extensive post-processing disadvantages and lengthy production duration (Chakravarty et al. 2019). The interactive parametric effects of supercritical CO_2 on membrane porosity corresponded closely to pressure and temperature induced in the system (Matsuyama et al. 2001). The exposure of supercritical CO_2 and depressurization procedures in cellulose triacetate and polyimides membranes investigated by Scholes and Kanehashi (2018) led to the alterations in polymer morphology and gas permselectivity. Apart from tuning of membrane properties, Reverchon and Cardea (2004) produced copolymer membrane poly(vinylidene fluoride) with hexafluoropropylene that possessed immense biomedical applications with various filtration processes. While efforts to push forward for the concept of green synthesis to replace conventional toxic organic solvents are applauded, only a small proportion was made up of green synthesis methods. The use of SF technology eliminates the need for additional removal of organic solvents as well as the ability to control pore sizes and structures of the membranes.

One of the more particular successful areas in membrane synthesis technology is the introduction of biological membranes. Material developments of biological membranes are highly based on bio-additives as well as de novo design of

TABLE 4.1.1
Summary of Gaps and Future Perspectives of Enzymatic Reactions in Supercritical CO_2 Medium

Knowledge Gaps	Description	Remarks
Enzymatic stability in supercritical fluids	Effect of temperature, pressure and pH conditions	Determination of optimum temperature, pressure and pH conditions for sustenance of enzyme activity
	Physical form of enzymes	Immobilized enzymes are more stable in supercritical media to retain enzymatic activity
	Possible formation of carbonic acid by water presence	Utilization of non-green stable gases such as ethylene, ethane, propane and sulphur hexafluoride
Effect of water on enzyme activity	Water concentration requirement in reaction system	Excess water may induce lower reaction rates, hydrolysis of reactant and agglomeration of enzymes
	Acidification in reaction media	Stabilize enzyme activity by controlling pH activity in the system through addition of organic and inorganic buffers
Effect of pressurization-depressurization on enzyme activity	Long-term stability of enzyme	Rapid pressurization may destroy enzyme structure while rapid depressurization causes inability of solvent to diffuse out from the enzymes and inadvertently self-destruct
Future Directions		
Development of bioreactors	Sustainability and practicality aspects	Reduction of bioreactor sizes and elimination of large pressure drops to minimize costs
Development of newer supercritical solvent	Limitations of supercritical CO_2	Current limitations of CO_2 include formation of carbonic acid and preferential dissolution with non-polar solutes only
Development of newer enzyme species	Stability of enzymatic activity at elevated conditions	Research of newer enzyme species by bioengineering techniques to deliver similar performances at unconventional supercritical conditions
Development of biomimetic enzyme in supercritical fluids	Application of biomimetic enzyme	Better control and less stability problems for enzymatic reactions in supercritical solvents

membrane functionalities depicting biological molecular structures (Ghadiri Reza et al. 1991). A notable utilization of biological membranes, in particular the plant aquaporin, a major intrinsic protein, is seen mainly in water purification disciplines due to its selective properties and permeability for water molecules while completely obviating transfers of ions and impurities (Fuwad et al. 2019). Furthermore, biological membranes possessing super-hydrophobic surface properties have also recently garnered research interests due to its high efficacy in oil/water mixture separations (Peng and Guo 2016). However, some of the limitations for the synthesis of hydrophobic properties including robustness, membrane fouling by chemical and mechanical stress induction, control of emulsion droplet size and large-scale synthesis production method were highlighted (Hélix-Nielsen 2018). Thus, supercritical CO_2 technology can be potentially applied in biological membrane production due to its non-polar attributes, low thermophysical properties, ability to control pore structures and its ease of technological scalability to industrial scale. Although not widely reported, it is worth investigating the active role supercritical CO_2 for membrane production by phase separation induction as a potential solution to the mechanical instability of lipid bilayer in biological membranes to hold protein molecules effectively (Fuwad et al. 2019).

4.1.6 BIOALCOHOL RECOVERY

Bioalcohols are an emerging source of alternative fuel or fuel additives given that the greatest challenge to sustain energy supply chains to meet increasing energy demands in the last few decades or so. The major concern lies ultimately in producing attractive renewable energy sources while competing with lower costs of fossil fuel-based energy. The production of bioalcohols is by means of fermentation of sugar and starch based raw materials, where simple sugars are readily converted to ethanol while starch is required to undergo hydrolysis prior to fermentation (Jacobson and Delucchi 2016). Although bioethanol contains 33% lesser energy per gallon (Zaldivar 2001), it boasts higher octane content, thus making it suitable as an fuel additive for gasolines. Bioethanol can also be integrated into the current fuel system with by mixture addition ranging between 5–15% bioethanol/gasoline mixtures (Vázquez-ojeda et al. 2013). To date, three generations of bioethanol are seen where first and second generations involved fermentation of edible food crops and non-food biomass, respectively, while third-generation bioethanol is produced by algae cultivation (to be discussed below).

Metabolic by-products from fermentation of biomass feedstocks produced extensive quantities of ethanol and CO_2 where production of ethanol are inhibited when ethanol concentration above 20 wt% (Utama et al. 2016) in the fermentation media. Thus, various separation and purification techniques such as pervaporation, gas stripping, vacuum filtration, adsorption and solvent extraction were proposed (Zentou et al. 2019). Moreover, the costs of these technologies alone make up of 40 to 80% of the current bioethanol production costs (Le et al. 2011). Therefore, a more viable solution, such as the utilization of supercritical fluids for the recovery of bioalcohols, is proposed. Table 4.1.2 summarizes the overview comparison of current separation technologies in bioalcohol treatment.

TABLE 4.1.2
Comparison of Current Separation Technologies for Recovery of Alcohol

Technology	Description	Advantages	Disadvantages
Pervaporation	• Reliance of non-porous membrane for separation dependent on concentration gradient by vacuum pressure	• Easy separation depending on properties of membrane used • Versatile in separation of azeotropic mixtures and dissolved organic mixtures	• Loss of productivity by fouling • Contamination problems by repetitive cleaning due to fouling
Gas stripping	• Anaerobic gas is recycled throughout the bioreactor and evaporates recovered bioethanol by condensation	• Simple process • Minimal investment costs • Requires less complex equipment and little to no plant modifications	• Possible inhibition of yeast growth in fermentation broth • Fluctuation in gas stripping performances
Vacuum fermentation	• Application of vacuum pressure under fermenter to evaporate ethanol at fermentation temperature	• Boiling point temperature of ethanol is reduced to range of fermentation temperature	• High energy requirements • Require high volumes of bioreactors
Adsorption	• Adsorption of ethanol solution followed by desorption for recovery of ethanol	• Simple and easy process	• Selectivity of adsorbent affinity towards ethanol • Regeneration of adsorbent and associated costs
Solvent extraction	• Continuous mixing of fermentation broth and extractant solvent	• Does not require modifications to equipment • Enhanced fermentation rate	• Compatibility of suitable solvent against yeast growth • Compatibility of suitable solvent for ethanol solubilization • Additional separation process of liquid extracts required

The extraction of alcohols from alcohol and water mixtures by supercritical CO_2, butane and propane was carried out by Brignole and Fredenslund (1987) with the latter two solvents associated with ethanol preferentially compared to CO_2. A promising result was obtained by De Lucas et al. (2007) in their pilot plant study for the recovery of long-chain alcohols from sugarcane wax by supercritical CO_2. Simultaneous recovery of aromatic compounds and removal of ethanol was applied in a two-step separation process of rose wine in the presence of supercritical CO_2 by Ruiz-Rodríguez et al. as well (Ruiz-rodríguez et al. 2012). Similarly, Silva et al. (2017) had successfully reduced the ethanol content in red wine by membrane-based supercritical fluid extraction technique.

Although the technological concept for the recovery of bioalcohol by supercritical fluids are still immature, the integration of such process seems promising and feasible. The metabolic by-product CO_2 from alcoholic fermentation is recoverable and can be recycled as potential solvent feedstock. Furthermore, the low critical points of supercritical CO_2 do not pose detrimental effects towards generation of bioalcohols and selective extraction of ethanol from the fermentation broth makes it a viable conceptual technology too. In addition, combination of supercritical CO_2 in the presence of water can also form carbonic acid to acidify the supercritical medium for enhanced hydrolysis of lignocellulosic materials as well. Waibel and Krukonis (2012) had also patented the use of supercritical CO_2 for the dissolution of ethanol from ethanol-water mixture where clean separation of ethanol can be obtained. Furthermore, both Hashi et al. (2010) and Sonego et al. (2014) carried out CO_2 stripping for the recovery of ethanol from fermentation broth to obtain favourable results. Similarly, supercritical CO_2 can be used in a counter-current fractionation separator unit to selectively recover ethanol in the supercritical medium and converted into vapour phase by condensation of the carrier solvent. Figure 4.1.4 illustrates the conceptual design of the separation technology for bioethanol recovery.

Nevertheless, deployment of mature technology is often dependent on the operating costs and the scale of production intended in order to realize technical feasibility of supercritical fluid technology.

4.1.7 ALGAE TECHNOLOGY

Algae are photoautotrophic organisms that can grow in a range of habitats including wastewater. It functions to thrive either alone or symbiotically with other organisms at wide range of temperature, salinities and pH values as well as varying light intensity conditions. Macroalgae (seaweeds) are multi-cellular organisms visible to the naked eye while microalgae are photosynthetic organisms that may be prokaryotic or eukaryotic (Khan et al. 2018). Furthermore, microalgae are able to divide their cells once every three to four hours, but mostly divide every one to two days under favourable growing conditions (Williams and Laurens 2010). This is basically due to their simple cellular structure and large surface to volume ratio that give them the ability to uptake large amount of nutrients from water sources and thus, promoting their growth rate (Khan et al. 2009). Currently, microalgae such as *Chlorella vulgaris*, *Botryococcus braunii* and *Scenedesmus obliquus* have been

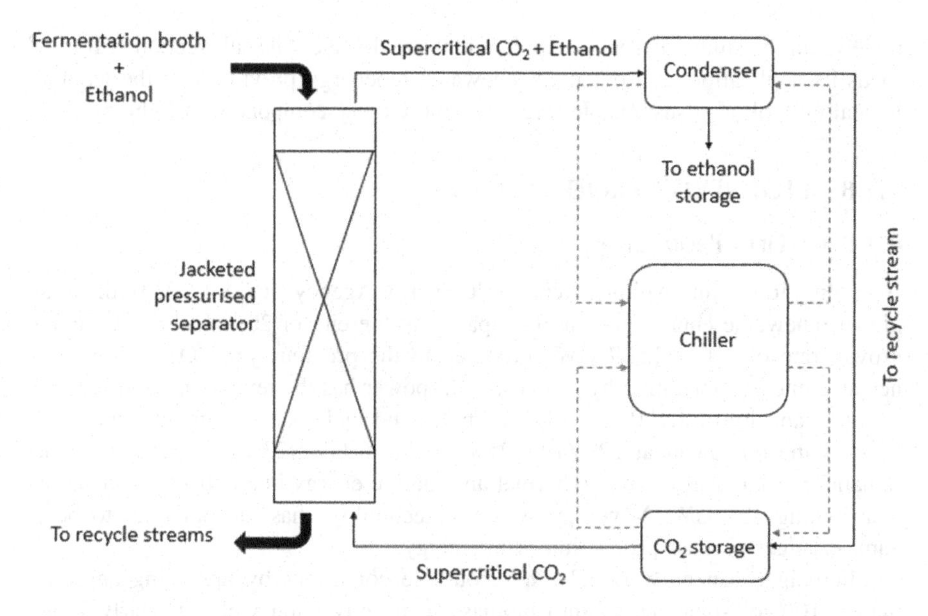

FIGURE 4.1.4 Schematic illustration of supercritical CO_2 stripping for bioethanol recovery.

identified as one of the most attractive renewable energy sources, mainly due to their rapid growth rate approximately 100 times faster than terrestrial plant to double their biomass in less than a day (Tredici 2010).

In essence, microalgae contain high concentrations of carbon compounds that can be utilized for biofuel, pharmaceuticals and cosmetics in addition to wastewater treatment and anthropogenic CO_2 mitigation. Microalgae can retain a significant amount of lipid for as high as 75% of their total weight and subsequent converts accumulated lipid into biodiesel (Vadillo et al. 2013). Cultivation of microalgae biomass for biodiesel production is relatively a new field in renewable biofuel industry. The emerging of this new field is further encouraged by the investment of world giant oil companies, such as Sinopec (SINOPEC) and CNPC from China, ExxonMobil (ExxonMobil 2018) and Chevron (Chevron 2015) from the United States, and BP from England. To date, research in microalgae biofuels have been intensified in several countries, particularly the United States, Canada and Australia. These companies anticipated that microalgae biofuels could potentially reduce carbon emission and increase renewable energy supply in the future.

Microalgae cells also contain carbohydrates that can be further hydrolyzed to simple reducing sugar for bioethanol production by fermentation process (Biswas et al. 2009). In addition, microalgae are also capable to fix CO_2 from the atmosphere, flue gases or soluble carbonate into their cells while simultaneously capturing solar energy with efficiency 10 to 50 times greater than terrestrial plants which presents a golden opportunity for carbon credit programmes (Tredici 2010). Hence, microalgae can act as a strong backbone in bio-fixing the CO_2 from atmosphere while producing renewable fuels, thus making it possible to integrate microalgae technology into a feasible biorefinery concept. Although literature reviews on the study microalgae applications are diverse, this sub-section will only focus its application as a potential renewable bioenergy provider and the technological outlook as a sustainable integrated biorefinery component in Industry 5.0.

4.1.8 BIOENERGY PRODUCTION

4.1.8.1 Lipid Production

According to the International Renewable Energy Agency (IRENA 2020), the total global renewable energy generation capacity at the end of 2019 had a substantial growth rate of 7.4 at 2,537 GW compared to the previous year. Of the total renewable energy generation by sources, hydropower has the remaining largest share of total capacity of 1,190 GW (47%) while wind and solar energy accounted for most of the remainder at 623 GW (25%) and 586 GW (23%), respectively. The remaining 5% consisted of geothermal and marine energy in addition to bioenergy contributing 124 GW. Nevertheless, algae technology has the potential to be a game-changer in mass production of bioenergy.

Microalgae can grow rapidly in favourable conditions by absorbing approximately 10% of solar energy into biomass with conversion yield of nearly 77 g/biomass/m^2/day to generate 280 tonne/ha/year of biomass that requires a smaller cultivation area compared to land crops (Formighieri et al. 2012). Furthermore, microalgae do not directly compete in energy-water-food nexus compared to second-generation biofuels (terrestrial plants) utilizing food crops as source of energy. Another given advantage is the absence of the lignocellulosic component in microalgae cell walls to mitigate additional pretreatment procedures. Microalgae undergo a photosynthesis process to store lipids, such as glycerophospholipids and triacylglycerols, as energy storage in microalgal cells. Extracted lipids from microalgal cells are converted into fatty acid methyl esters by the transesterification process to produce biodiesel (Zhu et al. 2016). There have been studies showing capabilities of microalgae producing more than 12,000 m^3/km^2 area volume of biodiesel from lipid oil (Medipally et al. 2015). Nevertheless, efficient large-scale cultivation of microalgae in a controlled environment favourable for lipid production is still required compared to wild-type microalgae.

Several approaches in effort to promote lipids production have been carefully studied. The effects of different light wavelengths such as blue lights (400–500 nm) and red lights (600–700 nm) on microalgae growth and its associated metabolism were studied. Furthermore, research efforts to investigate the effects of light intensity produced diverse reaction with regards to the type of microalgae species. In addition, other cultivation conditions such as CO_2 levels, temperature, nutrient concentrations and salinity concentrations are considered as well. Recently, the use of water treatment in lipid recovery after initial solvent extraction of microalgae was found to be significantly enhanced without altering fatty acids composition (Ren et al. 2017). Table 4.1.3 summarizes some of the comparative findings of the various cultivation conditions in the production of lipid from microalgae species.

In addition, genetic modification offers an alternative approach in bid to increase lipid production from microalgae. Genes related to production of lipid, such as

TABLE 4.1.3
Findings Summary of the Effects of Cultivation Conditions on Lipid Production by Microalgae

Microalgae Species	Parameters	Range	Findings	References
Chlorella sp.	Light wavelength	600–700 nm 520–700 nm	Lipid production by two-folds from 30% (w/w) to 60% (w/w) without altering functional groups or chemical compositions.Green light produced negative effect on lipid production while red light yielded highest lipid production.	Severes et al. (2017)Rai et al. (2015)
Chlorella sp. and *Monoraphidium sp.*	Light intensity	40–400 μE photons m^2/s	Maximum high light intensity stimulates lipid production by decreasing protein, carbohydrate and chlorophyll contents.	He et al. (2015)
Desmodesmus sp. and *Scenedesmus obliquus*		50–300 μE photons m^2/s	Increasing light intensity improves overall fatty acid contents but lower oleic and linolenic acid concentrations.	Nzayisenga et al. (2020)
Chlorella vulgaris	CO_2 concentration	30%	The highest lipid content obtained was 45.68%, and the highest lipid productivity was 86.03 $mg/day^{-1}L^{-1}$.	Huang and Su (2014)
Heterochlorella luteoviridis	Temperature	22–32 °C	Lower temperature improved biosynthesis of ω3 type fatty acids.	Menegol et al. (2017)
Dunaliella tertiolecta	Nutrients concentration	10-fold nitrogen concentration	Maximum lipid productivity obtained was three-fold more at standard conditions to yield 33.5%.	Mata et al. (2013)
C. vulgaris and *A. obliquus*	Salinity concentrations	0.4 M NaCl	Highest lipid content obtained was 49% and 43% in *C. vulgaris* and *A. obliquus*, respectively.	Pandit et al. (2017)

photosynthetic process, biomass growth rate and durable resistances against extreme cultivation conditions can be modified to adapt to the environmental stress while producing similar if not better biomass production. Nevertheless, the main limitation of such methodology requires reliance on available genome sequencing information to obtain greater detail and accuracy for different genes for their related metabolic pathways (Aratboni et al. 2019). Other disadvantages of genetic modification are often associated to its high production costs, low transformation success or incomplete genetic sequencing (Tabatabaei et al. 2011). Assessments on the environmental impacts of genetically modified microalgae such as potential threats against ecological food systems, competitive displacement of native species and harmful algal blooms as well as associated ethical issues must be considered prior to its release (Aratboni et al. 2019).

4.1.8.2 Algae Derived Bioalcohol Production

Bioalcohol is another form of bioenergy that can be easily mass produced from microalgae. During photosynthesis, microalgae produced monosaccharide glucose (simple sugars) as a form of energy to supplement production of carbohydrates, lipids and proteins. Excess glucose can be converted into polysaccharides by inducing high irradiation source or limiting nutrient supply as excess production of glucose cannot be stored. The conversion of glucose into polysaccharides is relatively faster rather than conversion to lipid, in which subsequent accumulation of carbohydrates are carried out first and lipids afterwards (Ho et al. 2012). Typical carbohydrate content stored in microalgae can range widely from 6–64% depending on the species. Some of the carbohydrate, protein and lipid contents of major microalgae species are outlined in Table 4.1.4.

Nutrient starvation that limits certain nutrient uptakes, such as nitrogen, phosphorus, sulphur, potassium and manganese, is an effective method to accumulate carbohydrate concentration (Martın-Juarez et al. 2017). There are numerous studies on the effects of nitrogen and phosphorus supply on the diversifications in biochemical compositions to yield up to more than 60% carbohydrate accumulation (Markou 2012; Sassano et al. 2010). The effects of nitrogen starvation alters the metabolic pathways towards lipid and carbohydrate synthesis from protein synthesis

TABLE 4.1.4
Carbohydrate, Protein and Lipid Contents of Some Major Microalgae

Microalgae Species	Carbohydrate (%)	Protein (%)	Lipid (%)	References
Chlorella sp.	12–17	51–58	14–22	Renaud et al. (1994)
Dunaliella sp.	4–32	49–57	6–8	Parsons et al. (1961)
Porphyridium sp.	50–57	28–39	–	Becker (1994)
Scenedesmus sp.	10–52	50–56	12–14	Becker (1994)
Spirogyra	33–64	6–20	11–21	Becker (1994)

instead while phosphorus starvation disables inhibition of 3-phosphoglycerate enzyme to synthesize carbohydrates (Martın-Juarez et al. 2017). Other treatment methods to maximize recovery of polysaccharides includes mechanical methods, such as bead milling and pretreatments, and chemical methods for pH adjustment via acid/alkali treatment. Other methods like ozonolysis mainly used for delignification of lignocellulosic biomass are applied in microalgae treatment as a more energy-efficient process compared to others (Kadir et al. 2018). Nevertheless, it should be noted that detrimental effects of stress conditions imposed may also hinder the biomass growth of microalgae instead.

The conversion of simple sugars into bioethanol and by-product CO_2 by fermentation process is carried out in the presence of microorganisms such as bacteria, yeasts and fungi. Chng et al. (2017) obtained more than 50% ethanol yield of the total carbohydrate content in *S. dimorphus* with sugar conversion carried out by hydrothermal acidic hydrolysis treatment at 125 °C and 4% v/v acid concentration. Sivaramakrishnan and Incharoensakdi (2018) had obtained 86% of ethanol yield using *S. cerevisiae* for fermentation of *Scenedesmus sp.*

The current outlook on the implementation of industrial scale production of bioalcohol by fermentation of carbohydrate-enriched microalgae is mainly deterred by present hydrolysis and fermentation technologies in addition to the high cultivation costs of microalgae. The competitive pricing of fossil fuels remained to be the significant factor to discourage investments and governmental subsidies from potential stakeholders (Eduardo et al. 2016). The present industrial-size bioethanol production plant is owned by Algenol (Bonita Springs, FL, USA: http://www.algenol.com/) with ethanol productivity of more than 60,000 L ha^{-1} $year^{-1}$ with engineered microorganisms such as *Cyanobacterium sp.* reported to have tolerance of 1% of bioethanol in 16 weeks (Wang et al. 2014). Furthermore, another project by Joule Unlimited (Bedford, MA, USA: http://www.jouleunlimited.com/news) to build an industrial plant for bioethanol production from engineered cyanobacterium by light, carbonic gas, water and salts. The company reported good photosynthetic conversion efficiency of 6–7% compared to open-pond system of 1.5% at outdoor conditions. Production capacity for bioethanol production is estimated to be more than 230,000 L ha^{-1} $year^{-1}$ with $0.16/L ethanol with subsidies.

4.1.8.3 Biohydrogen Production

A report by International Renewable Energy Agency (2018) highlighted one-third of global energy emissions are derived from economic sectors with no present economic alternatives to fossil fuels. Energy intensive industry sectors and transportation sectors are made up most of those emissions. The notion that hydrogen (H_2) will play an important role in decarbonization of these sectors, integration of substantial amount of variable renewable energy (VRE) and production of transportable H_2 is perceptible as production of hydrogen is not economically viable at present.

The generation of H_2 fuel is considered cleanest renewable fuel due to zero emission of CO_2 and only water vapour by-products. H_2 contains comparatively high specific energy content (142 MJ/kg) than methane (56 MJ/kg), natural gas

(54 MJ/kg) and gasoline (47 MJ/kg) combined (Srirangan et al. 2011). To date, 95% of total hydrogen productions are fossil-fuel based with steam-methane reforming (SMR) being the most common process available, apart from oil and coal gasification processes. Production of H_2 by SMR is an effective and timesaving method but the technology itself requires moderate to high reaction temperatures to undergo endothermic reaction to produce H_2, CO and a minute amount of CO_2 (Xin et al. 2019). Furthermore, utilization of non-renewable fossil-based methane in SMR technology is unsustainable in the long-term.

With regards to this, biohydrogen production (BHP) is considered as one of the most promising alternatives to the unsustainable fossil based H_2 while considering the climate and energy crisis. In comparison to BHP by biomass waste gasification, BHP by biological route is less energy intensive and can be carried out at ambient temperature instead. Furthermore, biological production of H_2 does not interfere with the food supply chain and compete with agricultural land for food production. In general, BHP by algae biomass can be classified into direct and indirect biophotolysis, photofermentation and dark fermentation (Rittmann and Herwig 2012). Figure 4.1.5 illustrates an overview on the types of technological classifications for the H_2 production methods available.

Direct and indirect biophotolysis by microalgae involves thermochemical reaction to split water into a single molecule of H_2 and a ½ molecule of O_2 in the presence or absence of sunlight as energy source respectively. For direct biophotolysis, light is absorbed by photosynthetic green microalgae as it possess photosynthetic systems and chlorophylls – namely Photosystem (PS) I and Photosystem (PS) II respectively (Das and Veziroglu 2008). However, the presence of oxygen could inhibit the monomeric enzyme hydrogenases to consequently stop producing H_2 in addition to the significant amount requirement of free energy available (high light intensity) are some of the technological bottlenecks for BHP via direct biophotolysis. The inhibition of hydrogenase enzymes is eliminated for indirect

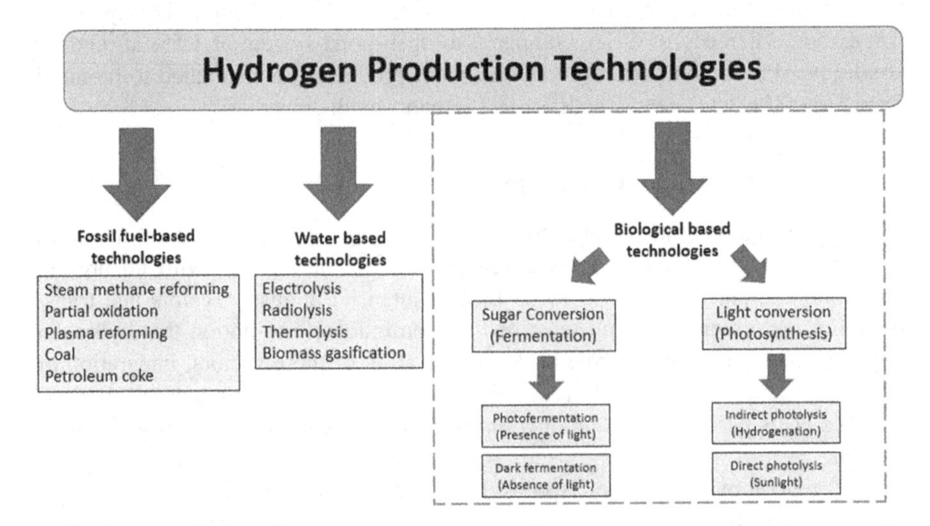

FIGURE 4.1.5 Overview of the hydrogen production technologies available.

biophotolysis by means of temporal or spatial separation of O_2 and H_2 generated. A two-step process is observed in direct biophotolysis – firstly, water molecules are allowed to be split in the presence of sunlight to produce carbohydrates within microalgae cells and by-product O_2. The second step, termed anaerobic dark fermentation, utilized nitrogenase enzymes (nitrogen fixation) or hydrogenase enzymes (carbon dioxide fixation) to convert stored carbohydrates into H_2 and by-product CO_2. Comparative studies had shown conversion efficiency by carbon dioxide fixation to H_2 to be more favourable at 27.1% compared to nitrogen fixation at 16.3% (Prince and Kheshgi 2005). Cyanobacteria, or blue-green microalgae, are microorganisms often employed for BHP via indirect biophotolysis due to its filamentous properties and the presence of heterocysts (nitrogen-fixing cells) (Eroglu and Melis 2011). Unlike direct biophotolysis route, significant amount of adenosine triphosphate (ATP) requirement by nitrogenase enzymes and application of continuous light source at larger-scale processes are some of the drawbacks of this method (Sharma and Arya 2017).

Photofermentation converts organic acid substrates into H_2 and CO_2 by utilizing solar energy as the substrates are oxidized via tricarboxylic acid cycle (TCA) to produce electrons, protons and carbon dioxide. Nevertheless, dark fermentation is superior for H_2 production, but the limitation lies mainly on the use of fermentative bacteria instead of green microalgae. Moreover, substrate conversion in the dark fermentation process is relatively low and expensive. A viable solution was proposed to utilize industrial food wastes or wastewater as a source for low-cost substrates, although effluent toxicity, additional pretreatment steps and inconsistent substrate concentrations may compromise production of H_2. A recent study for the conversion of organic wastewater by sequential dark fermentation and algal lipid accumulation had shown remarkably improvement in energy conversion efficiency up to 37.4% (Ren et al. 2014). Lam et al. (2019) had proposed a novel integrated system between direct biophotolysis by microalgae and dark fermentation by fermentative bacteria to mitigate the discreet disadvantages of each technological routes outlined earlier. BHP is carried out conventionally by direct biophotolysis route until saturated production of H_2 by microalgae is achieved and the remaining biomass is taken advantage of as a substrate for fermentative bacteria to resume BHP via the dark fermentation route. The resulting H_2 and by-product CO_2 produced in the second stage can be separated via gas separation unit to recycle CO_2 back into the first stage as a carbon source for microalgae cultivation. In essence, a cyclical process is obtained with better energy conversion efficiency and CO_2 utilization (Lam et al. 2019).

Nevertheless, the debottlenecking aspects of BHP by microalgae biomass technologies in order for the technology to succeed at larger scale must be carefully considered and overcome. Limitations such as low substrate conversion efficiency, inhibition of enzymatic activities, photobioreactor designs and harvesting methods should be considered prior scaling-up. Exploitation of hybrid bioreactors that integrates two or more systems may improve the overall energy balance and economic feasibility, Furthermore, recycling of unwanted by-product CO_2 stream as a value-added source into microalgae cultivation ecosystem instead of open emission into environment should be considered in line with the sustainable management in bioeconomy concept.

4.1.9 BIOREFINERY INTEGRATION PARADIGM

The versatility of microalgae technology allows them not only to produce bioenergy sources, such as lipid, bioalcohols and biohydrogen, but also as a potential green component to remove unwanted gaseous greenhouse gases (GHGs) and depollution of wastewaters in a sustainable biorefinery framework. The definition of biorefinery is defined as "the sustainable processing of biomass into a spectrum of bio-based products (food, feed, chemicals, materials) and bioenergy (biofuel, power and/or heat)" (Cherubini 2010). The concept of integrated microalgae technology is analogous to a separator or a carbon capture and storage (CCS) mechanism that exploits unwanted emissions from traditional refinery processes in the form of solid, liquid or gas as a form of nutrient source for metabolic growth of microalgae to produce by-product bioenergy resources as represented in Figure 4.1.6. In essence, this framework allows closer realization towards a circular energy economy by converting environmental problems into sustainable economic opportunities.

The growth of microalgae is spurred by the absorbance and utilization of nitrogen, phosphorus and trace elements nutrients as well as gaseous CO_2 to produce energy in the presence of light source. These intrinsic microalgae properties and characteristics alone make them the ideal candidate for biological wastewater treatment and CO_2 bioremediation in addition to the various value-added bioproducts generation by them (Schiano et al. 2019). However, the given climate of commercialization technology maturation in microalgae industry as a stand-alone algal biofuel refinery to at a competitive cost with fossil-based fuel is still infeasible, owing to the high capital and operating costs as well as questionable profitable return of investment from the investor's perspective (Subhandra 2020). Therefore, an alternative approach to such a scenario is to diversify microalgae utilization efficiently such as low-volume but high-value bioproducts (namely biomaterials, pharmaceutical products, etc.) or high-volume but low-value liquid transportation fuel (namely biodiesel, biogas, etc.) to achieve twofold improvements in terms of economic and environmental performances.

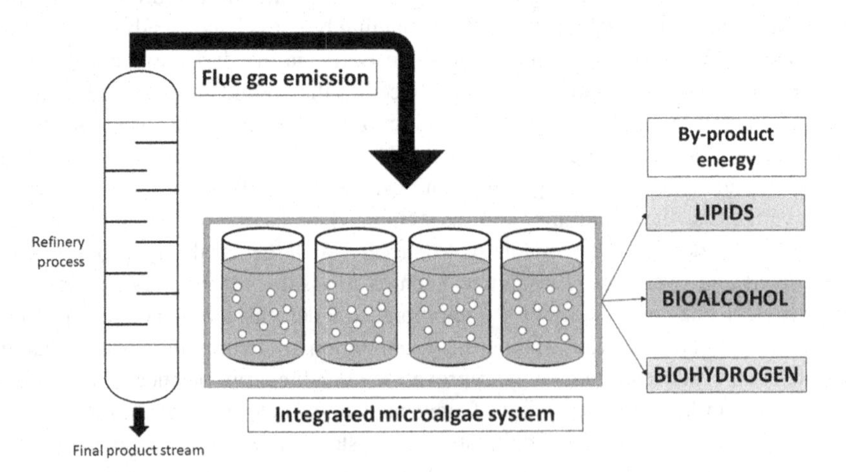

FIGURE 4.1.6 Schematic representation of an integrated microalgae biorefinery system.

A comprehensive case study conducted by Posada et al. (2016) to integrate microalgae-based biorefineries using flue gases from CO_2-intensive industries with regards to environmental performance and potential environmental impacts reduction via life cycle assessment (LCA) study. The key takeaway points from Posada et al.'s study (Posada et al. 2016) are (i) oil conversion to green diesel does not offer positive impacts in terms of energy and GHG emissions and (ii) poor economic and environmental performances for production of biogas from oil-free cake. In all scenarios studied, the recommended energy products are only favourable towards lipid production only. Supercritical fluid extraction (SFE) offered lesser non-renewable energy use and GHG emission compared to organic solvent extraction methods for extraction of lipids, thus highlighting synergistic combination of SFE and microalgae-based lipid production in a sustainable biorefinery integration (Posada et al. 2016). *Botryococcus braunii, Chlorella sp., Chlorella vulgaris, Scenedesmus obliquus* and *Scenedesmus sp.* were some of the prominent microalgae strains identified to be able to assimilate large quantity of CO_2 to produce substantial amount of lipid for biodiesel (Ho et al. 2010; Yoo et al. 2010; Yeh et al. 2010). Low CO_2 concentration in flue gas reduces life cycle energy efficiency for microalgae biodiesel production associated to the low mass transfer of CO_2 in water and subsequent higher energy consumption needed for air pump operations (Lam and Lee 2011). Increasing CO_2 concentration from 5% to 12.5% can reduce up to 72.6% of the overall fossil-energy input required for microalgae biodiesel production (Stephenson et al. 2010). Similar past performances were obtained where flue gas emissions positively improved growth of microalgae with removal efficiency up to 67% in pilot scale system (Li et al. 2011; Yoo et al. 2010) to indicate microalgae's superior role as a natural carbon sink. Park et al. (2019) investigated effects of direct injection of exhaust gas from thermal power plant on pilot scale microalgae cultivation of *Nephroselmis sp.* growth to obtain lipid content at 39.4%. Olofsson et al. (2015) used cement industrial flue gas on Brackish Baltic Sea to yield favourable lipid and carbohydrate content of 15–30% range with no toxic side effects. Aslam et al. (2017) had demonstrated successful cultivation of *Desmodesmus* spp. by 100% unfiltered flue gas from coal-fired power plant via step-wise increment and reactors-in-series arrangements.

Depending on the emission source, flue gas may contain other compounds apart from CO_2 such as NO_x, SO_x and HCl as well as heavy metals and particulate matter that are detrimental towards microalgae growth. The effects of NO_x and SO_x towards microalgae growth inhibition are dependent on the different types of strains although the concentration implication of harmful compounds remained pivotal. Nevertheless, studies have shown NO_x and SO_x concentration below 100 ppm and 50 ppm respectively are insignificant towards inhibition growth of various microalgae species such as *Chlorella sp., Dunaliella tertiolecta*, and *Scenesdesmus obliquus* (Lam et al. 2012). The removal of NO_x compounds is largely carried out through its consumption as a form of nutrient by microalgae although it is only effective in the presence of light and oxygen (Nagase et al. 1997). Furthermore, the dissolution of NO_x in aqueous solution is often considered to be the rate-limiting step. By increasing residence time or introducing complexing agent, NO molecules can be converted into NO_3^- to improve biofixation potential of algae to remove NO_x

effectively from flue gas emissions (Huang et al. 2016). Literary studies have shown presence of SO_x compounds at high concentrations (>100 ppm) severely inhibits microalgae growth due to the high dissolution activity of SO_x compounds in water to form either H_2SO_3 or H_2SO_4 acidic solutions (Vuppaladadiyam et al. 2018). Green algae species such as *Chlorella sp.* were reported to have better SO_2 tolerance although inhibition of growth was observed (Lee et al. 2002). Nevertheless, Kao et al. reported nearly two-fold in growth rate when flue gas from steel plant was used to aerate *Chlorella sp.* cultivation medium with presence of NO_x (8–80 ppm), SO_x (15–80 ppm) and CO_2 (24–25 vol%).

Microalgae are also capable microorganisms adaptable by mixotrophic growth by absorbing organic and inorganic carbon from biomass wastewater effluents for the production of carbohydrates, lipids and proteins in the presence of light. The current commercialized wastewater treatment strategies utilize conventional anaerobic-aerobic treatment systems although physical and energy constraints, such as large space requirements, open emissions in populated environment, low process efficiencies, formation of sludge and high energy consumption, were indicated (Sikosana et al. 2019). These constraints can be mitigated through incorporation of microalgae technology for wastewater treatment due to its low energy requirements, reduction activities in GHG emission and sludge formations as well as cost-effective treatment in addition to valuable biomass production via nutrient remediation from wastewater (Batista et al. 2015). Furthermore, the applications of microalgae in wastewater treatment functions to reduce biochemical oxygen demand (BOD), chemical oxygen demand (COD), coliform bacteria and heavy metals are present in industrial and municipal effluent sources.

The implementation of microalgae in agriculture-produced industrial wastewater effluent is highly practical due to the presence of rich carbon nutrients available. Waste effluent from distillery industries are one of the most polluting industries that contributes high BOD and COD content in its effluent. Depending on the type of wastewater, the high BOD (210–35,000 mg L^{-1}) and COD (3100–110,000 mg L^{-1}) content were attributed to the presence of organic compounds such as polysaccharides, reduced sugars, lignin, waxes and proteins (Kharayat 2012; Sankaran et al. 2014). Furthermore, dark in colour distillery effluent discharges inhibits light penetration into local aquatic system to subsequently deplete oxygenation of water by photosynthesis to endanger aquatic life. In regard to this, microalgae struggle to consume organic and inorganic nutrients presence as light is an essential parameter for mixotrophic growth. Batch dilution, ozonation or wet air oxidation are some of the alternative workarounds to reduce colour of the wastewater (Gupta et al. 2019) although few studies on bioremediation activities by microalgae on undiluted distillery effluents were reported. de Mattos and Bastos (2015) reported COD and nitrogen removals up to 36.2% and 52.1% respectively in lieu of lower organic and inorganic nutrients removal using *Desmodesmus sp.* in stirred batch reactor. Santana et al. (2017) reported similar responses with *Micractinium sp.* with only TOC removal at 7.2%, nitrate at (46.7%) and ammonical nitrogen at (39%). Nevertheless, bioremediation activities by microalgae found greater success when applied in brewery wastewater effluents. Subramaniyam et al. (2016) achieved total removal of nitrogen, phosphorus and organic carbon compounds in addition to the substantial growth of *Chlorella sp.* Lutzu et al. (2015) had reported total removal of more than 99% of nitrogen and phosphorus compounds to below 0.2 mg L^{-1} concentration by *Scenedesmus dimorphus* microalgae.

Textile industry is another important industrial sector that consumes substantial amount of water everyday and produces proportionate amount of wastewater. The presence of organic dyes, phosphates and nitrates are detrimental to the aquatic environment and can be bioremediated by microalgae wastewater treatment via bioconversion or bioaccumulation processes (Fazal et al. 2018). Microalgae readily consumes and converts dyes into metabolites while concurrently acting as biosorbent to adsorb dyes on cell wall surfaces due to its high surface area and strong binding affinity towards azo dyes (Pathak et al. 2015). The resultant microalgae growth is then used to convert carbohydrates into lipids and subsequently be used to produce biodiesel. The transition of electric usage in Pakistan from national grid to diesel-based electric generator had contributed a significant amount of CO_2 emission in bid to reduce financial loss in textile industries (Khan and Khan 2010). Therefore, algae-produced biodiesel can be used to replace fossil-based diesel while emission of CO_2 from electric generators can be channelled back as a carbon source for the cultivation of microalgae to attain a circular energy economy setting. Furthermore, other applications for the bioremediation of wastewater discharges by microalgae to be converted into bioenergy resources can also be applied but not limited to food processing industries, such as soybean processing (Hongyang et al. 2011), snacks processing (Gupta and Pawar 2018), dairy wastewater effluents (Brar et al. 2019; Choi 2016), municipal wastewater treatment plants (Menger-krug et al. 2012; Nayak et al. 2016) and agriculture wastewater effluents (Cheah et al. 2018, 2020; De Carvalho et al. 2018).

This section had discussed on the roles of microalgae technology with its potential in delivering renewable bioenergy and circular energy economy approach by integration as biocomponent in the current traditional production or refinery processes. External factors such as industry scale biophotoreactor designs, harvesting and drying methods of microalgae biomass, solubility of gases in water and other technological breakthroughs including the use of microbubble and membrane technologies which had been studied extensively elsewhere were not discussed in this sub-section. Nevertheless, with the perpetual advances in biotechnology pushing boundaries in innovating technological solutions to the present challenges, the industrial interest in a microalgae-inspired future remains a viable proposition.

4.1.10 CONCLUSION

This chapter discussed extensively the potential roles of supercritical fluid and algae biomass technologies with regards to Industry 5.0. Although well-established in their respective field, the progress of both technologies continues to be outweighed by conventional technological approaches. The inter-related elements of bioeconomy concept will continue to play a pivotal role to transition the current economy towards Industry 5.0 that encompasses sustainable resources management and environmental considerations. Furthermore, the current lack of representation and implementation of circular energy economy concept, especially to developing countries, are recognized around the globe, thus imposing limitations on state-of-the-art technology advancement. To do so, it is imperative to search relentlessly for practical solutions on the associated challenges and limitations imposed of the present technologies and make them viable for commercialization.

ACKNOWLEDGEMENT

The authors would like to gratefully express their sincere appreciation for the financial support from Fundamental Research Grant Scheme (015MA0-004) awarded by Ministry of Higher Education, Malaysia and the conferment of HICoE award by Ministry of Higher Education, Malaysia to Centre for Biofuel and Biochemical Research (HICoE-CBBR), Universiti Teknologi PETRONAS is acknowledged.

REFERENCES

Abbas, K., A. Mohamed, A. Abdulamir, and H. Abas. 2008. "A review on supercritical fluid extraction as new analytical method." *American Journal of Biochemistry and Biotechnology* 4: 345–353. https://doi.org/10.3844/ajbbsp.2008.345.353.

Aguilar, A., T. Twardowski, and R. Wohlgemuth. 2019. "Bioeconomy for sustainable development." *Biotechnology Journal* 14: 1–11. https://doi.org/10.1002/biot.201800638.

Aratboni, A., M. Cell, H.A. Aratboni, N. Rafiei, R.G. Granados, and A. Alemzadeh. 2019. "Biomass and lipid induction strategies in microalgae for biofuel production and other applications." *Microbial Cell Factories* 18: 1–17. https://doi.org/10.1186/s12934-019-1228-4.

Aslam, A., S.R. Thomas-hall, T. Aziz, and P.M. Schenk. 2017. "Selection and adaptation of microalgae to growth in 100% unfiltered coal-fired flue gas." *Bioresource Technology* 233: 271–283. https://doi.org/10.1016/j.biortech.2017.02.111.

Badgujar, V.C., K.C. Badgujar, P.M. Yeole, and B.M. Bhanage. 2019. "Enhanced biocatalytic activity of immobilized steapsin lipase in supercritical carbon dioxide for production of biodiesel using waste cooking oil." *Bioprocess and Biosystems Engineering* 42: 47–61. https://doi.org/10.1007/s00449-018-2013-1.

Batista, A.P., L. Ambrosano, S. Graça, C. Sousa, P.A.S.S. Marques, B. Ribeiro, E.P. Botrel, P. Castro, and L. Gouveia. 2015. "Combining urban wastewater treatment with biohydrogen production – An integrated microalgae-based approach." *Bioresource Technology* 184: 230–235. https://doi.org/10.1016/j.biortech.2014.10.064.

Becker, E.W. 1994. *Microalgae: Biotechnology and Microbiology*. Cambridge: Cambridge University Press.

Biswas, A., R.L. Shogren, and J.L. Willett. 2009. "Ionic liquid as a solvent and catalyst for acylation of maltodextrin." *Industrial Crops and Products* 30: 172–175. https://doi.org/10.1016/j.indcrop.2009.02.003.

Brar, A., M. Kumar, and N. Pareek. 2019. "Comparative appraisal of biomass production, remediation, and bioenergy generation potential of microalgae in dairy wastewater." *Frontiers in Microbiology* 10: 1–12. https://doi.org/10.3389/fmicb.2019.00678.

Brignole, E.A., and A. Fredenslund. 1987. "Supercritical fluid extraction of alcohols from water." *Industrial & Engineering Chemistry* 26: 254–261.

Caniaz, R.O., and C. Erkey. 2014. "Process intensification for heavy oil upgrading using supercritical water." *Chemical Engineering Research and Design* 92: 1845–1863. https://doi.org/10.1016/j.cherd.2014.06.007.

Chakravarty, P., A. Famili, K. Nagapudi, and M.A. Al-sayah. 2019. "Using supercritical fluid technology as a green alternative during the preparation of drug delivery systems." *Pharmaceutics* 11: 629

Cheah, W.Y., P.L. Show, J.C. Juan, J. Chang, and T.C. Ling. 2018. "Microalgae cultivation in palm oil mill effluent (POME) for lipid production and pollutants removal." *Energy Conversion and Management* 174: 430–438. https://doi.org/10.1016/j.enconman.2018.08.057.

Cheah, W.Y., P.L. Show, Y.J. Yap, H. Fatimah, M. Zaid, M.K. Lam, J.W. Lim, Y. Ho, and Y. Tao. 2020. "CY-1 biomass and lipid production in palm oil mill effluent (POME) using novel-designed photobioreactor." *Bioengineered.* 11: 61–69. https://doi.org/10.1080/21655979.2019.1704536.

Cherubini, F. 2010. "The biorefinery concept: Using biomass instead of oil for producing energy and chemicals." *Energy Conversion and Management* 51: 1412–1421. https://doi.org/10.1016/j.enconman.2010.01.015.

Chevron. 2015. *Biofuels.* https://www.chevron.com/stories/biofuels.

Chng, L.M., K.T. Lee, and D.C.J. Chan. 2017. Evaluation on microalgae biomass for bioethanol production. In *29th Symposium of Malaysian Chemical Engineers 2016.* https://doi.org/10.1088/1757-899X/206/1/012018.

Choi, H. 2016. "Dairy wastewater treatment using microalgae for potential biodiesel application." *Environmental Engineering Research* 21: 393–400.

Darani, K.K., and M.R. Mozafari. 2009. "Supercritical fluids technology in bioprocess industries: A review." *Journal of Biochemical Technology* 2: 144–152.

Das, D., and T.N. Veziroglu. 2008. "Advances in biological hydrogen production processes." *International Journal of Hydrogen Energy.* 33: 6046–6057. https://doi.org/10.1016/j.ijhydene.2008.07.098.

De Carvalho, J.C., I.A. Borghetti, L.C. Cartas, A.L. Woiciechowski, V.T. Soccol, and C.R. Soccol. 2018. "Biorefinery integration of microalgae production into cassava processing industry: Potential and perspectives." *Bioresource Technology* 247: 1165–1172. https://doi.org/10.1016/j.biortech.2017.09.213.

De Lucas, A., A. Garc, A. Alvarez, and I. Gracia. 2007. "Supercritical extraction of long chain n-alcohols from sugar cane crude wax." *The Journal of Supercritical Fluids* 41: 267–271. https://doi.org/10.1016/j.supflu.2006.09.013.

de Mattos, L.F.A., and R.G. Bastos. 2015. "COD and nitrogen removal from sugarcane vinasse by heterotrophic green algae Desmodesmus sp." *Desalination and Water Treatment* 57: 1–9. https://doi.org/10.1080/19443994.2015.1028454.

Demir, K.A., and Cicibas, H. 2017. "Industry 5.0 and a Critique of Industry 4.0." In 4th international management information systems conference, Istanbul, Turkey (pp. 17–20).

Eduardo, C., D.F. Silva, and A. Bertucco. 2016. "Bioethanol from microalgae and cyanobacteria: A review and technological outlook." *Process Biochemistry* 51: 1833–1842. https://doi.org/10.1016/j.procbio.2016.02.016.

Ekinci, M.S., and M. Gürü. 2014. "Extraction of oil and β-sitosterol from peach (*Prunus persica*) seeds using supercritical carbon dioxide." *Journal of Supercritical Fluids* 92: 319–323. https://doi.org/10.1016/j.supflu.2014.06.004.

Eroglu, E., and A. Melis. 2011. "Photobiological hydrogen production: Recent advances and state of the art." *Bioresource Technology* 102: 8403–8413. https://doi.org/10.1016/j.biortech.2011.03.026.

ExxonMobil. 2018. *Advanced biofuels and algae research: Targeting the technical capability to produce 10,000 barrels per day by 2025.* https://corporate.exxonmobil.com/Research-and-innovation/Advanced-biofuels/Advanced-biofuels-and-algae-research.

Fazal, T., A. Mushtaq, F. Rehman, A. Ullah, N. Rashid. 2018. "Bioremediation of textile wastewater and successive biodiesel production using microalgae." *Renewable and Sustainable Energy Reviews* 82: 3107–3126. https://doi.org/10.1016/j.rser.2017.10.029.

Folayan, A.J., P.A.L. Anawe, A.O. Ayeni. 2019. "Synthesis and characterization of *Salicornia bigelovii* and *Salicornia brachiata* halophytic plants oil extracted by supercritical CO_2 modified with ethanol for biodiesel production via enzymatic transesterification reaction using immobilized *Candida antarctica* lipase catalyst in tert-butyl alcohol (TBA) solvent." *Cogent Engineering* 6:1. https://doi.org/10.1080/23311916.2019.1625847.

Formighieri, C., F. Franck, and R. Bassi. 2012. "Regulation of the pigment optical density of an algal cell: Filling the gap between photosynthetic productivity in the laboratory and in mass culture." *Journal of Biotechnology* 162: 115–123. https://doi.org/10.1016/j.jbiotec.2012.02.021.

Fuwad, A., H. Ryu, N. Malmstadt, S.M. Kim, and T.J. Jeon. 2019. "Biomimetic membranes as potential tools for water purification: Preceding and future avenues." *Desalination* 458: 97–115. https://doi.org/10.1016/j.desal.2019.02.003.

Ghadiri Reza, M., J.R. Granja, and L.K. Buehler. 1991. "Artificial transmembrane ion channels from self-assembling peptide nanotubes." *Nature* 369354: 301.

Gupta, S., S.B. Pawar, and R.A. Pandey. 2019. "Current practices and challenges in using microalgae for treatment of nutrient rich wastewater from agro-based industries." *Science of The Total Environment* 687: 1107–1126. https://doi.org/10.1016/j.scitotenv.2019.06.115.

Gupta, S., and S.B. Pawar. 2018. "An integrated approach for microalgae cultivation using raw and anaerobic digested wastewaters from food processing industry." *Bioresource Technology* 269: 571–576. https://doi.org/10.1016/j.biortech.2018.08.113.

Hashi, M., F.H. Tezel, and J. Thibault. 2010. "Ethanol recovery from fermentation broth via carbon dioxide stripping and adsorption." *Energy Fuels* 24: 4628–4637. https://doi.org/10.1021/ef901130q.

He, Q., H. Yang, L. Wu, and C. Hu. 2015. "Effect of light intensity on physiological changes, carbon allocation and neutral lipid accumulation in oleaginous microalgae." *Bioresource Technology* 191: 219–228. https://doi.org/10.1016/j.biortech.2015.05.021.

Hélix-Nielsen, C. 2018. "Biomimetic membranes as a technology platform: Challenges and opportunities." *Membranes (Basel)* 8: 44. https://doi.org/10.3390/membranes8030044.

Heng, Y., P. Zhang, J. Sun, and Y. Ma. 2016. "Biomanufacturing: History and perspective." *Journal of Industrial Microbiology & Biotechnology*. https://doi.org/10.1007/s10295-016-1863-2.

Ho, S., C. Chen, and J. Chang. 2012. "Effect of light intensity and nitrogen starvation on CO_2 fixation and lipid/carbohydrate production of an indigenous microalga *Scenedesmus obliquus* CNW – N." *Bioresource Technology* 113: 244–252. https://doi.org/10.1016/j.biortech.2011.11.133.

Ho, S., C. Chen, K. Yeh, W. Chen, C. Lin, and J. Chang. 2010. "Characterization of photosynthetic carbon dioxide fixation ability of indigenous Scenedesmus obliquus isolates." *Biochemical Engineering Journal* 53: 57–62. https://doi.org/10.1016/j.bej.2010.09.006.

Hongyang, S., Z. Yalei, Z. Chunmin, Z. Xuefei, and L. Jinpeng. 2011. "Cultivation of *Chlorella pyrenoidosa* in soybean processing wastewater." *Bioresource Technology* 102: 9884–9890. https://doi.org/10.1016/j.biortech.2011.08.016.

Huang, G., F. Chen, and Y. Kuang. 2016. "Current techniques of growing algae using flue Gas from exhaust gas industry: A review." *Applied Biochemistry and Biotechnology* 178: 1220–1238. https://doi.org/10.1007/s12010-015-1940-4.

Huang, Y.-T., and C.-P. Su. 2014. "High lipid content and productivity of microalgae cultivating under elevated carbon dioxide." *International Journal of Environmental Science and Technology* 11: 703–710. https://doi.org/10.1007/s13762-013-0251-y.

IRENA. 2020. Renewable capacity highlights. https://www.irena.org/-/media/Files/IRENA/Agency/Publication/2019/Mar/RE_capacity_highlights_2019.pdf.

Jacobson, M.Z., and M.A. Delucchi. 2016. "A path to sustainable energy by 2030." *Scientific American* 58–65. https://doi.org/10.1038/scientificamerican1109-58.

Kadir, W.N.A., M.K. Lam, Y. Uemura, J.W. Lim, and K.T. Lee. 2018. “Harvesting and pre-treatment of microalgae biomass via ozonation for lipid extraction: A preliminary study.” *AIP Conference Proceedings* 2016: 020064.

Khan, A.A., and M. Khan. 2010. “Pakistan textile industry facing new challenges.” *Research Journal of International Studies* 21–29.

Khan, M.I., J.H. Shin, and J.D. Kim. 2018. “The promising future of microalgae: Current status, challenges, and optimization of a sustainable and renewable industry for biofuels, feed, and other products.” *Microbial Cell Factories* 17: 1–21. https://doi.org/10.1186/s12934-018-0879-x.

Khan, S.A., M.Z. Hussain, S. Prasad, and U.C. Banerjee. 2009. “Prospects of biodiesel production from microalgae in India.” *Renewable and Sustainable Energy Reviews* 13: 2361–2372. https://doi.org/10.1016/j.rser.2009.04.005.

Kharayat, Y. 2012. “Distillery wastewater: Bioremediation approaches.” *Journal of Integrative Environmental Sciences* 9: 69–91. https://doi.org/10.1080/1943815X.2012.688056.

Kim, S., K.S. Jang, H.D. Choi, S.H. Choi, S.J. Kwon, I.D. Kim, J.A. Lim, and J.M. Hong. 2013. “Porous polyimide membranes prepared by wet phase inversion for use in low dielectric applications.” *International Journal of Molecular Sciences* 14: 8698–8707. https://doi.org/10.3390/ijms14058698.

Knez, E., Markočič, M., Leitgeb, M., Primožič, M., and Knez Hrnčič, M. 2014. “Škerget, Industrial applications of supercritical fluids: A review.” *Energy* 77: 235–243. https://doi.org/10.1016/j.energy.2014.07.044.

Knez, Ž., M. Leitgeb, and M. Primožič. 2014. “Enzymatic reactions in supercritical fluids.” In *High Pressure Fluid Technology for Green Food Processing*, 185–215. New York: Springer.

Lam, M.K., A. Chun, M. Loy, S. Yusup, and K.T. Lee. 2019. “Biohydrogen production from algae.” In *Biohydrogen,* 2nd edition, edited by A. Pandey, S.V. Mohan, J.-S. Chang, P.C. Hallenbeck, and C. Larroche, 219–245. United Kingdom: Elsevier B.V. https://doi.org/10.1016/B978-0-444-64203-5.00009-5.

Lam, M.K., K.T. Lee, and A.R. Mohamed. 2012. “Current status and challenges on microalgae-based carbon capture.” *International Journal of Greenhouse Gas Control* 10: 456–469. https://doi.org/10.1016/j.ijggc.2012.07.010.

Lam, M.K., and K.T. Lee. 2011. “Renewable and sustainable bioenergies production from palm oil mill effluent (POME): Win – win strategies toward better environmental protection.” *Biotechnology Advances* 29: 124–141. https://doi.org/10.1016/j.biotechadv.2010.10.001.

Lang, Q., and C.M. Wai. 2001. “Supercritical fluid extraction in herbal and natural product studies – A practical review.” *Talanta* 53: 771–782. https://doi.org/10.1016/S0039-9140(00)00557-9.

Le, N.L., Y. Wang, and T. Chung. 2011. “Pebax/POSS mixed matrix membranes for ethanol recovery from aqueous solutions via pervaporation.” *Journal of Membrane Science* 379: 174–183. https://doi.org/10.1016/j.memsci.2011.05.060.

Lee, H.J., M. Haq, P.S. Saravana, Y.N. Cho, and B.S. Chun. 2017. “Omega-3 fatty acids concentrate production by enzyme-catalyzed ethanolysis of supercritical CO_2 extracted oyster oil.” *Biotechnology and Bioprocess Engineering* 22: 518–528. https://doi.org/10.1007/s12257-017-0293-y.

Lee, J., D. Kim, J. Lee, S. Park, J. Koh, H. Cho, and S. Kim. 2002. “Effects of SO_2 and NO_2 on growth of Chlorella sp. KR-1.” *Bioresource Technology* 82: 2–5.

Li, F., Z. Yang, R. Zeng, G. Yang, X. Chang, J. Yan, and Y. Hou. 2011. “Microalgae capture of CO_2 from actual flue gas discharged from a combustion chamber.” *Industrial & Engineering Chemistry Research* 50: 6496–6502.

Lutzu, G.A., W. Zhang, T. Liu, G.A. Lutzu, W. Zhang, and T. Liu. 2015. "Feasibility of using brewery wastewater for biodiesel production and nutrient removal by *Scenedesmus dimorphus*." *Environmental Technology* 37: 1–14. https://doi.org/10.1080/09593330.2015.1121292.

Marillán, C., and E. Uquiche. 2020. "Inhibition of α-amylase activity by extracts from *Leptocarpha rivularis* stalks obtained with supercritical CO_2." *Journal of Supercritical Fluids* 161: 104849. https://doi.org/10.1016/j.supflu.2020.104849.

Markou, G. 2012. "Alteration of the biomass composition of *Arthrospira (Spirulina) platensis* under various amounts of limited phosphorus." *Bioresource Technology* 116: 533–535. https://doi.org/10.1016/j.biortech.2012.04.022.

Martın-Juarez, J., G. Markou, K. Muylaert, A. Loreno-Hernando, and S. Bolado. 2017. "Breakthroughs in bioalcohol production from microalgae: Solving the hurdles." In *Microalgae-Based Biofuels and Bioproducts*, edited by C. Gonzalez-Fernandez and R. Muñoz, 183–207. Cambridge, United Kingdom: Elsevier. https://doi.org/10.1016/B978-0-08-101023-5.00008-X.

Mata, T.M., R. Almeida, and N.S. Caetano. 2013. "Effect of the culture nutrients on the biomass and lipid productivities of microalgae *Dunaliella tertiolecta*." *Chemical Engineering Transactions* 32: 973–978.

Matsuyama, H., H. Yano, T. Maki, M. Teramoto, K. Mishima, and K. Matsuyama. 2001. "Formation of porous flat membrane by phase separation with supercritical CO_2." *Journal of Membrane Science* 194: 157–163. https://doi.org/10.1016/S0376-7388(01)00436-7.

Mcgovern, P.E., J. Zhang, J. Tang, Z. Zhang, G.R. Hall, R.A. Moreau, E.D. Butrym, M.P. Richards, C. Wang, G. Cheng, Z. Zhao, and C. Wang. 2004. "Fermented beverages of pre- and proto-historic China." *Proceedings of the National Academy of Sciences of the United States of America* 101: 17593–17598.

Medipally, S.R., F. Yusoff, S. Banerjee, and M. Shariff. 2015. "Microalgae as sustainable renewable energy feedstock for biofuel production." *BioMed Research International* 2015: 1–13.

Melgosa, R., M.T. Sanz, Ó. Benito-Román, A.E. Illera, and S. Beltrán. 2019. "Supercritical CO_2 assisted synthesis and concentration of monoacylglycerides rich in omega-3 polyunsaturated fatty acids." *Journal of CO_2 Utilization* 31: 65–74. https://doi.org/10.1016/j.jcou.2019.02.015.

Menegol, T., A.B. Diprat, E. Rodrigues, and R. Rech. 2017. "Effect of temperature and nitrogen concentration on biomass composition of *Heterochlorella luteoviridis*." *Food Science and Technology* 37: 28–37.

Menger-krug, E., J. Niederste-hollenberg, T. Hillenbrand, and H. Hiessl. 2012. "Integration of microalgae systems at municipal wastewater treatment plants: Implications for energy and emission balances." *Environmental Science & Technology* 46: 11505–11514.

Nagase, H., K. Yoshihara, K. Eguchi, Y. Yokota, R.I.E. Matsui, K. Hirata, and K. Miyamoto. 1997. "Characteristics of biological NOx removal from flue gas in a *Dunaliella tertiolecta* culture system." *Journal of Fermentation and Bioengineering* 83: 461–465.

Nahavandi, S. 2019. "Industry 5.0 – A human-centric solution." *Sustainability* 11. https://doi.org/10.3390/su11164371.

Nargund, S., and K. Guenther. 2019. "The move toward Biopharma 4.0." *Genetic Engineering and Biotechnology News*. https://www.genengnews.com/resources/tutorial/the-move-toward-biopharma-4-0/ (accessed April 10, 2020).

Nayak, M., A. Karemore, and R. Sen. 2016. "Sustainable valorization of flue gas CO_2 and wastewater for the production of microalgal biomass as a biofuel feedstock in closed and open." *RSC Advances* 6: 91111–91120. https://doi.org/10.1039/C6RA17899E.

Nlandu, H., K. Belkacemi, N. Chorfa, S. Elkoun, M. Robert, and S. Hamoudi. 2020. "Flax nanofibrils production via supercritical carbon dioxide pre-treatment and enzymatic hydrolysis." *Canadian Journal of Chemical Engineering* 98: 84–95. https://doi.org/10.1002/cjce.23596.

Nzayisenga, J.C., X. Farge, S.L. Groll, and A. Sellstedt. 2020. "Effects of light intensity on growth and lipid production in microalgae grown in wastewater." *Biotechnology for Biofuels* 13: 1–8. https://doi.org/10.1186/s13068-019-1646-x.

Oliveira, J.V., and D. Oliveira. 2000. "Kinetics of the enzymatic alcoholysis of palm kernel oil in supercritical CO_2." *Industrial & Engineering Chemistry Research* 39: 4450–4454. https://doi.org/10.1021/ie990865p.

Olofsson, M., E. Lindehoff, B. Frick, F. Svensson, and C. Legrand. 2015. "Baltic Sea microalgae transform cement flue gas into valuable biomass." *Algal Research* 11: 227–233. https://doi.org/10.1016/j.algal.2015.07.001.

Pandit, P.R., M.H. Fulekar, M. Sri, and L. Karuna. 2017. "Effect of salinity stress on growth, lipid productivity, fatty acid composition, and biodiesel properties in *Acutodesmus obliquus* and *Chlorella vulgaris*." *Environmental Science and Pollution Research* 24: 13437–13451. https://doi.org/10.1007/s11356-017-8875-y.

Park, S., Y. Ahn, K. Pandi, M.-K. Ji, H.-S. Yun, and J. Choi. 2019. "Microalgae cultivation in pilot scale for biomass power plants." *Energies* 12: 3497.

Parsons, T.R., K. Stephens, and J.D.H. Strickland. 1961. "On the pigment composition of eleven species of marine phytoplankters." *Journal of the Fisheries Research Board of Canada* 18: 1001–1016. https://doi.org/10.1139/f61-064.

Pathak, V.V., R. Kothari, A.K. Chopra, and D.P. Singh. 2015. "Experimental and kinetic studies for phycoremediation and dye removal by *Chlorella pyrenoidosa* from textile wastewater." *Journal of Environmental Management* 163: 270–277. https://doi.org/10.1016/j.jenvman.2015.08.041.

Peng, Y., and Z. Guo. 2016. "Recent advances in biomimetic thin membranes applied in emulsified oil/water separation." *Journal of Materials Chemistry A* 4: 15749–15770. https://doi.org/10.1039/c6ta06922c.

Pollardo, A.A., H. shik Lee, D. Lee, S. Kim, and J. Kim. 2017. "Effect of supercritical carbon dioxide on the enzymatic production of biodiesel from waste animal fat using immobilized *Candida antarctica* lipase B variant." *BMC Biotechnology* 17: 1–6. https://doi.org/10.1186/s12896-017-0390-1.

Posada, J.A., L.B. Brentner, A. Ramirez, and M.K. Patel. 2016. "Conceptual design of sustainable integrated microalgae biore fineries: Parametric analysis of energy use, greenhouse gas emissions and techno-economics." *Algal Research* 17: 113–131. https://doi.org/10.1016/j.algal.2016.04.022.

Prince, R.C., and H.S. Kheshgi. 2005. "The photobiological production of hydrogen: Potential efficiency and effectiveness as a renewable fuel." *Critical Reviews in Microbiology* 31:19–31. https://doi.org/10.1080/10408410590912961.

Putrino, F.M., M. Tedesco, R.B. Bodini, and A.L. De Oliveira. 2020. "Study of supercritical carbon dioxide pretreatment processes on green coconut fiber to enhance enzymatic hydrolysis of cellulose." *Bioresource Technology* 309: 123387. https://doi.org/10.1016/j.biortech.2020.123387.

Rai, M.P., T. Gautom, and N. Sharma. 2015. "Effect of salinity, pH, light intensity on growth and lipid production of microalgae for bioenergy application." *OnLine Journal of Biological Sciences* 15: 260–267. https://doi.org/10.3844/ojbsci.2015.260.267.

Raynie, D.E. 1993. "Warning concerning the use of nitrous oxide in supercritical fluid extractions." *Analytical Chemistry* 65: 3127–3128. https://doi.org/10.1021/ac00069a028.

Reinhardt, I.C., D.J.C. Oliveira, and D.D.T. Ring. 2020. "Current perspectives on the development of industry 4.0 in the pharmaceutical sector." *Journal of Industrial Information Integration* 18: 100131. https://doi.org/10.1016/j.jii.2020.100131.

Ren, H., B. Liu, F. Kong, L. Zhao, D. Xing, and N. Ren. 2014. "Enhanced energy conversion efficiency from high strength synthetic organic wastewater by sequential dark fermentative hydrogen production and algal lipid accumulation." *Bioresource Technology* 157: 355–359. https://doi.org/10.1016/j.biortech.2014.02.009.

Ren, X., X. Zhao, F. Turcotte, J.S. Deschênes, R. Tremblay, and M. Jolicoeur. 2017. "Current lipid extraction methods are significantly enhanced adding a water treatment step in *Chlorella protothecoides*." *Microbial Cell Factories* 16: 1–13. https://doi.org/10.1186/s12934-017-0633-9.

Renaud, S.M., D.L. Parry, and L. Van Thinh. 1994. "Microalgae for use in tropical aquaculture I: Gross chemical and fatty acid composition of twelve species of microalgae from the Northern Territory, Australia." *Journal of Applied Phycology* 6: 337–345. https://doi.org/10.1007/BF02181948.

Reverchon, E., and S. Cardea. 2004. "Formation of cellulose acetate membranes using a supercritical fluid assisted process." *Journal of Membrane Science* 240: 187–195. https://doi.org/10.1016/j.memsci.2004.04.020.

Rittmann, S., and C. Herwig. 2012. "A comprehensive and quantitative review of dark fermentative biohydrogen production." *Microbial Cell Factories* 11: 20–25.

Ruiz-rodríguez, A., T. Fornari, L. Jaime, E. Vázquez, B. Amador, J. Antonio, M. Yuste, M. Mercader, and G. Reglero. 2012. "Supercritical CO_2 extraction applied toward the production of a functional beverage from wine." *Journal of Supercritical Fluids* 61: 92–100. https://doi.org/10.1016/j.supflu.2011.09.002.

Sankaran, K., M. Premalatha, M. Vijayasekaran, and V.T. Somasundaram. 2014. "DEPHY project: Distillery wastewater treatment through anaerobic digestion and phycoremediation—A green industrial approach." *Renewable and Sustainable Energy Reviews* 37: 634–643. https://doi.org/10.1016/j.rser.2014.05.062.

Santana, H., C.R. Cereijo, V.C. Teles, R.C. Nascimento, M.S. Fernandes, P. Brunale, R.C. Campanha, I.P. Soares, F.C.P. Silva, P.S. Sabaini, F.G. Siqueira, and B.S.A.F. Brasil. 2017. "Microalgae cultivation in sugarcane vinasse: Selection, growth and biochemical characterization." *Bioresource Technology* 228: 133–140. https://doi.org/10.1016/j.biortech.2016.12.075.

Sassano, C.E.N., L.A. Gioielli, L.S. Ferreira, M.S. Rodrigues, S. Sato, A. Converti, and J.C.M. Carvalho. 2010. "Evaluation of the composition of continuously-cultivated *Arthrospira (Spirulina) platensis* using ammonium chloride as nitrogen source." *Biomass and Bioenergy* 34: 1732–1738. https://doi.org/10.1016/j.biombioe.2010.07.002.

Schiano, G., A. Spicer, C.J. Chuck, and M.J. Allen. 2019. "The microalgae biorefinery: A perspective on the current status and future opportunities using genetic modification." *Applied Sciences* 9: 4793.

Scholes, C.A., and S. Kanehashi. 2018. "Polymeric membrane gas separation performance improvements through supercritical CO_2 treatment." *Journal of Membrane Science* 566: 239–248. https://doi.org/10.1016/j.memsci.2018.09.014.

Severes, A., S. Hegde, L.D. Souza, and S. Hegde. 2017. "Use of light emitting diodes (LEDs) for enhanced lipid production in micro-algae based biofuels." *Journal of Photochemistry and Photobiology B: Biology* 170: 235–240. https://doi.org/10.1016/j.jphotobiol.2017.04.023.

Sharma, A., and S.K. Arya. 2017. "Hydrogen from algal biomass: A review of production process." *Biotechnology Reports* 15: 63–69. https://doi.org/10.1016/j.btre.2017.06.001.

Sikosana, M.L., K. Sikhwivhilu, R. Moutloali, M. Daniel, R. Moutloali, and M. Daniel. 2019. "Municipal wastewater treatment technologies: A review." *Procedia Manufacturing* 35: 1018–1024. https://doi.org/10.1016/j.promfg.2019.06.051.

Silva, W., J. Romero, E. Morales, R. Melo, L. Mendoza, and M. Cotoras. 2017. "Red wine extract obtained by membrane-based supercritical fluid extraction: Preliminary characterization of chemical properties." *Brazilian Journal of Chemical Engineering* 34: 567–581.

SINOPEC. New energy, (n.d.). http://www.sinopecgroup.com/group/en/technologicalinnovation/Newenergy/.

Sivaramakrishnan, R., and A. Incharoensakdi. 2018. "Utilization of microalgae feedstock for concomitant production of bioethanol and biodiesel." *Fuel* 217: 458–466. https://doi.org/10.1016/j.fuel.2017.12.119.

Sonego, J.L.S., D.A. Lemos, G.Y. Rodriguez, A.J.G. Cruz, and A.C. Badino. 2014. "Extractive batch fermentation with CO_2 stripping for ethanol production in a bubble column bioreactor: Experimental and modeling." *Energy & Fuels* 28: 7552–7559

Srirangan, K., M.E. Pyne, and C.P. Chou. 2011. "Bioresource technology biochemical and genetic engineering strategies to enhance hydrogen production in photosynthetic algae and cyanobacteria." *Bioresource Technology* 102: 8589–8604. https://doi.org/10.1016/j.biortech.2011.03.087.

Stephenson, A.L., E. Kazamia, J.S. Dennis, C.J. Howe, S.A. Scott, and A.G. Smith. 2010. "Life-cycle assessment of potential algal biodiesel production in the United Kingdom: A comparison of raceways and air-lift tubular bioreactors." *Energy & Fuels* 24: 4062–4077. https://doi.org/10.1021/ef1003123.

Subhandra, B. 2020. "Environmental benefits of integrated algal biorefineries conversion." In *New and Future Developments in Catalysis*, edited by S.L. Suib, 229–251. Elsevier B.V. https://doi.org/10.1016/B978-0-444-53878-9.00011-4.

Subramaniyam, V., S. Ramraj, and V. Ganeshkumar. 2016. "Cultivation of chlorella on brewery wastewater and nano-particle biosynthesis by its biomass." *Bioresource Technology* 211: 698–703. https://doi.org/10.1016/j.biortech.2016.03.154.

Tabatabaei, M., M. Tohidfar, G. Salehi, M. Safarnejad, and M. Pazouki. 2011. "Biodiesel production from genetically engineered microalgae: Future of bioenergy in Iran." *Renewable and Sustainable Energy Reviews* 15: 1918–1927. https://doi.org/10.1016/j.rser.2010.12.004.

Tredici, M.R. 2010. "Photobiology of microalgae mass cultures: Understanding the tools for the next green revolution." *Biofuels* 1: 143–162.

Utama, G.L., T. Benito, A. Kurnani, and R.L. Balia. 2016. "The isolation and identification of stress tolerance ethanol-fermenting yeasts from mozzarella cheese whey." *International Journal on Advanced Science, Engineering and Information Technology* 6: 252–257.

Vadillo, V., J. Sa, J. Ramo, E.J. Mart, and D. Ossa. 2013. "Problems in supercritical water oxidation process and proposed solutions." *Industrial & Engineering Chemistry Research* 52: 7617–7629. https://doi.org/10.1021/ie400156c.

Vadillo, V., J. Sánchez-Oneto, J.R. Portela, and E.J. Martinez de la Ossa. 2013. "Problems in supercritical water oxidation process and proposed solutions." *Industrial & Engineering Chemistry Research* 52 (23): 7617–7629

Vázquez-ojeda, M., J.G. Segovia-hernández, S. Hernández, A. Hernández-aguirre, and A. Alexandru. 2013. Design and optimization of an ethanol dehydration process using stochastic methods. *Separation and Purification Technology* 105: 90–97. https://doi.org/10.1016/j.seppur.2012.12.002.

Von Braun, J. 2018. "Bioeconomy – The global trend and its implications for sustainability and food security," *Global Food Security* 19: 81–83. https://doi.org/10.1016/j.gfs.2018.10.003.

Vuppaladadiyam, A.K., J.G. Yao, N. Florin, A. George, P. Ralph, P.S. Fennell, and M. Zhao. 2018. "Impact of Flue Gas Compounds on Microalgae and Mechanisms for Carbon Assimilation and Utilization." *ChemSusChem* 11: 334–355. https://doi.org/10.1002/cssc.201701611.

Waibel, B.J.J., and V.J. Krukonis. 2012. Energy efficient separation of ethanol from aqueous solution, US8,263,814 B2.

Wang, K., T. Shi, I. Piven, M. Inaba, F. Uliczka, D. Kramer, H. Enke, K. Baier, A. Friedrich, and U. Duehring. 2014. Cyanobacterium sp. for production of compounds, WO 2014/100799 A2. https://patents.google.com/patent/WO2014100799A2/pt.

Williams, P.J.B., and L.M.L. Laurens. 2010. "Microalgae as biodiesel & biomass feedstocks: Review & analysis of the biochemistry, energetics & economics." *Energy & Environmental Science* 3: 554–590. https://doi.org/10.1039/b924978h.

Xin, A., Y. Mah, W. Shin, C. Phun, C. Bong, M. Johari, and N.G. Chemmangattuvalappil. 2019. "Review of hydrogen economy in Malaysia and its way forward." *International Journal of Hydrogen Energy* 44: 5661–5675. https://doi.org/10.1016/j.ijhydene.2019.01.077.

Yeh, K.-L., J. Chang, and W. Chen. 2010. "Effect of light supply and carbon source on cell growth and cellular composition of a newly isolated microalga *Chlorella vulgaris*." *Engineering in Life Sciences* 10: 201–208. https://doi.org/10.1002/elsc.200900116.

Yoo, C., S. Jun, J. Lee, C. Ahn, and H. Oh. 2010. "Selection of microalgae for lipid production under high levels carbon dioxide." *Bioresource Technology* 101: S71–S74. https://doi.org/10.1016/j.biortech.2009.03.030.

Zaldivar, M.J. 2001. "Fuel ethanol production from lignocellulose: A challenge for metabolic engineering and process integration." *Applied Microbiology and Biotechnology* 56: 17–34. https://doi.org/10.1007/s002530100624.

Zentou, H., Z.Z. Abidin, R. Yunus, D.R.A. Biak, and D. Korelskiy. 2019. "Overview of alternative ethanol removal techniques for enhancing bioethanol recovery from fermentation broth." *Processes* 7: 1–16.

Zhang, Q., M. Zhao, Q. Xu, H. Ren, and J. Yin. 2019. "Enhanced enzymatic hydrolysis of sorghum stalk by supercritical carbon dioxide and ultrasonic pretreatment." *Applied Biochemistry and Biotechnology* 188: 101–111. https://doi.org/10.1007/s12010-018-2909-x.

Zhang, S., Z. Zhang, R. Zhao, J. Gu, J. Liu, B. Ormeci, and J. Zhang. 2016. "A review of challenges and recent progress in supercritical water oxidation of wastewater." *Chemical Engineering Communications* 204: 265–282.

Zhao, M.J., Q.Q. Xu, G.M. Li, Q.Z. Zhang, D. Zhou, J.Z. Yin, and H.S. Zhan. 2019. "Pretreatment of agricultural residues by supercritical CO_2 at 50–80 °C to enhance enzymatic hydrolysis." *Journal of Energy Chemistry* 31: 39–45. https://doi.org/10.1016/j.jechem.2018.05.003.

Zhu, L.D., Z.H. Li, and E. Hiltunen. 2016. "Strategies for lipid production improvement in microalgae as a biodiesel feedstock. "*BioMed Research International* 2016: 7–9.

4.2 Sustainability and Development of Industry 5.0

Hui Shi Saw, Abdul Azim bin Azmi,
Kit Wayne Chew, and Pau Loke Show

CONTENTS

4.2.1 SUSTAINABLE PROCESSES IN BIOMANUFACTURING

4.2.1.1 Principles of Biomanufacturing

Biomanufacturing has branched out in the paradigm of manufacturing, possessing an increasing trend in the sustainable development of the industry. As a growing field necessary to meet society's demand, reshaping the industry of production, which is currently heavily built on the basis of utilizing the natural resources has brought to attention. The feasibility of current chemical manufacturing methods, in the long run, is questionable. The complexity of such large-scale production involves high consumption of energy in the setup of mega infrastructures, as well as fossil-based feedstock.

While the expense is not only in regard to the production cost, permanent damage to the environment, including being the root cause of pollution should not be taken lightly. Aside from industrial use chemicals, food production closely related to livestock contributes greatly to the emission of greenhouse gas, which eventually leads to climate change (Rojas-Downing, Nejadhashemi, Harrigan, and Woznicki 2017).

The surge of the global population with a potential increase in household income could accelerate the depletion of natural resources, as demand for material resources will also increase. While the threshold of Earth to sustain our consumption remains unchanged, this represents a bigger threat to the balance of the ecosystem in the future (Devezas, Vaz, and Magee 2017). A new transformation is therefore much needed to revolutionize the production of goods to meet the current needs without compromising the ability of future generations to meet their own needs (Dresner 2003).

4.2.1.2 DNA Sequencing, the Onset of Systematic Biomanufacturing

The address of driving Industry 5.0 towards a stable environment has shed light on biomanufacturing. The history of utilizing the biological system as a factory to manufacture raw materials have been explored thousand years ago prior modernization, with the onset of solid-state fermentation (Zhang, Sun, and Ma 2017). The evolution of bioproduction has occurred in parallel with the progress in technology. Trial and error method used in tracking as the reason behind the occurrence of the early discovery of fermentation in milk has now been replaced. Instead of the random event by chance, the understanding of the expression system has allowed researchers to target the production of targeted compounds, which is closely tied to the advancement of DNA sequencing. The understanding of genetic code has unlocked potentials in manipulating the existing biological systems, bringing desired design into the act.

Whole-genome sequencing project has been helpful in determining the model systems, including the microorganism *Escherichia coli* and plant model *Arabidopsis thaliana* (Theologis 2001). With the known sequence, these complete map of the genome could be understood and the restrictions to manipulate with the uncertainty is greatly reduced. The better understanding of evolution process, gene function and gene expression control has attributed to propel the advancement in biomanufacturing.

Redesign of biological systems can be done in unicellular or multicellular organisms, ranging from microorganisms, insect, plant and animal cell lines, to a fully grown plant. Techniques on the transfer of genetic material across different organisms differ, where the basic method includes obeying the transformation concept of using plasmid for gene insertion. Plasmid, an extrachromosomal genetic element not essential for growth obtained from prokaryotes is redesigned to serve as a vehicle that ferries target gene into a host, which could be a different species (Madigan et al. 2018). Under heat shock, the mechanism of plasmid DNA enters chemically induced competent *E. coli*, for instance in the presence of calcium chloride, would be established. Another natural tool commonly used in plants can be demonstrated by agrobacterium-mediated gene transfer. Development of binary plasmid of *Agrobacterium tumefaciens* T-DNA carrying desired new trait can be transferred into a grown plant by agroinfiltration based on the syringe and vacuum infiltration (Chen et al. 2013).

Aside from the use of a plasmid vector to add a new gene that does not naturally exist, direct delivery of exogenous DNA into the cell is available as well. Biolistic, also known as a gene gun, applies pressure from helium gas to bombard gold-coated DNA particles to force the entry of genetic material into the plant cell. Whereas in electroporation, temporary pores in the plasma are created by electric shock, allowing uptake of nucleic acid into protoplast.

4.2.1.3 Protein Synthesis through Central Dogma

At the cellular level, deletion of a gene that hampers overexpression, or generation of a by-product that inhibits the synthesis of a target product can be performed by targeting a known gene. Gene to add or remove can be based on genotype, which is the known sequence, or phenotype, from the traits and characteristics of protein with an unknown sequence. To exemplify, *in silico* analysis with the establishment of bioinformatics tools and database enables hypothetical protein sequence to be generated, where the potential gene product model can be predicted. Having access to the structure of a protein can help to determine a suitable feature, for example, the hydrophobicity and function of the protein, that needs to be employed via genetic manipulation. The available tools, such as BLAST, ExPASy and Entrez are helpful in increasing the success rate of an experiment, which might reduce the waste of resources as compared to the traditional trial and error approach.

Compared to the rational design mentioned earlier, directed evolution emphasizes the selection of successful mutants with desired traits, without prior structural or mechanistic information (McCullum et al. 2010). A large "mix and match" library of sequences from a single parent DNA could be generated with the advantage of directed evolution, where the combined sequence that drives the synthesis of ideal proteins could be identified. A naturally occurring DNA repairing mechanism is useful to generate base change in the sequence, which could alter the characteristic of amino acid produced. Error-prone polymerase chain reaction (epPCR) therefore plays a role in performing random mutagenesis, an approach of conducting directed evolution. The standard polymerase chain reaction (PCR) was modified by increasing the concentration of Taq DNA polymerase and concentration of magnesium chloride ions to create an intentional error in the amplification process. Such a change of condition is effective in creating a rate of random mutagenesis at ~2% per nucleotide in a PCR reaction (Leung 1989).

In the effort of maximizing the potential of biological systems in manufacturing, researchers have established gene-editing techniques helpful in studying gene function that drives the key to highly productive strain. Manipulation at the DNA level, either a presence or absence of a gene affecting the metabolism of an organism can be described as an absolute, 0 or 1 binary relationship. Instead of addition or removal of a gene, researchers have also looked into the RNA level by "tuning" the expression of a targeted gene. Unlike DNA sequence, the study on transcriptome stands an advantage in understanding the pattern of gene regulation, and how the final product can be synthesized, especially in eukaryotes where alternative splicing occurs (Ozsolak and Milos 2011). RNA interference (RNAi) in animals, or known as transcriptional gene silencing (PTGS) in plants, are mediated gene silencing processes induced by double-stranded DNA (dsDNA) which could be introduced exogenously (Mello and Conte 2004; Tian et al. 2004). With a similar concept in suppressing gene expression by blocking translation, antisense RNA binds to a 5′ untranslated region (5′-UTR), and/or open reading frame (ORF) of a transcript (Thomason and Storz 2010). For instance, antisense RNA has been demonstrated to downregulate squalene synthase, encoded by an essential gene in baker's yeast, *Saccharomyces cerevisiae*. This repression has been reported by

Scalcinati et al., whereby the enhancement of α-santalene, a compound commonly used in perfumery and aromatherapy industries was achieved.

Interestingly, the choice of expression system is no longer limited to a single host system. This is made possible by the use of a shuttle vector, which is a cloning vector that can replicate in two widely different species. Even though gene cloning techniques are often transferable, they might be limited for some organisms, and therefore requires the advantage of shuttle vector to carry out initial cloning, commonly using *E. coli* before attempting on other host organisms (Dale 2010). This follows the concept of gene insertion into an *E. coli* plasmid with an origin of replication that enables the function in another host, as presented in *Bacillus subtilis* for the protein secretory expression (Guo et al. 2014).

4.2.1.4 Synthesis of Metabolites

While most manipulation focuses on the three main processes in central dogma-replication, transcription and translation of the gene product, i.e., protein, biomanufacturing of other metabolites often does not follow the same, direct biochemical pathway as protein synthesis (Krebs, Lewin, Goldstein, and Kilpatrick 2014). In place of a direct target on the final product, intermediate in the biochemical pathway is aimed. Biomanufacturing plays an advantage in producing compounds that are harvested from nature, such as vinblastine, vincristine, paclitaxel (Taxol®), docetaxel, camptothecin, colchicine, demecolcine and podophyllotoxin. These anticancer compounds are not economical to synthesize chemically owing to their structure with chiral molecules (Wink et al. 2005). Biosynthesis of a potent anticancer drug, paclitaxel (Taxol®) depicts the approach of deriving natural product using microbial systems of *E. coli* and *S. cerevisiae*. Obtaining this compound from the natively produced paclitaxel in the bark or leaves of the slow-growing Pacific yew tree (*Taxus brevifolia*) is less sustainable and impractical in the long run as it involves deforestation activities. On the contrary, the heterologous microbial expression could achieve high growth result within a shorter cell cycle (Kemper et al. 2017; Jiang, Stephanopoulos, and Pfeifer 2012). In the attempt of engineering the partitioned synthesis of paclitaxel in *E. coli*, polyisoprene units are generated using units of isopentenyl diphosphate (IPP) through an upstream methylerythritol-phosphate (MEP) pathway is a starting substrate, which then condensed with dimethylallyl diphosphate (DMAPP) via heterologous downstream terpenoid – forming a pathway to form the final active compound in a divided route to optimize the yield of Taxol biosynthesis (Ajikumar et al. 2010). Alternatively, semi-synthesis of the intermediate in Taxol synthesis, the Baccatin III could also be converted to paclitaxel through the inclusion of chemical reactions in the presence of sunlight (Patel et al. 2018).

4.2.1.5 The Harvesting of End Product

Downstream processing can be energy consuming when involving mechanical or chemical cell lysis to release fermentation product accumulated in the cytoplasm which in turn elevates the cost of production as well (Gao et al. 2013). Membrane translocation to secrete desired target proteins into culture supernatant possesses a benefit in the simplification of product recovery as cell disintegration is not required, significantly reducing the subsequent purification and downstream processing steps (Freudl 2018).

Short amino-terminal parts of exported precursor proteins, the signal peptides direct the export of respective proteins in the cytoplasmic membrane. Gram-positive bacteria, bacillus species that usually possess only a single cytoplasmic membrane can therefore export a target protein tagged with the corresponding signal across this major permeable barrier into the growth medium. In the effort of increased secretion of heterologous proteins by bacterial host organism, research on modification of existing signal peptides or *de novo* design of synthetic signal peptides is reported.

A similar attempt was also exhibited in the introduction of lysis genes from bacteriophage into bacteria that produces short-chain length and medium chain length polyhydroxyalkanoates (PHA) (Jung et al. 2005; Martínez et al. 2011). Instead of exporting target proteins out from the cell, this approach utilizes the holin-endolysin lysis mechanism of most bacteriophages, in which oligomerization of holins, the small proteins that allow endolysins to disrupt the host bacterial wall. Permeabilization of a membrane can be controlled by the change in culture conditions, exemplified by success cell lysis provoked by a switch in temperature upon completion of fermentation (Resch et al. 1998). Whereas in the study conducted by Zhang et al., the cell wall collapse was auto-induced when the magnesium concentration of the cell solution dropped upon transfer.

4.2.2 DEVELOPMENT OF AUTOMATED SYSTEMS AND NOVEL TECHNOLOGIES

4.2.2.1 Synthetic Biology

Being the newly emerged field, the cyber-biological system is a potential in catalyzing the progression of the Fifth Industrial Revolution in the second half of the 21st century. In contrast to Industrial Revolution 4.0, the main emphasis switches from cyber-physical systems that use a software-controlled algorithm, to a more complex cyber-biological system. With the existing technology of engineering organisms that can reproduce, encoding control algorithms within DNA in place of the physical electronic devices is possible. This field of study, termed *synthetic biology,* could leverage model-driven biology to go beyond the achievements with cyber-physical systems (Peccoud 2016).

Within the vast applications of synthetic biology, lies the cell-free system as a platform to revolutionize the production of high-value commodities (Tinafar, Jaenes, and Pardee 2019). Cell-free gene expression (CFE) is a system that uses crude cell extract instead of an intact cell to mimic transcription and/or translation of a living cell. This foundational principle made the synthesis of complex biomolecules possible as native cellular transcriptional and translational machinery is being retained in cellular extracts (Silverman, Karim, and Jewett 2020). The requirement of cellular viability, as well as undesirable genetic regulation is eliminated, allowing a bigger degree of freedom in experimental design.

Manipulation of the substrate in reaction, such as supplementing cofactors, ionic liquids, organic solvents exogenously to protein synthesis can be accurately monitored (Wang et al. 2011). Modelling a biological system can be conducted under lesser restriction, in comparison to when growth and maintenance are crucial for cell survival. A wider range of reaction conditions can be adapted, as demonstrated by thermostable enzymes (You and Zhang 2012). Higher levels of organic solvents or toxic chemical compounds can be tolerated by enzymes, subsequently lead to high product titers. Cell-free systems also pose the advantage of yielding a high concentration of product as compared to the living system. This could be demonstrated in a significant increase to 0.95 mol/mol of 1,3-propanediol production from glycerol due to the ability of avoiding by-product losses associated with traditional fermentation (0.6 mol/mol) (Rieckenberg, Ardao, Rujananon, and Zeng 2014).

The absence of a cellular membrane in transporting might overcome the Thauer limit. In a living organism where ATP support is needed, hydrogen yield is capped at four moles per mole of glucose, which an oxidation of glucose with water as an oxidant is often incomplete. In contrast, when transport of substrate across the cellular membrane is no longer necessary, a closer theoretical value of nearly 12 moles of hydrogen per mole of glucose can be yielded (Maeda, Sanchez-Torres, and Wood 2012; Ye et al. 2009). Hence, utilization of carbohydrate as the source of energy can be more efficient if not diverted for cell duplication and by-product formation in a cell (Zhang et al. 2012; Huang and Zhang 2011).

Feasibility of the cell-free system has showcased in the advances for scaling up the reaction volumes of 100 litres with consistency achieved from the same stockpile of reagents (Dudley, Karim, and Jewett 2015; Bundy et al. 2018). Aside from using this system in rapid prototyping of a small-scale design, it is a potential for high-value pharmaceuticals to be produced with this approach. Among the therapeutics expressed in cell-free systems, antibodies and antibody fragments, vaccine antigens, virus-like particles and antimicrobials are essential in drug discovery and development. Coupled with high-throughput feedstock preparation techniques, synthetic biology is poised to accelerate and meet the United Nation's sustainable development goal 3: good health and well-being (Tinafar, Jaenes, and Pardee 2019; Didovyk et al. 2017). As part of the effort to achieve sustainability, accessible treatment for transmissible diseases is crucial in the face of environmental issues and poverty that impacts the quality of many lives. These factors will bring forward the trend of increase in communicable diseases worldwide, hence technologies in tackling an outbreak should be readily available ahead of the occurrence. The ability of synthetic biology could therefore be explored to make it an ideal candidate in speeding up the process of biomanufacturing, especially the application in therapeutics production.

With the advantages poses by synthetic biology, this platform has been further expanded to creating biobatteries. While having the features of smaller environmental footprints, its energy storage densities are superior to the current lithium-ion devices. This biodegradable electrobiochemical cell, known as an enzymatic fuel cell, works by converting chemical energy into electricity using low-cost biocatalyst enzymes (Zhu et al. 2014). The cell is powered by a renewable source, using sugar obtained from starch catabolism. Similar artificial construct is also seen in the production of ATP photosynthetically in a cell-free protein system. These studies are helpful in creating biodevices capable of synthesizing its own constituents by self-sufficient energy (Berhanu, Ueda, and Kuruma 2019; Perez, Stark, and Jewett 2016). Apart from energy storage, a cell-free system stands at an advantage in synthesizing biomaterials. In an example reported by Bawazer et al. 2012, the team successfully synthesized solid-state materials by tailoring *in vitro* protein expression and enzymatic mineralization. The variants were later chosen for their silica or titanium dioxide deposition onto microbeads in the oil-water emulsion, showing the potential of using green chemistry for the deposition of semiconductor materials (Tinafar, Jaenes, and Pardee 2019). In the future, utilizing low-cost, renewable energy from waste or biomass could make industrial manufacturing more environmentally friendly, at the same time lowering its cost.

4.2.2.2 High Throughput and Automation in Processing

In recent years, high throughput and automation have been important additions to the picture of bioproduct manufacturing. The higher success rate is relevant to the reduction of carbon footprint, and the ability to launch a product within a short period of time to meet the sudden growth in demand, for example, mass production of a vaccine upon disease outbreak is crucial. The realization of these goals often starts with experimental design, prior to the upscaling for mass production. One of the strategies, the high throughput screening is useful in optimizing the conditions for recombinant enzyme production. Traditionally, the method of screening relies on the use of shaken flask, fed-batch or chemostat (Büchs 2001). In order to achieve yield upscalable experimental models that could return a quantitative result for analysis, a high throughput strategy combines the control and monitor of microbial strain, medium composition and culture conditions optimization simultaneously (Duetz 2007). This approach utilizes monitored microtiter plate cultivations, including microfluidic (up to 1 mL) and miniscale bioreactors (2 to 100 mL) (Rohe et al. 2012; Lattermann and Büchs 2015).

The microtiter plate is a device that integrates online monitoring of parameters, such as pH, agitation rate, biomass, dissolved oxygen, oxygen transfer, temperatures and humidity through noninvasive optical sensors. On top of that, fluorescently tagged proteins can be used as a marker for gene expression, detectable and controllable online (Bhambure, Kumar, and Rathore 2011; Käß et al. 2014). Parallelization of the microbioreactor stands at an advantage in enabling the incorporation of automated platforms to high-throughput screening and production processes, for instance, Robo-Lector® (M2p-Labs, Aachen, Germany) or in Robotic System (JANUS Integrator, PerkinElmer) (Rohe et al. 2012; Huber et al. 2009; Jacques et al. 2017). Automation of the media preparation, sample tracking and storage in controlling microfluidic bioprocesses has shown to mimic the similar condition when duplicated in larger bioreactors (Oliveira et al. 2016, Blesken et al. 2016). It was reported that the growth behaviour of *E. coli* cultures in 2L laboratory-scale fermenter resembles that of microfluidic microtiter plates, even when fed-batch cultivation is applied (Funke et al. 2010). Success in fed-batch and continuous cultivation of *S. cerevisiae* are also observed with the development of a new microfluidic device which allows 48 stirred tank bioreactors to operate in parallel (Puskeiler et al. 2005; Gebhardt et al. 2011). Process optimization done at a microtiter plate scale showed promising results and potential to be a widespread application at the developmental stage of industrial manufacturing in the near future.

The maturing of bioprocessing technology alone is not sufficient to provide the thrust force necessary to expand biomanufacturing through sustainable approaches. The emergence of new, highly precise genome sequencing and editing tool is of colossal importance to meet the pace of evolution in bioprocessing technologies. In any bioproduction pipeline, the choice of a biological system is the major determinant of the product quality. Nature of a strain used, whether obtained naturally or manipulated has to be driven to its maximum potential by understanding the underlying genetic codes. Characterization of the regulatory architecture of transcriptional networks can be facilitated through advancement in DNA affinity purification sequencing, known as DAP-Seq or DAP-chip (Bartlett et al. 2017; Brown et al. 2019; Hussey et al. 2019). Coupling of next-generation sequencing of a whole genomic library with affinity-purified transcription factors leads to the design of a high throughput profiling method (Bartlett et al. 2017). This fast, low-cost and easily scaled method is an *in vitro* transcription factor binding site discovery assay. It enables a better understanding of individual transcription factor, subsequently allow discovery to accurately control transcriptional changes and gene expression associated with product yield.

The aforementioned high-throughput DNA analysis is also being applied in proteomic analysis. In common, these analyses are capable of processing samples quickly, close to a hundred samples per day (Vowinckel et al. 2018). Improvement in the robustness is required to satisfy the need for a large sample size analysis. Enlargement of sample size might often lead to amplified effects of measurement noise, leading to the effect of batch effects becoming prevalent and stochastic elements that could greatly reduce the number of consistently quantifiable peptides (Vowinckel et al. 2018). Time taken to develop a novel protein discovery pipeline could therefore be shortened with the aid of tools to automate proteomic sample preparation and product validation by data analysis (Chen et al. 2020).

4.2.2.3 Breakthrough of CRISPR-Cas9

The breakthrough of molecular biology was surfaced upon discovery of a genomic tool named CRISPR-Cas9. Based on genomic Clustered Regularly Interspaced Short Palindromic Repeats (CRISPR) and CRISPR-associated proteins (Cas), this technology originated from a prokaryotic defence system (Barrangou et al. 2007; Garneau et al. 2010). It comprises two main components, which the CRISPR RNAs (crRNAs) bind to DNA or RNA sequences of an invader by complementary base pairing, then allows the Cas protein to remove the recognized genetic material (Luo, Leenay, and Beisel 2016). Despite first being unveiled to function as "immunity" in a microorganism, this mechanism is exploited for genomic editing due to the unique feature of spacer sequences that are homologous to foreign plasmid and bacteriophage sequences (Bolotin et al. 2005; Mojica, García-Martínez, and Soria 2005). Among many Cas proteins, Cas9 has been widely accepted in site-specific DNA binding and cleavage in genomic manipulation (Jinek et al. 2013). This nuclease is guided by sgRNA, consisting of a 20 nucleotide guide sequence (Garneau et al. 2010; Gasiunas et al. 2012). The pairing of guide sequence with target DNA, recognized directly upstream of a requisite 5′ protospacer adjacent motif (PAM) associated with protospacer within the DNA target (Barrangou et al. 2007). Subsequently, a double-strand break was stimulated to the targeted genomic locus, mediated by Cas9. Introduction of double-strand breaks gives rise to sequence alterations when repaired by endogenous repair pathway (Horwitz et al. 2015; Ronda et al. 2015; Mans et al. 2015). This is beneficial for researchers to modify and manipulate genomic DNA, in addition to controlling gene expression via the assembly of synthetic transcription factors (Donohoue, Barrangou, and May 2018; Gilbert et al. 2013; Qi et al. 2013).

This programmable tool has fuelled the construction and screening of *in silico* designed strains. In the context of industrial manufacturing, CRISPR-Cas mediated metabolic engineering is applicable in enhancing the performance of a wide range of bacterial species as a cell factory (Mougiakos et al. 2018). This idea is supported by the study in the editing of yeast with CRISPR-Cas9. CRISPR-Cas9 is chosen over other conventional tools due to its capability in introducing double-stranded breaks, which in turn significantly increases the rate of recombination when used in concurrence with an appropriate DNA donor (Jacobs et al. 2014; Min et al. 2016). This could overcome the limitation of lacking robust homologous recombination machinery, or unavailability of suitable selection markers and stable plasmids for the exogenous insertion of DNA in certain yeast strains (Mans et al. 2015; Chen et al. 2020). Furthermore, CRISPR-Cas9 enables multiplexing, which is the targeting of multiple loci simultaneously. Although multiple selection marker is available, the actual practice of multiple recombination events in a single transformation is proven arduous even in model yeast strains. However, with the use of CRISPR-Cas9 along with multiple sgRNAs and donor cassettes, biosynthetic production pathways have been successfully incorporated into *S. cerevisiae* and *Kluyveromyces lactis* via a single transformation event (Horwitz et al. 2015; Mans et al. 2015; Ronda et al. 2015).

Strain engineering using CRISPR-Cas9 is also developed for other industrial used strains, including *Bacillus subtilis* commonly used for the production of the industrial enzyme, improve succinate titer in cyanobacteria and *Streptomyces* species in the discovery of natural products with antimicrobial activity (Li et al. 2016; Altenbuchner 2016; Huang et al. 2015; Tong et al. 2015). Moreover, lactic acid bacterium *Lactobacillus reuteri* has also be engineered using CRISPR-Cas9 due to its probiotic properties, likewise *Clostridium beijerinckii* is capable of producing biochemicals; for instance, acetone and ethanol are also exploited (Oh and van Pijkeren 2014; Wang et al. 2016). The wide application has justified the potential of CRISPR-Cas9 to be a scalable, pragmatic tool for comprehensive modifications of genetic makeup across species of microorganisms (Donohoue, Barrangou, and May 2018).

4.2.3 TOWARDS A CLEANER ENVIRONMENT

The translational of the advances in biotechnology have nurtured the growth of the manufacturing sector towards sustainability. The large scale of biomanufacturing involves the cultivation of microorganisms that requires feedstocks, which mainly are carbon sources. Achieving sustainability can start from the upstream bioprocess, using raw materials that do not have a conflict of interest with human and animal consumption as food or feed.

Proteinaceous whey can be separated from a lactose-rich substrate with a pre-processed step by ultrafiltration, followed by enzymatic hydrolysis which is purposed to concentrate the blend. These additional processes can transform this surplus product from cheese production to raw materials for microbe cultivation (Koller et al. 2012; Ahn, Park, and Lee 2001). Recycling of useful compounds considerably reduces environmental risks connected to disposal of these salty waste streams, preventing the cause of potential eutrophication. Pais et al., 2016 successfully used the surplus as a medium in a batch bioreactor cultivation of *Haloferax mediterranei*, an extremely halophilic organism. This strain could utilize carbon sources in the production of poly(3-hydroxybutyrate-*co*-3-hydroxyvalerate), P(3HB-*co*-3HV), or commonly known as bioplastic. The use of halophilic archaea also stands at an advantage in the recovery of biopolymer, simplifying the downstream processing, in turn potentially reduce the consumption of energy. Therefore, creating an ecosystem conducive for the growth of the strain using waste as a medium of culture is a pivotal strategy to produce an eco-friendly product achieved through sustainable processes. Sustainable production chain was also demonstrated by Kraus et al., where waste extruded from carbohydrate-rich rice bran and starch is used as a substrate for *H. mediterranei*–based PHBHV production. Similarly for cereal-producing industry, wheat milling by-products in the form of hydrolysate contains glucose and maltose beneficial for the growth of *Aspergillus succinogenes* to produce succinic acid (Dorado et al. 2009).

Meanwhile in the agricultural industry, value-addition of waste from apple pomace and apple pomace sludge generated from fruit processing was investigated. The increase in these biodegradable waste is raising concern due to the surge of demand in fruit products. To tackle this issue, employing the waste in microbe cultivation is deemed innovative. Solid-state fermentation is widely implemented in filamentous fungi as they showed efficient growth on complex solid substrates and produce an extensive variety of extracellular products. Nutrient-enriched fruit waste contains a high content of polysaccharides, of which the cellulose, hemicellulose and lignin present could act as natural inducers. These sugar rich compound serve as residues to promote fungal growth, leading to economical production of cellulo- and ligninolytic enzymes (Oberoi et al. 2010; Dhillon, Oberoi, et al. 2011). Instead of supplementing fermentation media with artificial nutrients, utilization of waste provides a good supply of vitamins and other mineral ions, on top of the naturally present citric and malic acid that can be metabolized by cultures (Dhillon, Kaur, and Brar 2013). With the nature of apple pomace to be acidic (pH 3–3.5), it creates a suitable cultivation condition for *Aspergillus niger* (Dhillon, Brar, et al. 2011a,b). Bioproduction of citric acid from this strain can be achieved using readily available apple pomace as substrate, without the need of pretreatment, greatly reducing the environmental footprint in such production. Citric acid is known as a natural metabolic intermediate with GRAS (generally recognized as safe) status, biodegradable and biocompatible. Its market value is considerable by the wide usage across multiple sectors, for instance in the pharmaceutical industry for synthesis of biopolymers for drug delivery and human cell line culture. Additionally, this idea is also expanded to microbiological production of lactic acid using *Lactobacillus rhamnosus* (Dhillon, Oberoi, et al. 2011). Production of enzymes and natural antioxidants that are suitable for commercial use are demonstrated from other types of microorganisms too (Dhillon, Kaur, and Brar 2013).

It is with the hope that industrial use microorganisms can play a dual role in bioremediation, at the same time utilizing the waste as a substrate to generate valuable outputs. Microalgae have been extensively studied from the prospects of cultivation with sewage water, dairy wastewater, swine effluent, anaerobic digestate and brewery effluent (Ummalyma and Sukumaran 2014; Ji et al. 2014; Wu et al. 2013; Cho et al. 2013; Mata et al. 2014). In a research conducted by Usha et al., 2016, microalgae are effective in the removal of nitrate, phosphate, iron and zinc when treated with pulp and paper mill effluent. Accumulation of major fatty acids, including palmitic acid, oleic acid, linoleic acid and α-linolenic acid in harvested biomass suggested their ideal characteristics for biofuel production. Apart from lipid, the presence of protein, vitamins and minerals of microalgae makes them an ideal alternative for fishmeal to improve animal growth in the aquaculture sector (Shah et al. 2018). In this regard, microalgae could be utilized as a platform for several streams of industrial usage while perpetuating the carbon cycle.

4.2.4 CONCLUDING REMARKS

Biomanufacturing of products with industrial value has marked a milestone in the spectrum of sustainable development. In the outlook of the Fifth Industrial Revolution, technologies in molecular biology can be leveraged to expand the study of conventionally manufactured molecules. High throughput and automation strategies need to be further enhanced in post-experimental stages with the aim of running large-scale production in a cost-effective manner. Even though numerous studies had inferred the advantages of biological production, it cannot be denied that the feasibility of these applications is also dependent on public acceptance. Ultimately, the products synthesized using biological systems have to be reviewed in ensuring the product safety, especially to the human body. Upon reaching this goal, greater confidence towards the product can be instilled in consumers, encouraging more producers to adopt the new mode of biomanufacturing while minimizing the adverse effect on the environment.

REFERENCES

Ahn, Woo Suk, Si Jae Park, and Sang Yup Lee. 2001. "Production of poly (3-hydroxybutyrate) from whey by cell recycle fed-batch culture of recombinant *Escherichia coli*." *Biotechnology Letters* 23 (3): 235–240.

Ajikumar, Parayil Kumaran, Wen-Hai Xiao, Keith E. J. Tyo, Yong Wang, Fritz Simeon, Effendi Leonard, Oliver Mucha, Too Heng Phon, Blaine Pfeifer, and Gregory Stephanopoulos. 2010. "Isoprenoid pathway optimization for Taxol precursor overproduction in *Escherichia coli*." *Science (New York, N.Y.)* 330 (6000): 70–74. doi: 10.1126/science.1191652.

Altenbuchner, Josef. 2016. "Editing of the *Bacillus subtilis* genome by the CRISPR-Cas9 system." *Applied and Environmental Microbiology* 82 (17): 5421–5427.

Barrangou, Rodolphe, Christophe Fremaux, Hélène Deveau, Melissa Richards, Patrick Boyaval, Sylvain Moineau, Dennis A. Romero, and Philippe Horvath. 2007. "CRISPR provides acquired resistance against viruses in prokaryotes." *Science* 315 (5819): 1709–1712.

Bartlett, Anna, Ronan C. O'Malley, Shao-Shan Carol Huang, Mary Galli, Joseph R. Nery, Andrea Gallavotti, and Joseph R. Ecker. 2017. "Mapping genome-wide transcription-factor binding sites using DAP-seq." *Nature Protocols* 12 (8): 1659–1672. doi: 10.1038/nprot.2017.055.

Bawazer, Lukmaan A., Michi Izumi, Dmitriy Kolodin, James R. Neilson, Birgit Schwenzer, and Daniel E. Morse. 2012. "Evolutionary selection of enzymatically synthesized semiconductors from biomimetic mineralization vesicles." *Proceedings of the National Academy of Sciences* 109 (26): E1705. doi: 10.1073/pnas.1116958109.

Berhanu, Samuel, Takuya Ueda, and Yutetsu Kuruma. 2019. "Artificial photosynthetic cell producing energy for protein synthesis." *Nature Communications* 10 (1): 1325. doi: 10.1038/s41467-019-09147-4.

Bhambure, Rahul, Kaushal Kumar, and Anurag S. Rathore. 2011. "High-throughput process development for biopharmaceutical drug substances." *Trends in Biotechnology* 29 (3): 127–135.

Blesken, Christian, Till Olfers, Alexander Grimm, and Niklas Frische. 2016. "The microfluidic bioreactor for a new era of bioprocess development." *Engineering in Life Sciences* 16 (2): 190–193.

Bolotin, Alexander, Benoit Quinquis, Alexei Sorokin, and S. Dusko Ehrlich. 2005. "Clustered regularly interspaced short palindrome repeats (CRISPRs) have spacers of extrachromosomal origin." *Microbiology* 151 (8): 2551–2561.

Brown, Katrien, Lazarus T. Takawira, Marja M. O'Neill, Eshchar Mizrachi, Alexander A. Myburg, and Steven G. Hussey. 2019. "Identification and functional evaluation of accessible chromatin associated with wood formation in *Eucalyptus grandis*." *New Phytologist* 223 (4): 1937–1951.

Büchs, Jochen. 2001. "Introduction to advantages and problems of shaken cultures." *Biochemical Engineering Journal* 7 (2): 91–98.

Bundy, Bradley C., J. Porter Hunt, Michael C. Jewett, James R. Swartz, David W. Wood, Douglas D. Frey, and Govind Rao. 2018. "Cell-free biomanufacturing." *Current Opinion in Chemical Engineering* 22: 177–183. doi: https://doi.org/10.1016/j.coche.2018.10.003.

Chen, Qiang, Huafang Lai, Jonathan Hurtado, Jake Stahnke, Kahlin Leuzinger, and Matthew Dent. 2013. "Agroinfiltration as an effective and scalable strategy of gene delivery for production of pharmaceutical proteins." *Advanced Techniques in Biology & Medicine* 1 (1): 103. doi: 10.4172/atbm.1000103.

Chen, Yan, Deepanwita Banerjee, Aindrila Mukhopadhyay, and Christopher J. Petzold. 2020. "Systems and synthetic biology tools for advanced bioproduction hosts." *Current Opinion in Biotechnology* 64: 101–109. doi: https://doi.org/10.1016/j.copbio.2019.12.007.

Cho, Sunja, Nakyeong Lee, Seonghwan Park, Jaecheul Yu, Thanh Thao Luong, You-Kwan Oh, and Taeho Lee. 2013. "Microalgae cultivation for bioenergy production using wastewaters from a municipal WWTP as nutritional sources." *Bioresource Technology* 131: 515–520.

Dale, Jeremy. 2010. *Molecular Genetics of Bacteria/Jeremy W. Dale and Simon F. Park*, 5th edition, edited by Simon Park. Chichester: Wiley-Blackwell.

Dhillon, Gurpreet Singh, Satinder Kaur Brar, Mausam Verma, and Rajeshwar Dayal Tyagi. 2011a. "Apple pomace ultrafiltration sludge—A novel substrate for fungal bioproduction of citric acid: Optimisation studies." *Food Chemistry* 128 (4): 864–871.

Dhillon, Gurpreet Singh, Satinder Kaur Brar, Mausam Verma, and Rajeshwar Dayal Tyagi. 2011b. "Recent advances in citric acid bio-production and recovery." *Food and Bioprocess Technology* 4 (4): 505–529.

Dhillon, Gurpreet Singh, Surinder Kaur, and Satinder Kaur Brar. 2013. "Perspective of apple processing wastes as low-cost substrates for bioproduction of high value products: A review." *Renewable and Sustainable Energy Reviews* 27: 789–805. doi: https://doi.org/10.1016/j.rser.2013.06.046.

Dhillon, Gurpreet Singh, Harinder Singh Oberoi, Surinder Kaur, Sunil Bansal, and Satinder Kaur Brar. 2011. "Value-addition of agricultural wastes for augmented cellulase and xylanase production through solid-state tray fermentation employing mixed-culture of fungi." *Industrial Crops and Products* 34 (1): 1160–1167.

Didovyk, A., T. Tonooka, L. Tsimring, and J. Hasty. 2017. "Rapid and scalable preparation of bacterial lysates for cell-free gene expression." *ACS Synthetic Biology* 6 (12): 2198–2208. doi: 10.1021/acssynbio.7b00253.

Donohoue, Paul D., Rodolphe Barrangou, and Andrew P. May. 2018. "Advances in industrial biotechnology using CRISPR-Cas systems." *Trends in Biotechnology* 36 (2): 134–146. doi: https://doi.org/10.1016/j.tibtech.2017.07.007.

Dorado, M. Pilar, Sze Ki Carol Lin, Apostolis Koutinas, Chenyu Du, Ruohang Wang, and Colin Webb. 2009. "Cereal-based biorefinery development: Utilisation of wheat milling by-products for the production of succinic acid." *Journal of Biotechnology* 143 (1): 51–59. doi: https://doi.org/10.1016/j.jbiotec.2009.06.009.

Dresner, Simon. 2003. "The principles of sustainability." *Management of Environmental Quality: An International Journal* 14 (3): 423.

Dudley, Quentin M., Ashty S. Karim, and Michael C. Jewett. 2015. "Cell-free metabolic engineering: Biomanufacturing beyond the cell." *Biotechnology Journal* 10 (1): 69–82. doi: 10.1002/biot.201400330.

Duetz, Wouter A. 2007. "Microtiter plates as mini-bioreactors: Miniaturization of fermentation methods." *Trends in Microbiology* 15 (10): 469–475.

Freudl, Roland. 2018. "Signal peptides for recombinant protein secretion in bacterial expression systems." *Microbial Cell Factories* 17 (1): 52. doi: 10.1186/s12934-018-0901-3.

Funke, Matthias, Andreas Buchenauer, Uwe Schnakenberg, Wilfried Mokwa, Sylvia Diederichs, Alan Mertens, Carsten Müller, Frank Kensy, and Jochen Büchs. 2010. "Microfluidic biolector—Microfluidic bioprocess control in microtiter plates." *Biotechnology and Bioengineering* 107 (3): 497–505.

Gao, Yongqiang, Xinjun Feng, Mo Xian, Qi Wang, and Guang Zhao. 2013. "Inducible cell lysis systems in microbial production of bio-based chemicals." *Applied Microbiology and Biotechnology* 97 (16): 7121–7129. doi: 10.1007/s00253-013-5100-x.

Garneau, Josiane E., Marie-Ève Dupuis, Manuela Villion, Dennis A. Romero, Rodolphe Barrangou, Patrick Boyaval, Christophe Fremaux, Philippe Horvath, Alfonso H. Magadán, and Sylvain Moineau. 2010. "The CRISPR/Cas bacterial immune system cleaves bacteriophage and plasmid DNA." *Nature* 468 (7320): 67–71.

Gasiunas, Giedrius, Rodolphe Barrangou, Philippe Horvath, and Virginijus Siksnys. 2012. "Cas9–crRNA ribonucleoprotein complex mediates specific DNA cleavage for adaptive immunity in bacteria." *Proceedings of the National Academy of Sciences* 109 (39): E2579–E2586.

Gebhardt, Gabi, Ralf Hortsch, Klaus Kaufmann, Matthias Arnold, and Dirk Weuster-Botz. 2011. "A new microfluidic concept for parallel operated milliliter-scale stirred tank bioreactors." *Biotechnology Progress* 27 (3): 684–690.

Gilbert, Luke A., Matthew H. Larson, Leonardo Morsut, Zairan Liu, Gloria A. Brar, Sandra E. Torres, Noam Stern-Ginossar, Onn Brandman, Evan H. Whitehead, and Jennifer A. Doudna. 2013. "CRISPR-mediated modular RNA-guided regulation of transcription in eukaryotes." *Cell* 154 (2): 442–451.

Guo, Su, Jia-jie Tang, Dong-zhi Wei, and Wei Wei. 2014. "Construction of a shuttle vector for protein secretory expression in *Bacillus subtilis* and the application of the mannanase functional heterologous expression." *Journal of Microbiology and Biotechnology* 24 (4): 431–439.

Horwitz, Andrew A., Jessica M. Walter, Max G. Schubert, Stephanie H. Kung, Kristy Hawkins, Darren M. Platt, Aaron D. Hernday, Tina Mahatdejkul-Meadows, Wayne Szeto, and Sunil S. Chandran. 2015. "Efficient multiplexed integration of synergistic alleles and metabolic pathways in yeasts via CRISPR-Cas." *Cell Systems* 1 (1): 88–96.

Huang, He, Guosong Zheng, Weihong Jiang, Haifeng Hu, and Yinhua Lu. 2015. "One-step high-efficiency CRISPR/Cas9-mediated genome editing in Streptomyces." *Acta Biochimica et Biophysica Sinica* 47 (4): 231–243.

Huang, Wei-Dong, and Y.-H. Percival Zhang. 2011. "Analysis of biofuels production from sugar based on three criteria: Thermodynamics, bioenergetics, and product separation." *Energy & Environmental Science* 4 (3): 784–792.

Huber, Robert, Daniel Ritter, Till Hering, Anne-Kathrin Hillmer, Frank Kensy, Carsten Müller, Le Wang, and Jochen Büchs. 2009. "Robo-Lector–a novel platform for automated high-throughput cultivations in microtiter plates with high information content." *Microbial Cell Factories* 8 (1): 42.

Hussey, Steven G., Jacqueline Grima-Pettenati, Alexander A. Myburg, Eshchar Mizrachi, Siobhan M. Brady, Yasuo Yoshikuni, and Samuel Deutsch. 2019. "A standardized synthetic eucalyptus transcription factor and promoter panel for re-engineering secondary cell wall regulation in biomass and bioenergy crops." *ACS Synthetic Biology* 8 (2): 463–465.

Jacobs, Jake Z., Keith M. Ciccaglione, Vincent Tournier, and Mikel Zaratiegui. 2014. "Implementation of the CRISPR-Cas9 system in fission yeast." *Nature Communications* 5 (1): 1–5.

Jacques, Philippe, Max Béchet, Muriel Bigan, Delphine Caly, Gabrielle Chataigné, François Coutte, Christophe Flahaut, Egon Heuson, Valérie Leclère, Didier Lecouturier, Vincent Phalip, Rozenn Ravallec, Pascal Dhulster, and Rénato Froidevaux. 2017. "High-throughput strategies for the discovery and engineering of enzymes for biocatalysis." *Bioprocess and Biosystems Engineering* 40 (2): 161–180. doi: 10.1007/s00449-016-1690-x.

James M. Clomburg, Anna M. Crumbley, Ramon Gonzalez. 2017. "Industrial biomanufacturing: The future of chemical production." *Science* 355 (6320): 1–10

Ji, Min-Kyu, Akhil N. Kabra, El-Sayed Salama, Hyun-Seog Roh, Jung Rae Kim, Dae Sung Lee, and Byong-Hun Jeon. 2014. "Effect of mine wastewater on nutrient removal and lipid production by a green microalga Micratinium reisseri from concentrated municipal wastewater." *Bioresource Technology* 157: 84–90.

Jiang, Ming, Gregory Stephanopoulos, and Blaine A. Pfeifer. 2012. "Toward biosynthetic design and implementation of *Escherichia coli*-derived paclitaxel and other heterologous polyisoprene compounds." *Applied and Environmental Microbiology* 78 (8): 2497–2504. doi: 10.1128/AEM.07391-11.

Jinek, Martin, Alexandra East, Aaron Cheng, Steven Lin, Enbo Ma, and Jennifer Doudna. 2013. "RNA-programmed genome editing in human cells." *eLife* 2: e00471.

Jocelyn, E. Krebs, Benjamin Lewin, Elliott S. Goldstein and Stephen T. Kilpatrick. 2014. *Lewin's Genes XI*. 11th ed. Burlington, MA: Jones & Bartlett Learning.

Jung, Il Lae, Ki Heon Phyo, Kug Chan Kim, Hyo Kook Park, and In Gyu Kim. 2005. "Spontaneous liberation of intracellular polyhydroxybutyrate granules in *Escherichia coli*." *Research in Microbiology* 156 (8): 865–873.

Käß, Friedrich, Arjun Prasad, Jana Tillack, Matthias Moch, Heiner Giese, Jochen Büchs, Wolfgang Wiechert, and Marco Oldiges. 2014. "Rapid assessment of oxygen transfer impact for *Corynebacterium glutamicum*." *Bioprocess and Biosystems Engineering* 37 (12): 2567–2577.

Kemper, K., M. Hirte, M. Reinbold, M. Fuchs, and T. Brück. 2017. "Opportunities and challenges for the sustainable production of structurally complex diterpenoids in recombinant microbial systems." *Beilstein Journal of Organic Chemistry* 13: 845–854. doi: 10.3762/bjoc.13.85.

Koller, Martin, Anna Salerno, Alexander Muhr, Angelika Reiterer, Emo Chiellini, Sergio Casella, Predrag Horvat, and Gerhart Braunegg. 2012. "Whey lactose as a raw material for microbial production of biodegradable polyesters." *Polyester* 347: 51–92.

Lattermann, Clemens, and Jochen Büchs. 2015. "Microscale and miniscale fermentation and screening." *Current Opinion in Biotechnology* 35: 1–6.

Leung, David W. 1989. "A method for random mutagenesis of a defined DNA segment using a modified polymerase chain reaction." *Technique* 1: 11–15.

Li, Hung, Claire R. Shen, Chun-Hung Huang, Li-Yu Sung, Meng-Ying Wu, and Yu-Chen Hu. 2016. "CRISPR-Cas9 for the genome engineering of cyanobacteria and succinate production." *Metabolic Engineering* 38: 293–302. doi: https://doi.org/10.1016/j.ymben.2016.09.006.

Luo, Michelle L., Ryan T. Leenay, and Chase L. Beisel. 2016. "Current and future prospects for CRISPR-based tools in bacteria." *Biotechnology and Bioengineering* 113 (5): 930–943. doi: 10.1002/bit.25851.

Madigan, Michael T., Kelly S. Bender, Daniel H. Buckley, W. Matthew Sattley, and David A. Stahl. 2018. *Brock Biology of Microorganisms*. 15th ed. United Kingdom: Pearson Education Limited.

Maeda, Toshinari, Viviana Sanchez-Torres, and Thomas K. Wood. 2012. "Hydrogen production by recombinant *Escherichia coli* strains." *Microbial Biotechnology* 5 (2): 214–225. doi: 10.1111/j.1751-7915.2011.00282.x.

Mans, Robert, Harmen M. van Rossum, Melanie Wijsman, Antoon Backx, Niels G.A. Kuijpers, Marcel van den Broek, Pascale Daran-Lapujade, Jack T. Pronk, Antonius J.A. van Maris, and Jean-Marc G. Daran. 2015. "CRISPR/Cas9: A molecular Swiss army knife for simultaneous introduction of multiple genetic modifications in *Saccharomyces cerevisiae*." *FEMS Yeast Research* 15 (2): 1–15.

Martínez, Virginia, Pedro García, José Luis García, and María Auxiliadora Prieto. 2011. "Controlled autolysis facilitates the polyhydroxyalkanoate recovery in *Pseudomonas putida* KT2440." *Microbial Biotechnology* 4 (4): 533–547.

Mata, Teresa M., Adélio M. Mendes, Nídia S. Caetano, and António A. Martins. 2014. "Sustainability and economic evaluation of microalgae grown in brewery wastewater." *Bioresource Technology* 168: 151–158.

McCullum, Elizabeth O., Berea A.R. Williams, Jinglei Zhang, and John C. Chaput. 2010. "Random mutagenesis by error-prone PCR." In *In Vitro Mutagenesis Protocols*, 103–109. Springer.

Mello, Craig C., and Darryl Conte. 2004. *Revealing the World of RNA Interference*. Nature Publishing Group.

Min, Kyunghun, Yuichi Ichikawa, Carol A. Woolford, and Aaron P. Mitchell. 2016. "*Candida albicans* gene deletion with a transient CRISPR-Cas9 system." *MSphere* 1 (3): 1–9.

Mojica, Francisco J.M., Jesús García-Martínez, and Elena Soria. 2005. "Intervening sequences of regularly spaced prokaryotic repeats derive from foreign genetic elements." *Journal of Molecular Evolution* 60 (2): 174–182.

Mougiakos, Ioannis, Elleke F. Bosma, Joyshree Ganguly, John van der Oost, and Richard van Kranenburg. 2018. "Hijacking CRISPR-Cas for high-throughput bacterial metabolic engineering: Advances and prospects." *Current Opinion in Biotechnology* 50: 146–157. doi: https://doi.org/10.1016/j.copbio.2018.01.002.

Oberoi, Harinder Singh, Yogita Chavan, Sunil Bansal, and Gurpreet Singh Dhillon. 2010. "Production of cellulases through solid state fermentation using kinnow pulp as a major substrate." *Food and Bioprocess Technology* 3 (4): 528–536.

Oh, Jee-Hwan, and Jan-Peter van Pijkeren. 2014. "CRISPR–Cas9-assisted recombineering in *Lactobacillus reuteri*." *Nucleic Acids Research* 42 (17): e131–e131. doi: 10.1093/nar/gku623.

Oliveira, Aline F., Amanda C.S.N. Pessoa, Reinaldo G. Bastos, and Lucimara G. de la Torre. 2016. "Microfluidic tools toward industrial biotechnology." *Biotechnology Progress* 32 (6): 1372–1389.

Ozsolak, Fatih, and Patrice M. Milos. 2011. "RNA sequencing: Advances, challenges and opportunities." *Nature Reviews Genetics* 12 (2): 87–98. doi: 10.1038/nrg2934.

Pais, Joana, Luísa S. Serafim, Filomena Freitas, and Maria A.M. Reis. 2016. "Conversion of cheese whey into poly(3-hydroxybutyrate-co-3-hydroxyvalerate) by *Haloferax mediterranei*." *New Biotechnology* 33 (1): 224–230. doi: https://doi.org/10.1016/j.nbt.2015.06.001.

Patel, Vikas K., Khan M. Sarim, Akash K. Patel, Prasant K. Rout, and Alok Kalra. 2018. "Chapter 14—Synthetic microbial ecology and nanotechnology for the production of Taxol and its precursors: A step towards sustainable production of cancer therapeutics." In *Design of Nanostructures for Theranostics Applications*, edited by Alexandru Mihai Grumezescu, 563–587. William Andrew Publishing.

Peccoud, Jean. 2016. "Synthetic biology: Fostering the cyber-biological revolution." *Synthetic Biology* 1 (1). doi: 10.1093/synbio/ysw001.

Perez, Jessica G., Jessica C. Stark, and Michael C. Jewett. 2016. "Cell-free synthetic biology: Engineering beyond the cell." *Cold Spring Harbor Perspectives in Biology* 8 (12): a023853. doi: 10.1101/cshperspect.a023853.

Puskeiler, Robert, Andreas Kusterer, Gernot T. John, and Dirk Weuster-Botz. 2005. "Miniature bioreactors for automated high-throughput bioprocess design (HTBD): Reproducibility of parallel fed-batch cultivations with *Escherichia coli*." *Biotechnology and Applied Biochemistry* 42 (3): 227–235.

Qi, Lei S., Matthew H. Larson, Luke A. Gilbert, Jennifer A. Doudna, Jonathan S. Weissman, Adam P. Arkin, and Wendell A. Lim. 2013. "Repurposing CRISPR as an RNA-guided platform for sequence-specific control of gene expression." *Cell* 152 (5): 1173–1183.

Resch, S., K. Gruber, G. Wanner, S. Slater, D. Dennis, and W. Lubitz. 1998. "Aqueous release and purification of poly (β-hydroxybutyrate) from *Escherichia coli*." *Journal of Biotechnology* 65 (2–3): 173–182.

Rieckenberg, Fabian, Inés Ardao, Rosarin Rujananon, and An-Ping Zeng. 2014. "Cell-free synthesis of 1, 3-propanediol from glycerol with a high yield." *Engineering in Life Sciences* 14 (4): 380–386.

Rohe, Peter, Deepak Venkanna, Britta Kleine, Roland Freudl, and Marco Oldiges. 2012. "An automated workflow for enhancing microbial bioprocess optimization on a novel microbioreactor platform." *Microbial Cell Factories* 11 (1): 1–14.

Rojas-Downing, M. Melissa, A. Pouyan Nejadhashemi, Timothy Harrigan, Sean A. Woznicki. 2017. "Climate change and livestock: Impacts, adaptation, and mitigation." *Climate Risk Management* 16: 145–163. doi: http://dx.doi.org/10.1016/j.crm.2017.02.001.

Ronda, Carlotta, Jérôme Maury, Tadas Jakočiūnas, Simo Abdessamad Baallal Jacobsen, Susanne Manuela Germann, Scott James Harrison, Irina Borodina, Jay D. Keasling, Michael Krogh Jensen, and Alex Toftgaard Nielsen. 2015. "CrEdit: CRISPR mediated multi-loci gene integration in *Saccharomyces cerevisiae*." *Microbial Cell Factories* 14 (1): 97.

Shah, Mahfuzur Rahman, Giovanni Antonio Lutzu, Asraful Alam, Pallab Sarker, M.A. Kabir Chowdhury, Ali Parsaeimehr, Yuanmei Liang, and Maurycy Daroch. 2018. "Microalgae in aquafeeds for a sustainable aquaculture industry." *Journal of Applied Phycology* 30 (1): 197–213. doi: 10.1007/s10811-017-1234-z.

Silverman, Adam D., Ashty S. Karim, and Michael C. Jewett. 2020. "Cell-free gene expression: An expanded repertoire of applications." *Nature Reviews Genetics* 21 (3): 151–170. doi: 10.1038/s41576-019-0186-3.

Tessaleno C. Devezas, António M. Vaz, Christopher L. Magee. 2017. "Global pattern in materials consumption: An empirical study." *Industry 4.0* 263–292. doi: https://doi-org.ezproxy.nottingham.ac.uk/10.1007/978-3-319-49604-7_14.

Theologis, Athanasios. 2001. "Goodbye to 'one by one' genetics." *Genome Biology* 2 (4): comment2004.1. doi: 10.1186/gb-2001-2-4-comment2004.

Thomason, Maureen Kiley, and Gisela Storz. 2010. "Bacterial antisense RNAs: How many are there, and what are they doing?" *Annual Review of Genetics* 44: 167–188.

Tian, Bin, Philip C. Bevilacqua, Amy Diegelman-Parente, and Michael B. Mathews. 2004. "The double-stranded-RNA-binding motif: Interference and much more." *Nature Reviews Molecular Cell Biology* 5 (12): 1013–1023.

Tinafar, Aidan, Katariina Jaenes, and Keith Pardee. 2019. "Synthetic biology goes cell-free." *BMC Biology* 17 (1): 64. doi: 10.1186/s12915-019-0685-x.

Tong, Yaojun, Pep Charusanti, Lixin Zhang, Tilmann Weber, and Sang Yup Lee. 2015. "CRISPR-Cas9 based engineering of actinomycetal genomes." *ACS Synthetic Biology* 4 (9): 1020–1029.

Ummalyma, Sabeela Beevi, and Rajeev K. Sukumaran. 2014. "Cultivation of microalgae in dairy effluent for oil production and removal of organic pollution load." *Bioresource Technology* 165: 295–301.

Usha, M.T., T. Sarat Chandra, R. Sarada, and V.S. Chauhan. 2016. "Removal of nutrients and organic pollution load from pulp and paper mill effluent by microalgae in outdoor open pond." *Bioresource Technology* 214: 856–860. doi: https://doi.org/10.1016/j.biortech.2016.04.060.

Vowinckel, Jakob, Aleksej Zelezniak, Roland Bruderer, Michael Mülleder, Lukas Reiter, and Markus Ralser. 2018. "Cost-effective generation of precise label-free quantitative proteomes in high-throughput by microLC and data-independent acquisition." *Scientific Reports* 8 (1): 4346. doi: 10.1038/s41598-018-22610-4.

Wang, Yi, Zhong-Tian Zhang, Seung-Oh Seo, Patrick Lynn, Ting Lu, Yong-Su Jin, and Hans P. Blaschek. 2016. "Bacterial genome editing with CRISPR-Cas9: Deletion, integration, single nucleotide modification, and desirable 'clean' mutant selection in *Clostridium beijerinckii* as an example." *ACS Synthetic Biology* 5 (7): 721–732.

Wang, Yiran, Weidong Huang, Noppadon Sathitsuksanoh, Zhiguang Zhu, and Y.-H. Percival Zhang. 2011. "Biohydrogenation from biomass sugar mediated by *in vitro* synthetic enzymatic pathways." *Chemistry & Biology* 18 (3): 372–380.

Wink, Michael, A. Wilhelm Alfermann, Rochus Franke, Bernhard Wetterauer, Melanie Distl, Jörg Windhövel, Oliver Krohn, Elisabeth Fuss, Hermann Garden, and Abdolali Mohagheghzadeh. 2005. "Sustainable bioproduction of phytochemicals by plant *in vitro* cultures: Anticancer agents." *Plant Genetic Resources* 3 (2): 90–100.

Wu, Pei-Fen, Jui-Chin Teng, Yun-Huin Lin, and Sz-Chwun John Hwang. 2013. "Increasing algal biofuel production using *Nannocholropsis oculata* cultivated with anaerobically and aerobically treated swine wastewater." *Bioresource Technology* 133: 102–108.

Ye, Xinhao, Yiran Wang, Robert C. Hopkins, Michael W.W. Adams, Barbara R. Evans, Jonathan R. Mielenz, and Y.-H. Percival Zhang. 2009. "Spontaneous high-yield production of hydrogen from cellulosic materials and water catalyzed by enzyme cocktails." *ChemSusChem: Chemistry & Sustainability Energy & Materials* 2 (2): 149–152.

You, Chun, and Y.-H. Percival Zhang. 2012. "Cell-free biosystems for biomanufacturing." In *Future Trends in Biotechnology*, 89–119. Springer.

Zhang, Yi-Heng Percival, Jibin Sun, and Yanhe Ma. 2017. "Biomanufacturing: History and perspective." *Industrial Microbiology and Biotechnology* 44: 773–784. doi: 10.1007/s10295-016-1863-2.

Zhang, Y. H. Percival, Chun You, Hongge Chen, and Rui Feng. 2012. "Surpassing photosynthesis: High-efficiency and scalable CO_2 utilization through artificial photosynthesis." In *Recent Advances in Post-Combustion CO_2 Capture Chemistry*, 275–292. American Chemical Society.

Zhu, Z., T. Kin Tam, F. Sun, C. You, and Y.H. Percival Zhang. 2014. "A high-energy-density sugar biobattery based on a synthetic enzymatic pathway." *Nature Communications* 5: 3026. doi: 10.1038/ncomms4026.

5.0 Industrial Perspective of Industry 5.0

Apurav Krishna Koyande, Vishno Vardhan Devadas, Kit Wayne Chew, and Pau Loke Show

CONTENTS

5.0.1 WHAT ARE THE MOST APPARENT CHANGES IN IR 5.0 FROM IR 4.0?

Industrial Revolution 4.0 (IR 4.0), was a revolution where data collected from machinery sensors was interpreted by a human. The data was often analyzed to find pattern similarities to predict future demands. Collecting pattern similarities helps an industry to optimize industrial operation toward sustainable plantwide control. Utilities such as electricity and water demand of an operation can be reduced effectively. Figure 5.0.1 depicts the timeline of Industrial Revolutions from the beginning. Industrial Revolution 5.0 (IR 5.0), is a parallel industrial revolution to IR 4.0, where artificial intelligence (AI) creates knowledge from thinking and learning autonomously from data collected from machines. In other words, synergy between artificial intelligence (AI) and humans will generate creative ideas with critical judgments in IR 5.0. However, IR 5.0 has an impact on the labor pool compared to IR 4.0 in employment as the workforce is replaced by AI-automated machines (Salimova et al. 2019).

Senior laborers of Baby Boomers and the X and Y generation will face difficulties in adapting to the new industrial revolution as the Z generation easily adapts to the digital environment (Berkup 2014). Furthermore, AI automation in IR 5.0 reduces the workforce infrastructure requirements by saving the environment from the exploitation of natural resources. It has also been stated that a country in IR 5.0 with AI-automated machines will eliminate revolution lags among growing countries within a short period compared to IR 4.0; 24-hour AI-operated machines

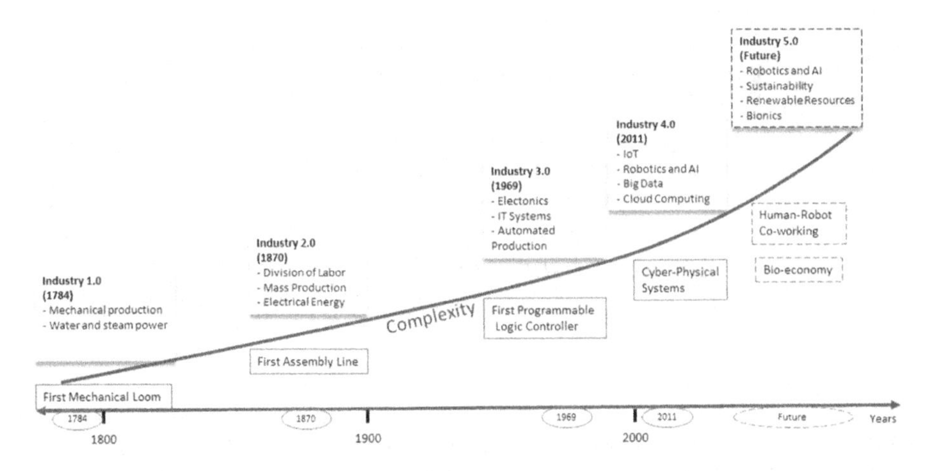

FIGURE 5.0.1 Timeline of every Industrial Revolution (Demir, Döven, and Sezen 2019).

results in higher and faster output efficiency compared to a conventional 8-hour labor force in IR 4.0 (Bahrin et al. 2016). Hence, the economic growth of a country in IR 5.0 will exponentially increase with the reduction of energy consumption using AI-automated machines in manufacturing eco-friendly sustainable products. Aside from economic changes in IR 5.0 from IR 4.0, AI also plays an important role in decision making on par with humans in the future. In other words, AI will refer in any decision-making situation to expand or improve an existing business; Deep Knowledge Ventures, Hong Kong, uses an AI algorithm called VITAL (Validating Investment Tool for Advancing Life Sciences) as a part of the board of directors to provide intelligent investment recommendations in the life science factor (Schwab 2017). This is because an AI algorithm makes future decisions faster by comparing the data collected previously in the system. It is also rational and less biased to the decision it makes in a problem-solving situation compared to humans. However, accountability must be taken into consideration by appointing chief officers with well-versed AI backgrounds to approve or execute decisions made by AI algorithms in business (Nahavandi 2019). In conclusion, the changes in IR 5.0 from IR 4.0 have positive and negative impacts in society as humans and AI collaborate to generate creative ideas with effective judgments by saving the environment from exploitation of natural resources.

5.0.2 WHAT IS THE DEMAND FROM THE COMMUNITY THAT CAN MAKE IR 5.0 SUCCESSFUL FROM AN INDUSTRIAL SCALE?

The demand from the community that can make IR 5.0 successful from an industrial scale is first by changing analog to a digital mindset of leaders. A traditional mindset of an analog leader about data and information management is more toward storing and centralizing. However, the modern mindset of a digital leader regarding data and information management should be toward open, transperant, shared and easily accessible data. Thus, an analog mindset leader processes his/her data sequentially slowly and a digital mindset processes data rapidly and multidimensionally (Kelly 2019). To make IR 5.0 successful, these leaders must quickly adapt to the technology by shaping their businesses toward a sustainable and fast and efficient goal by the synergy between artificial intelligence (AI) and humans to generate creative ideas with critical judgments (Daugherty and Wilson 2018). The second demand from the community that can make IR 5.0 successful from an industrial scale is by having a society that wants to make real-time decisions with a verified and validated concrete conclusion based on data collected. Humans usually solve problems with the analytical or intuitive decision based on their work experience, imagination and creativity but an AI solves the problem with an analytical decision involving in-depth data analysis that is most effective in overcoming complex problems (Jarrahi 2018). The third demand that can make IR 5.0 successful from an industrial scale is by having a society with a home automated system using AI. The benefits of home automation include interaction with monitoring of people 24/7, detection of suspicious activity, fire detection with emergency responses, shutting blinds, arranging work meetings, controling the temperature of rooms with AC and fan, speaking various languages and playing songs, etc. Thus, this technology allows humans to manage and collect data of the house that is useful in overall home security, saving electricity and water utilities efficiently. Home automation with AI can also replace conventional switches or RC remotes in the future, as it is very beneficial to elderly, disabled, injured and pregnant people (Tripathi et al. 2017). The last demand from the community that can make IR 5.0 successful from an industrial scale is having low and reliable cost benefits of AI automation in their daily lifestyle. Since AI automation will be the first generation in IR 5.0, the cost of installation and maintenance will be high, which makes the society use the traditional labor workforce for their business. In conclusion, AI automation in IR 5.0 can be successful if the algorithms are reliable and cheap and society has a digital mindset over analog, makes real-time decisions with a verified and validate concrete conclusion and home automation interests.

5.0.3 HOW CAN IR 5.0 BE IMPLEMENTED IN THE INDUSTRY WHILE MAINTAINING A GOOD COST-BENEFIT MARGIN?

A good cost-benefit margin in an industry indicates company or business sales have generated profit. To implement IR 5.0 in an industry while maintaining a good cost-benefit margin, first, the company needs to allocate a budget for a small project which will be fully operated using AI-automated machines to conduct cost-benefit margin analysis. This method allows the business leader to analyze the cost-benefit data obtained and compare the profit made before and after implementing IR 5.0 in the project. Thus, the leader can implement IR 5.0 technology in all the business operations while maintaining a good cost-benefit margin (Akdil, Ustundag, and Cevikcan 2018). Secondly, the government must have a local AI-automated machine service, which reduces the cost of investment for fast-growing local companies. Thus, the government can make Industrial 5.0 a strong job creation opportunity, which increases the local production rate of these machines and competes with other countries. Thirdly, the government must wave taxes for companies who implement

IR 5.0, as AI-automated machines operate efficiently, which saves energy and the environment (Kamble, Gunasekaran, and Sharma 2018). This allows an industry to cut down government taxes to allocate a budget on replacing production line to AI-automated machines (Sommer 2015). Fourthly, the government must form an IR 5.0 consultant firm to help industries by supporting them to adopt this technology in their business. This consultant firm must have software that can calculate the cost-benefit margin of a business if an IR 5.0 is implemented in the production line or services. Thus, this method gives a clear path for an industry to implement IR 5.0 in the business by keeping a good cost-benefit margin. Fifthly, an industry must carry out in-depth analysis as its research and development section of the company. An in-depth analysis must include the degree of AI automation required in the industry to maintain a good cost-benefit margin (Rao and Prasad 2018). Sixthly, an industry must conduct simulation at an early stage to implement IR 5.0 in business. This simulation provides details such as raw material usages and utility usages and compares the investment cost with cost-benefit margins. Thus, this method helps an industry to identify errors at the design state of the IR 5.0 implementation in business by maintaining a good cost-benefit margin (Ghobakhloo 2018). Lastly, an industry must use big data technology in their business, as this algorithm processes data accurately with an integrated sensor system. These data are then uploaded and stored in the cloud to further analyze the pattern obtained to optimize the production line of a business. Thus, this algorithm allows an industry to implement IR 5.0 while maintaining a good cost-benefit margin in the business (Zhou, Liu, and Zhou 2015).

5.0.4 HOW MUCH WILL INDUSTRIES BE WILLING TO ADAPT AND CHANGE TO IR 5.0?

The synergy between artificial intelligence (AI) and humans in IR 5.0 expands the capability of industry to monitor their automated production line to produce a customized product based on customers' demand in a most efficient way to speed up the production in the market by saving operational cost of utilities (Li, Hou, and Wu 2017). Thus, an industry who adapts and changes to IR 5.0 will be on par with service competitiveness in the market by keeping their products or services at high quality, have environmental savings and have their health safety managed using these AI algorithms (Berawi 2018). Furthermore, AI-automated robot and cobot in an industry is easy to set up, safe to operate for dangerous jobs and customizable depending on operation needs. They are capable of operating faster and most importantly efficient compared to a conventional labor workforce. Industries that are involved with simulation can save time by using an AI algorithm as it brings imagination into a 3D hologram model; mining and construction industries, geotechnical oil and gas industries, product research and development industries, automotive design and assembly industries and educational research institutes can use AI in their simulation to analyze and develop 3D models faster and efficiently to improve their products or services (Gerbert et al. 2015). The maritime industry is already using big data in most of their operations, such as manipulating the speed of vessels at optimum based on data patterns obtained to save fuel consumption. This industry also uses real-time tracking dashboards to predict the arrival of a vessel to manage onshore berth for loading-backloading services or maintenance work. Thus, the maritime industry will be willing to adapt and change to IR 5.0, as IR 4.0 is already being implemented in most of their operations, and besides, AI algorithms will make the industry operations efficient. In Malaysia, Malaysian Digital Economy Corporation (MDEC) and GRAB have collaborated to share real-time traffic data in Klang Valley. These data improve transportation issues in Klang Valley, such as increasing the emergency response time by detecting vehicle speed and lane-changing responses and reducing traffic congestion by manipulating traffic lights (Tariq 2018). This real-time data also increases the safety of people in Klang Valley as it collects information on a car's location with the registration number. Thus, this industry will be willing to adapt to IR 5.0, as IR 4.0 is already being implemented and besides, AI algorithms will ease their operation and indicate traffic activity faster and efficiently. The land development industry can increase the sales of people's investments by bringing IR 5.0 technology in the housing development. Technologies such as home automation can gain interest as it allows people to manage home devices in one place, maximizes home security and saves the usage of utilities. This industry also can use motion sensors in the malls to automate the AC depending on the most and least concentrated people movement to save electricity. Thus, land development industries will be willing to adapt to IR 5.0 as it saves the environment from exploitation and increases the sales of the development. In conclusion, industries are willing to adapt to IR 5.0 because AI automation can increase and improve the efficiency of the business operations.

REFERENCES

Akdil, Kartal Yagiz, Alp Ustundag, and Emre Cevikcan. 2018. "Maturity and Readiness Model for Industry 4.0 Strategy." In *Industry 4.0: Managing the Digital Transformation*, 61–94. Cham: Springer International Publishing. doi:10.1007/978-3-319-57870-5_4.

Bahrin, Mohd Aiman Kamarul, Mohd Fauzi Othman, Nor Hayati Nor Azli, and Muhamad Farihin Talib. 2016. "Industry 4.0: A review on industrial automation and robotic." *Jurnal Teknologi* 78 (6–13). doi:10.11113/jt.v78.9285.

Berawi, Mohammed Ali. 2018. "The fourth Industrial Revolution: Managing technology development for competitiveness." *International Journal of Technology* 1: 1–4. doi:10.14716/ijtech.v9i1.1504.

Berkup, Sezin Baysal. 2014. "Working with generations X and Y in generation Z period: Management of different generations in business life." *Mediterranean Journal of Social Sciences* 5 (19): 218–229. doi:10.5901/mjss.2014.v5n19p218.

Daugherty, Paul R., and James H. Wilson. 2018. *Human + Machine: Reimagining Work in the Age of AI*. 1st ed. Boston: Harvard Business Review Press.

Demir, Kadir Alpaslan, Gözde Döven, and Bülent Sezen. 2019. "Industry 5.0 and human-robot co-working." *Procedia Computer Science* 158: 688–695. doi:10.1016/j.procs.2019.09.104.

Gerbert, Philipp, Markus Lorenz, Michael Rüßmann, Manuela Waldner, Jan Justus, Pascal Engel, and Michael Harnisch. 2015. *Industry 4.0: The Future of Productivity and Growth in Manufacturing Industries*. Boston Consultation Group. https://www.bcg.com/publications/2015/engineered_products_project_business_industry_4_future_productivity_growth_manufacturing_industries.aspx.

Ghobakhloo, Morteza. 2018. "The future of manufacturing industry: A strategic roadmap toward Industry 4.0." *Journal of Manufacturing Technology Management* 29 (6): 910–936. doi:10.1108/JMTM-02-2018-0057.

Jarrahi, Mohammad Hossein. 2018. "Artificial intelligence and the future of work: Human-AI symbiosis in organizational decision making." *Business Horizons* 61 (4): 577–586. doi:10.1016/j.bushor.2018.03.007.

Kamble, Sachin S., Angappa Gunasekaran, and Rohit Sharma. 2018. "Analysis of the driving and dependence power of barriers to adopt Industry 4.0 in Indian manufacturing industry." *Computers in Industry* 101 (October): 107–119. doi:10.1016/j.compind.2018.06.004.

Kelly, Richard. 2019. *Constructing Leadership 4.0: Swarm Leadership and the Fourth Industrial Revolution*. Switzerland: Springer International Publishing AG. doi:10.1007/978-3-319-98062-1.

Li, Guoping, Yun Hou, and Aizhi Wu. 2017. "Fourth Industrial Revolution: Technological drivers, impacts and coping methods." *Chinese Geographical Science* 27 (August). Science Press: 626–637. doi:10.1007/s11769-017-0890-x.

Nahavandi, Saeid. 2019. "Industry 5.0—A human-centric solution." *Sustainability* 11 (16): 1–13. Article ID: 4371. doi:10.3390/su11164371.

Rao, Sriganesh K., and Ramjee Prasad. 2018. "Impact of 5G technologies on Industry 4.0." *Wireless Personal Communications* 100 (1): 145–159. doi:10.1007/s11277-018-5615-7.

Salimova, Tatyana, Nadezhda Guskova, Irina Krakovskaya, and Efim Sirota. 2019. "From Industry 4.0 to Society 5.0: Challenges for sustainable competitiveness of Russian industry." *IOP Conference Series: Materials Science and Engineering* 497 (April): 012090. doi:10.1088/1757-899X/497/1/012090.

Schwab, Klaus. 2017. *The Fourth Industrial Revolution*. 1st ed. Penguin Random House.

Sommer, Lutz. 2015. "Industrial Revolution – Industry 4.0: Are German manufacturing SMEs the first victims of this revolution?" *Journal of Industrial Engineering and Management* 8 (5): 1512–1532. doi:10.3926/jiem.1470.

Tariq, Qishin. 2018. "MDEC Collaborates with Grab to Beat KL Traffic." *The Star*. https://www.thestar.com.my/tech/tech-news/2018/04/13/mdec-and-grab-mou-on-malaysia-city-brain-project.

Tripathi, Garima, Melnita Dabre, Lyzanne Dsouza, and Tansy Fernandes. 2017. "Home automation system using artificial intelligence." *International Journal for Research in Applied Science & Engineering Technology (IJRASET)* 5 (8): 219–224.

Zhou, K., Taigang Liu, and Lifeng Zhou. 2015. "Industry 4.0: Towards Future Industrial Opportunities and Challenges." In *2015 12th International Conference on Fuzzy Systems and Knowledge Discovery (FSKD)*, 2147–2152. doi:10.1109/FSKD.2015.7382284.

Index

Printed in the United States
by Baker & Taylor Publisher Services